Principles of

MEASUREMENT AND TRANSDUCTION OF BIOMEDICAL VARIABLES

Principles of MEASUREMENT AND TRANSDUCTION OF BIOMEDICAL VARIABLES

VERA LUCIA DA SILVEIRA NANTES BUTTON

Department of Biomedical Engineering,
School of Electrical and Computing Engineering,
University of Campinas,
São Paulo, Brazil

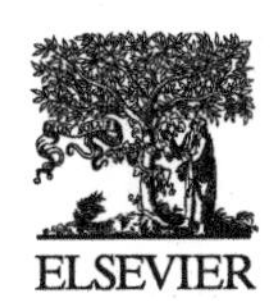

AMSTERDAM • BOSTON • HEIDELBERG • LONDON
NEW YORK • OXFORD • PARIS • SAN DIEGO
SAN FRANCISCO • SINGAPORE • SYDNEY • TOKYO
Academic Press is an imprint of Elsevier

Academic Press is an imprint of Elsevier
125 London Wall, London, EC2Y 5AS, UK
525 B Street, Suite 1800, San Diego, CA 92101-4495, USA
225 Wyman Street, Waltham, MA 02451, USA
The Boulevard, Langford Lane, Kidlington, Oxford OX5 1GB, UK

ISBN: 978-0-12-800774-7

British Library Cataloguing-in-Publication Data
A catalogue record for this book is available from the British Library.

Library of Congress Cataloging-in-Publication Data
A catalog record for this book is available from the Library of Congress.

For Information on all Academic Press publications
visit our website at http://store.elsevier.com/

Typeset by MPS Limited, Chennai, India
www.adi-mps.com

Printed and bound in the USA

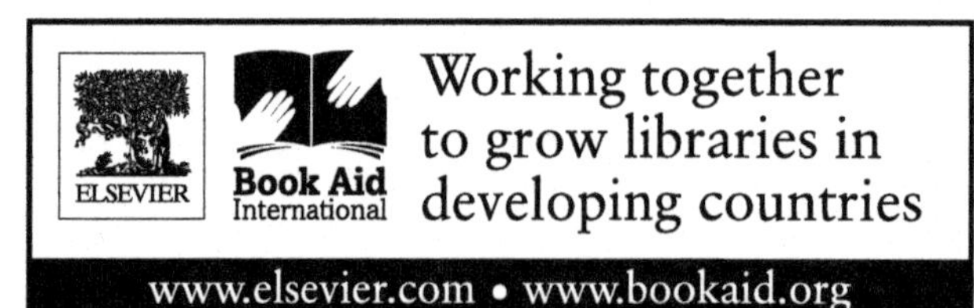

Publisher: Joe Hayton
Acquisition Editor: Fiona Geraghty
Editorial Project Manager: Cari Owen
Production Project Manager: Susan Li
Designer: Greg Harris

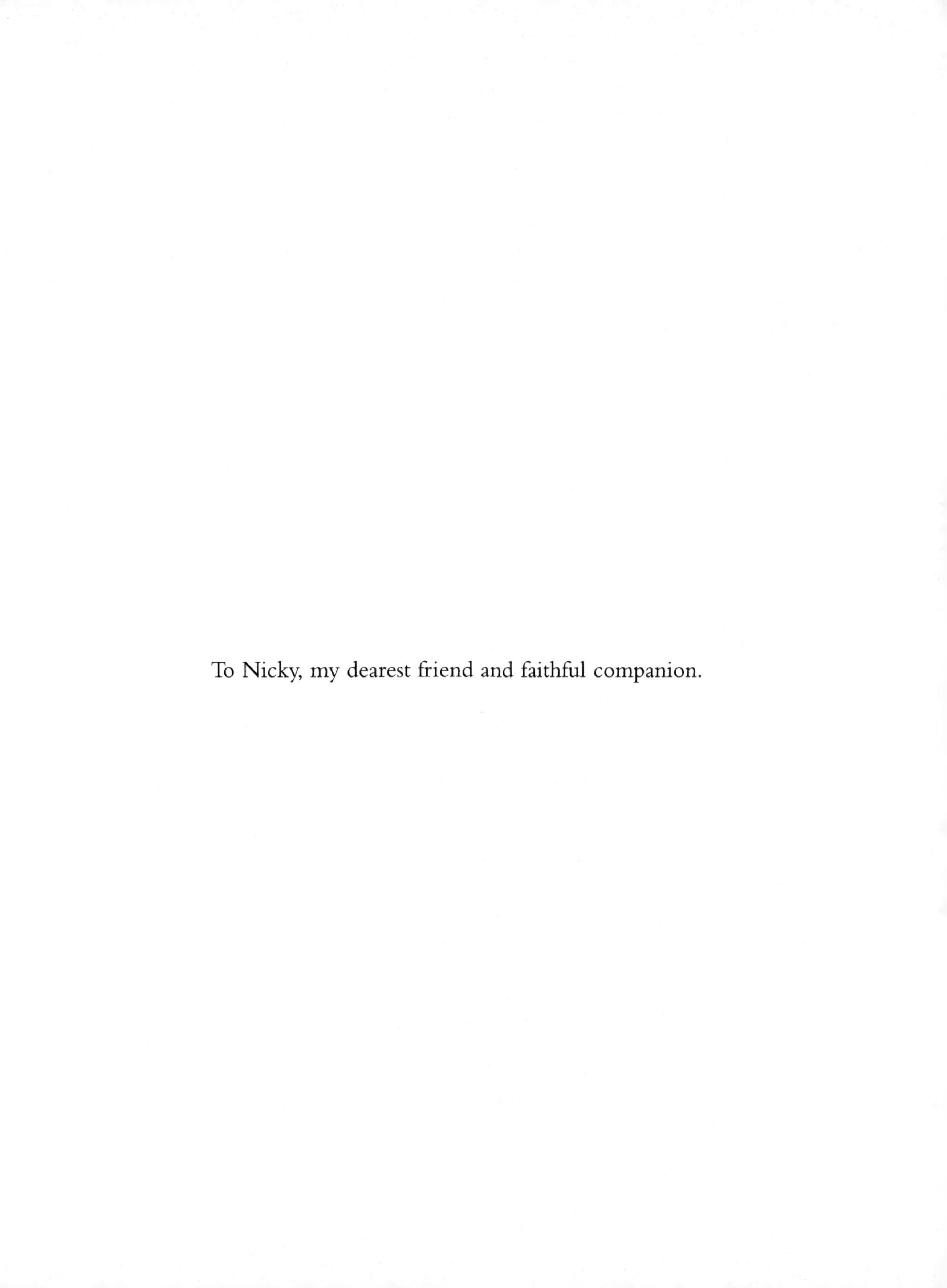

To Nicky, my dearest friend and faithful companion.

CONTENTS

PREFACE

After a few decades giving classes of biomedical instrumentation and transduction of biomedical variables for undergraduate and post-graduation students of electrical engineering at my university, came up the idea of bringing together the teachings on the operation of the main types of transducers used in biomedical engineering in a textbook. Transducers comprise virtually all devices and equipment used in biomedical engineering and in most cases, they are the interface between the biological tissue and electronic processing of the variable to be obtained for the purpose of diagnosis, monitoring, control, or study of biological systems.

The objective of this work is to provide a textbook to be used by students and professionals seeking careers in research and development in Biomedical Engineering and its related areas, for example, Medical and Biological Engineering, which deals with the development of electronic instrumentation and methods for processing signals and medical imaging; Bioengineering, which seeks the modeling and understanding of biological systems with the perspective of engineering on biological phenomena; Rehabilitation Engineering, which handles the development of instrumentation and techniques dedicated to the insertion of special needs patients in the society; and Clinical Engineering, which is dedicated to the management of health technology in all its levels, from the purchase of medical equipment, installation and maintenance until its deactivation. It will therefore be a textbook to be used by students in undergraduate and graduate courses and also for professionals working in Biomedical Engineering, willing to learn about the functioning of the transducers used in the measurement of biomedical variables.

The variety of types of transducers used in Biomedical Engineering is very large, and in the organization of this book some types of transducers were selected, the most commonly used in medical and biological instrumentation, to present their working principles and main applications. Chapter 1, Introduction to Biomedical Variables Transducing, presents some basic concepts useful to understand the particular characteristics of biomedical variables and transducers operation. Chapter 2, Electrodes for Biopotential Recording and Tissue Stimulation, explains the functioning of noninvasive and invasive electrodes, used in the biopotential detection and biological tissue stimulation; it also presents the functioning of standard electrodes and the importance of the electrode/electrolyte/skin interfaces in noninvasive measurements. Chapter 3, Electrodes for Measurement of Dissolved Gases and Ions Concentration in the Blood Plasma, is about the functioning of electrodes used for measurement of fundamental parameters of gasometry, pO_2, pCO_2, pH. Chapter 4, Temperature Transducers, presents the operating principle of the main temperature transducers used in biomedical procedures. Chapter 5, Displacement, Velocity, and Acceleration Transducers, starts explaining the functioning of main displacement transducers, which is fundamental to understand the transduction of velocity and acceleration quantities, as well as other biomedical variables, such as pressure, flow, and force. Chapter 6, Pressure and Force Transducers, presents the most important methods of blood pressure transduction, intra- and extravascular, direct and indirect, and the functioning of the transducers used; transduction methods for force measurement are also included in this chapter. Chapter 7, Flow Transducers, explains some of the methods to measure flow in biological systems and the functioning of transducers associated with them. Chapter 8, Optical Transducers for Oximetry and Capnography, explains the functioning of optical transducers used to determine oxygen saturation level of blood hemoglobin (SaO_2) in pulse oximetry, and the blood CO_2 concentration in capnography. The last chapter (Chapter 9), New Technological Advancements in Biomedical Variables Transducing, presents some of the contribution of the advancements in electronic devices, equipment and automation, material sciences, and signal and image processing for the biomedical transducers enhancement.

I want to thank my first teachers of Biomedical Engineering, Dr Maria Adélia Collier Farias, Dr Wang Binseng, and Dr José Wilson Magalhães Bassani, of whom I became a colleague in the Department of Biomedical Engineering of the School of Electrical and Computing Engineering at University of Campinas, for the teachings transmitted in motivating and inspiring classes. I also thank all department colleagues and students, who I met along more than thirty years of teaching.

CHAPTER 1

Introduction to Biomedical Variables Transducing

Contents

1.1 INTRODUCTION

When performing measurements on living organisms, it is necessary to understand the mechanisms involved in the generation of the signals to be measured, the effects of the devices involved in the measurement, and the best method to achieve the most possible reliable and accurate value of that variable or parameter. In this book, the functioning of the part of biomedical instrumentation required for the acquisition of biomedical variables, such as blood pressure, temperature, and blood flow, is studied: the transducers, which are responsible for transforming biomedical quantity into another physical quantity, usually electrical, more easily recorded, processed, and displayed by the instruments.

Biomedical equipment "see" the patients through transducers attached to their bodies. The biomedical variable is the quantity, condition, or physical property measured by the instrumentation system. Table 1.1 summarizes some of the biomedical variables, which are often obtained from patient body, for the purpose of either diagnosis, therapy, or monitoring.

Principles of Measurement and Transduction of Biomedical Variables.
DOI: http://dx.doi.org/10.1016/B978-0-12-800774-7.00001-5

Table 1.1 Biomedical variables measured by medical equipment

Biomedical variable	Description
ECG	Electrocardiogram
EEG	Electroencephalogram
HR	Heart rate (beats per minute)
CO	Cardiac output (liter per minute)
pH	H^+ concentration in blood plasma
paO_2	Oxygen partial pressure in blood plasma
$paCO_2$	Carbon dioxide partial pressure in blood plasma
SaO_2	Percentage of hemoglobin cells O_2 saturated
$ETCO_2$	End tidal CO_2
NIBP	Noninvasive blood pressure
BP	Invasive blood pressure
AA	Concentration of inspired anesthetic agent
N_2O	Concentration of inhaled nitrous oxide
Respiratory rate	Number of inspirations and expirations per minute
EMG	Electromyogram
EP	Evoked potentials
Temperature	Invasive or noninvasive body temperature

Biomedical variables can be obtained invasively or noninvasively. An invasive measurement needs to cut the biological tissues, as skin, muscles, and blood vessel wall, to insert a catheter or hypodermic needle, to get access to the variable. Most of the times, it is desirable to use noninvasive measurement methods due to the need of surgical procedures to implement invasive methods. Some biomedical variables, as pulmonary artery blood pressure, are obtained only through invasive methods; the temperature sensor is introduced from a periphery vein, through a catheter, to achieve the right ventricle output.

The method to obtain a medical variable can be either direct or indirect. When the variable is measured by a direct method, the transducer is connected with the biological medium where the variable is generated. One example is the body temperature measured with a surface temperature transducer (thermistor). Another example is to measure the pulmonary artery temperature with a thermistor placed in contact with the blood in the pulmonary artery. First example is a direct and noninvasive measurement, while the second is direct and invasive. Sometimes, the biomedical variable can be inferred from another, and in this case, the measurement is said indirect, as when the arterial blood pressure is inferred with a sphygmomanometer or the blood flow value is determined from the Doppler frequency difference.

Most of medical equipment are microcontrolled and microprocessed, and usually the biomedical variables need to be transduced to electric format (current or voltage)

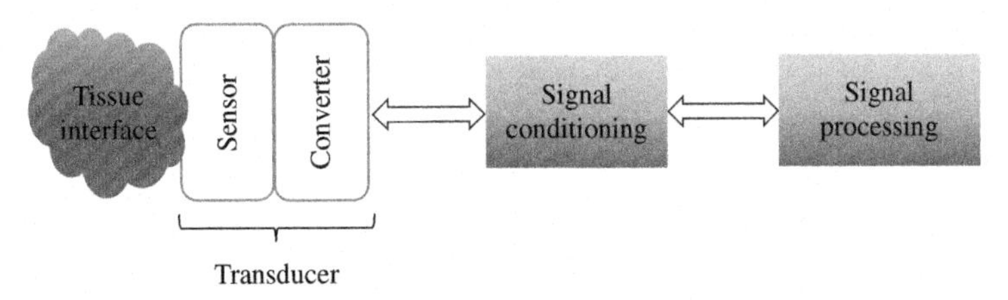

Figure 1.1 A transducer can be considered as having two parts: a sensor and a converter element.

before being amplified, filtered, digitized, and processed. When a thermocouple is used to measure an electrolytic solution temperature, thermal energy is transduced into electrical energy (EFM). When a metallic electrode is used to register the electric activity of heart, ionic current is transduced into electrical current at electrode/electrolyte/skin interfaces.

1.2 CHARACTERISTICS OF TRANSDUCERS

The transducer is a device that can convert a physical quantity into another. The most common transducers convert nonelectric physical quantities into electrical quantities, that is, act as energy converters. The transducer can be divided into primary sensor element, which detects the quantity to be measured, and converter element, which transforms the input power into another, usually an electric signal, which is processed by electronic circuits (Figure 1.1).

The transducer can be classified as passive/active or generator/modulator. The passive/generator transducer requires no external power source, and the energy of the input physical quantity is converted directly into the output signal. An example of this type of transducer is a thermocouple, whose operation is based on the combination of thermoelectric effects to produce an open circuit electromotive force when two metal junctions are maintained at different temperatures. The output energy (EMF) is fully provided by the physical input quantity (temperature) (Figure 1.2A). The active/modulator transducer uses an external power source, which is modulated by the input signal (variable), to produce the output signal. The auxiliary power source provides power to most of the output signal. Thermistor, photodiode, and *strain gages* are examples of active transducer (Figure 1.2B).

The performance of the transducer is defined by its static and dynamic characteristics. Static characteristics determine transducer response to time invariant inputs, according to environment conditions that it is submitted (temperature, humidity, vibration, atmospheric pressure, etc.). Dynamic characteristics determine transducer response to inputs that vary along time (sinusoidal, square wave, impulse, step, etc.).

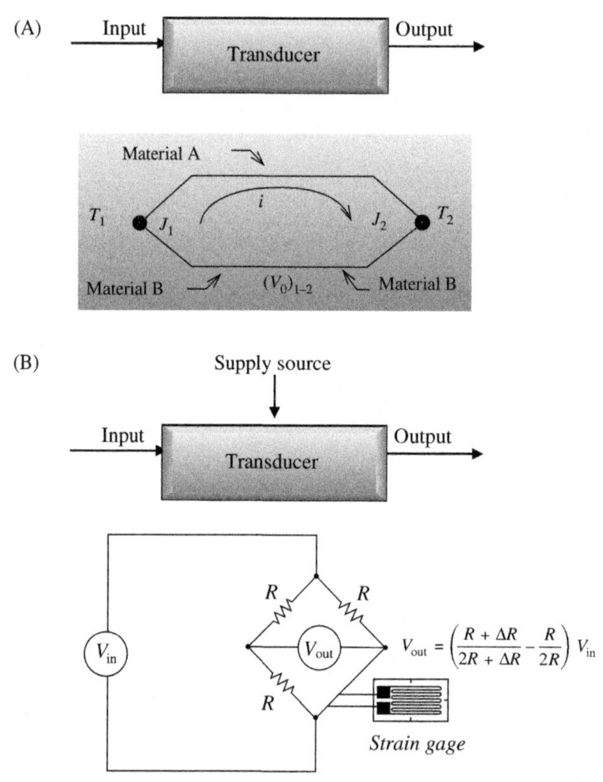

Figure 1.2 Examples of passive/generator (A) and active/modulator (B) transducers.

1.2.1 Static characteristics of transducers

A few static characteristics are presented below: static sensibility, linearity, working range, precision, accuracy, resolution, repeatability, reproducibility, hysteresis, and saturation.

1.2.1.1 Static sensitivity

The static sensitivity value of a transducer indicates how much the output varies to a certain amount of variation of the input variable (Figure 1.3):

$$S_s = \frac{\Delta V_{out}}{\Delta V_{in}} \tag{1.1}$$

For example, a blood pressure transducer with 1 mV per mmHg sensitivity shows an output of 80 mV to 80 mmHg pressure. The transducer has high sensitivity if a small variation in the blood pressure is indicated in its output as a large voltage variation. On the contrary, the sensitivity is low if a large variation in the input results in a small output variation (Figure 1.1). When the transducer output is related to the input

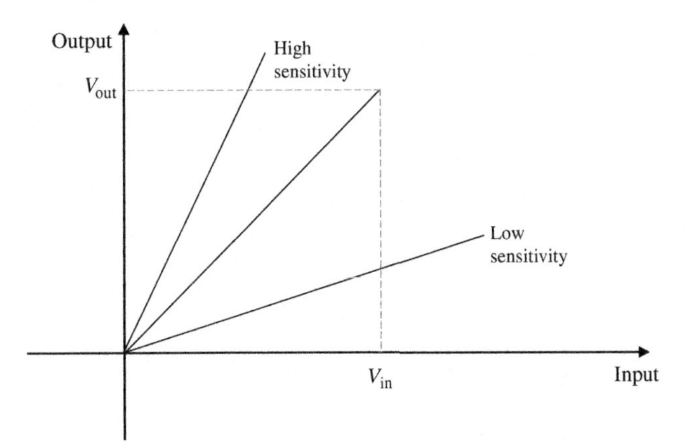

Figure 1.3 Sensitivity of a transducer.

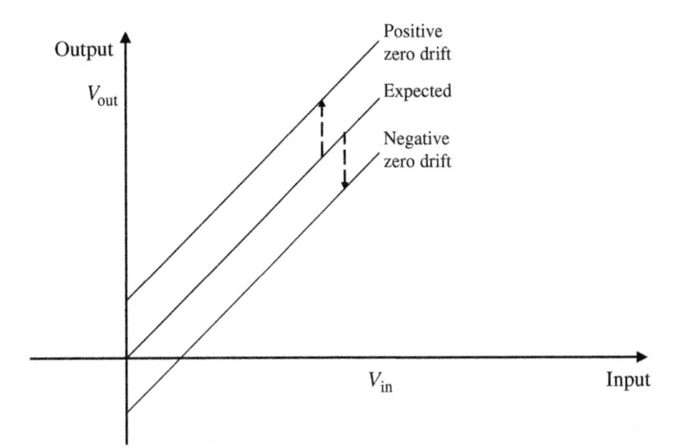

Figure 1.4 Zero drift.

by a function, $V_{\text{out}} = f(V_{\text{in}})$, sensitivity can also vary according to input value, and then sensitivity can be defined to a particular point:

$$S_s(x) = \frac{\mathrm{d}V_{\text{out}}}{\mathrm{d}V_{\text{in}}} / _{V_{\text{in}}=x} \tag{1.2}$$

The static calibration of a transducer is done varying the input in small steps or increments, over the working range, which results in a range of output increments. The zero drift is an undesirable change, due to environment influence or intrinsic characteristics of the transducer, which causes all the output values to be shifted upward or downward, i.e., all values are increased or decreased by the same amount, respectively, without slope changing (it does not change static sensitivity) (Figure 1.4).

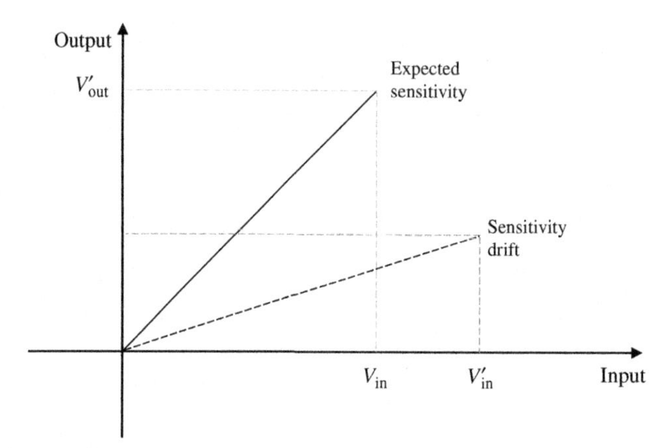

Figure 1.5 Sensitivity drift.

Ambient temperature variation, hysteresis, and vibration are possible causes of zero drift, as well as the displacement artifact, which changes the electrodes offset DC voltage during ECG measurement.

The sensitivity drift or span drift changes the slope of the static sensitivity curve; the output variation, compared to the expected values, is proportional to the input amplitude, as is shown in Figure 1.5.

Sensitivity drift causes loss of transducer sensitivity, because for the same input variation, the transducer responds with smaller variation than expected. It is usually due to changes in ambient conditions, as temperature and atmospheric pressure, and due to instability of the electronic circuit's power supply, which changes the voltage gain of biopotential amplifier, for example.

1.2.1.2 Linearity

Linearity is the transducer characteristic of providing proportional outputs to distinct inputs. If to an input V_{in1}, the output is V_{out1}, and for V_{in2}, is V_{out2}, then to an input $(a_1 V_{in1} + a_2 V_{in2})$ the output will be $a_1 V_{out1} + a_2 V_{out2}$; a_1 and a_2 are constants. The allowed maximum error of linearity for a transducer is defined by the values in the V_{out} versus V_{in} region delimited by linearity drift and zero drift, as is shown in Figure 1.6. Error of linearity specification describe a range around the expected best fit curve into which all measurements must fall. The magnitude of the range is equal to the worst case error throughout the transducer's measurement range. It is easily noticed that the value of the maximum output linearity error can be defined for distinct input ranges. The zero drift of a transducer is usually informed as a percentage of the full scale output (FSO) and the sensitivity drift, by a percentage of the variable value reading.

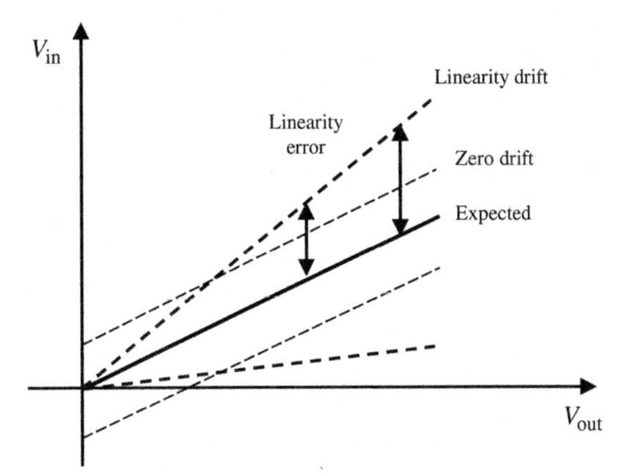

Figure 1.6 Linearity error.

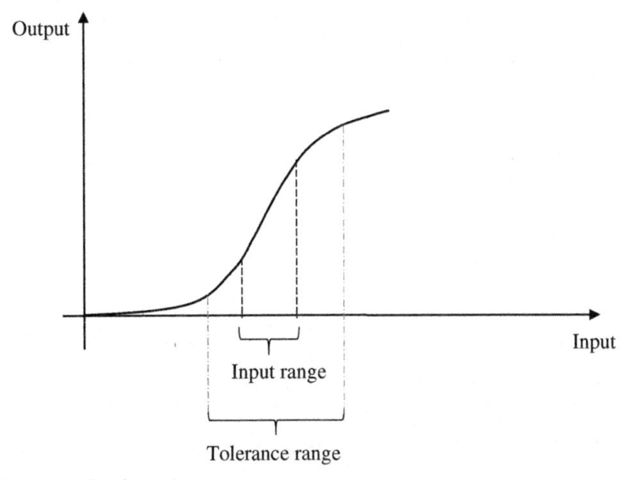

Figure 1.7 Input linear and tolerance ranges.

1.2.1.3 Input range

The input, working or operational range of a transducer is the range of the variable values that can be correctly converted by the transducer; it is limited by the minimum value that can be measured (inferior limit) and the maximum measured value that will not cause output saturation (superior limit). For example, the input range of a thermometer is $-18°C$ to $+70°C$, and of a displacement transducer is 0.1–100 μm. Span is the algebraic difference between superior and inferior limits of input range; in the last examples, span is 88°C and 99 μm, respectively. A linear input range guarantees transducer linear performance, while tolerance input range is the range of input values to which the linearity is not guaranteed, but it will not damage the transducer (Figure 1.7). For example, in the specifications of a blood pressure transducer, the manufacturer informs that the pressure range is −30 to +300 mmHg and the overpressure without damage is −100 to +500 mmHg.

1.2.1.4 Accuracy, resolution, threshold, and precision

Accuracy is the extent to which the result of a reading of a transducer approaches the true value of the measured variable, thus, is a comparison between true and measured values. It can be indicated as an error percentage value:

$$\text{Error}(\%) = \frac{y_t - y_m}{y_t} \tag{1.3}$$

where

y_t is the true value of the variable,

y_m is the transducer output or the measured value of the variable.

The closer to the real value, the smaller the error and more accurate is the measurement. Accuracy is indicated as a percentage of the reading, a percentage of full scale, ± the number of digits to digital outputs, or ± half of the smallest display division to analog scale.

Resolution is the smallest perceptible change in the variable value that the transducer can sense. If the variable input gradually increases from zero, there will be a minimum value required to give a detectable output change. This minimum value defines the threshold of the instrument. Thus, threshold is the smallest perceptible measurable input change. Precision is the degree of proximity between the results of successive measurements of the same variable, performed under the same conditions.

The output of a transducer can be precise, but not exact. For instance, a digital thermometer with 0.01°C resolution is used to measure ambient temperature, obtaining 25.64°C, 25.48°C, 25.62°C, 25.54°C, and 25.58°C. If the true value is 25.40°C, then the thermometer is precise, because the measured values are next to each other, but not exact, because they are different from the true temperature.

1.2.1.5 Repeatability and reproducibility

Repeatability is the degree of agreement between results of successive measurements of the same variable carried out under the same measurement conditions (same operator, same transducer). Repeatability of a transducer can vary along time, which does not necessarily indicate it is faulty, but rather that repeatability is a variable quantity.

Reproducibility is the degree of agreement between results of successive measurements of the same variable carried out under different measurement conditions (same operator but different transducers or same transducer but different operators).

Previous static characteristics presented here are named linear characteristics. The next two characteristics, hysteresis and saturation, are classified as nonlinear.

1.2.1.6 Hysteresis

Transducer output has hysteresis if the relation between the output value and the input variable depends on their previous state. In other words, if the input is monotonically incremented and then decremented, the output values do not coincide to the same input value in the upward and downward curves. Figure 1.8 shows a typical hysteresis loop. Hysteresis characteristic occurs because part of the input energy is not recovered, but is dissipated or stored in another type of energy. The loop area represents the amount of dissipated or stored energy. For example, the electric energy applied as AC current to the primary coil of an inductive displacement transducer is stored as magnetic energy and dissipated as heat.

1.2.1.7 Saturation

When the input variable exceeds the input range of the transducer, the output saturates, and even if the input value increases, the output remains at the same amplitude value. Figure 1.9 shows an example of saturation. Figure 1.9A shows a class B configuration circuit with bipolar junction transistors (BJT). NPN (Q_n) and PNP (Q_P) transistors are polarized at the conduction eminence at 25°C, by V_{pol}; base–emitter (BE) junctions act like temperature sensors and the V_{BE} necessary to transistors conduction decreases 2 mV/°C with each degree Celsius increase. Thus, as BE junction temperature increases, V_{BE} remains constant ($V_{pol} = V_{BEN} + V_{BEQ}$), but emitter current increases, as well as V_{out}, the voltage drop across R_L, until transistors saturate. From this point on, even with further temperature increase, emitter current does not increase and V_{out} remains constant. Dead zone is a static characteristic of the transducer, which corresponds to the input variables value that do not change the output value. In the example showed in Figure 1.9, dead zone corresponds to the subthreshold condition of bipolar transistor

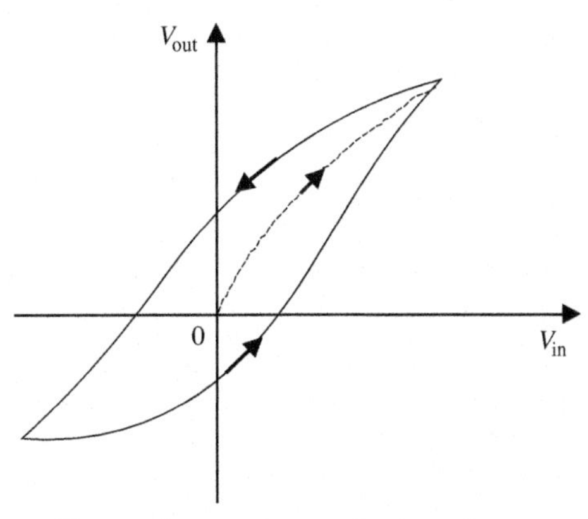

Figure 1.8 Typical V_{out} versus V_{in} transference curve of a transducer operation with hysteresis.

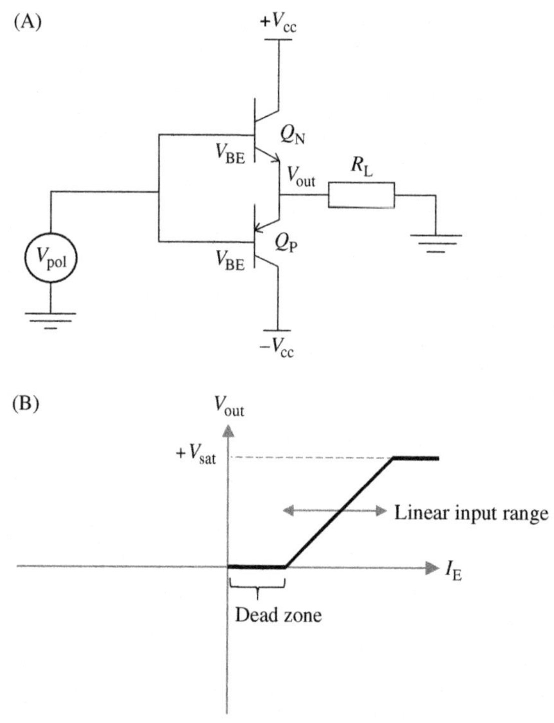

Figure 1.9 Example of transducer with hysteresis: PN junction-based temperature transducer in B class configuration (A) and V_{out} versus I_E showing dead zone, input range, and output saturation (B).

conduction ($V_{BE} < V_T$, threshold voltage), while voltage drop across BE junction does not achieve threshold value ($V_T \approx 0.7$ V for silicon transistor), transistor remains in the cut-off state.

1.2.2 Dynamic characteristics of transducers

Dynamic characteristics describe the performance of transducers when the measurable input variable is not constant, but varies with time. There are a few biomedical variables that have static behavior (constant) or quasi-static, for example, ionic concentration in blood plasma (pH, Ca^{2+}, etc.) and body temperature, except for the condition of malignant hyperthermia that may affect patients under volatile anesthetics effect. Many temperature measurements taken on the body surface, on the extra-corporeal blood circulation, or on an intravenous solution are executed under conditions where enough time is available for the temperature transducer to reach steady state, and there is no need to consider the device behavior under nonsteady state conditions. Static characteristics are sufficient. When variables that are treated by a measuring device, such as a flow transducer or an ECG electrode, exhibit rapid variation with time or at least noticeable to the measuring instruments, it is necessary to consider their dynamic response.

The dynamic characteristics describe the transient response and the frequency response of a measurement system. The transient response is the output transducer for an input variable in the format of a step. The frequency response determines the amplitude and phase of the transducer output for sinusoidal inputs of variable frequency and intensity. Biomedical variables are characterized by amplitude range and frequency content. Table 1.2 shows some examples of biomedical variables and their characteristics.

The transduction of dynamic biomedical variables will be considered after some important assumptions. First, the biomedical dynamic variables are treated as if they were electrical signals; second, the transducer performance is completely defined by its transfer function, which output can be determined to any input (biomedical variable); the transfer function is described by a linear, ordinary, time invariant differential equation of zero, first, or second order.

1.2.2.1 Dynamic variables

Dynamic variables can be represented by stationary signals (Figure 1.10A) and their spectral components do not change with time or nonstationary signals (Figure 1.10B), which means that spectral components change with time; there is also transient nonstationary classification (Figure 1.10C). They are signals that occur sporadically with sudden amplitude variations and the signal energy is contained in this transient variation.

Stationary variables can be deterministic or random. Deterministic means they are represented by mathematical functions and is possible to accurately determine the value of the variable at a given instant of time, for example, a sinusoidal function (Figure 1.11A):

$$f(t) = A\sin(\omega t) \tag{1.4}$$

where A and ω ($\omega = 2\pi f$ is the radial frequency) are constant.

Random stationary variables are represented by nonperiodic signals that happen along time with changing format and amplitude (Figure 1.11B).

Deterministic stationary variables can be periodic or nonperiodic. Periodic deterministic stationary variables are represented by signals, which amplitude varies with time

Table 1.2 Amplitude range and frequency content of biomedical variables

Variable	Amplitude range	Frequency range
ECG	0.5–5 mV	0.01–250 Hz
EEG	5–300 μV	DC—150 Hz
EMG	0.1–5 mV	DC—10 kHz
Blood pressure (indirect)	25–400 mmHg	DC—60 Hz
Blood pressure (direct)	10–400 mmHg	DC—50 Hz
Temperature	32–42°C	DC—0.1 Hz

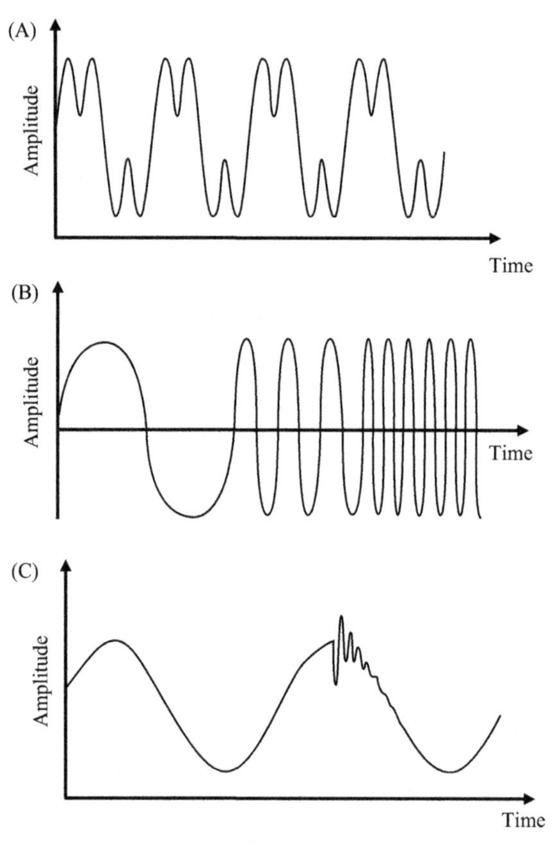

Figure 1.10 Dynamic variables classification: stationary (A), nonstationary (B), and transient nonstationary (C).

and their amplitude variation is repeated at constant time intervals (Figure 1.12A). Any periodic signal can be analyzed by means of its spectral components, that is, the sinusoids (with amplitudes, frequencies, and different lags) that compose it.

Transducers are used to measure biomedical variable, most of them can be explained as a combination of one or more signals of the following types:

1. *Random*. For example, the electroencephalogram (EEG) (Figure 1.13C) can be considered a random signal, although is possible to identify the rhythms of encephalic activity, known as alpha, beta, theta, and delta; electromyogram (EMG) registered with surface electrodes is another example of random signal.
2. *Periodic*. For example, the electrocardiogram signal (ECG); although little variation can occur from one cycle to another, QRS complex is repeated along time (Figure 1.13A)
3. *Transient*. For example, the EMG of the contraction of isolated muscle fiber (Figure 1.13D).

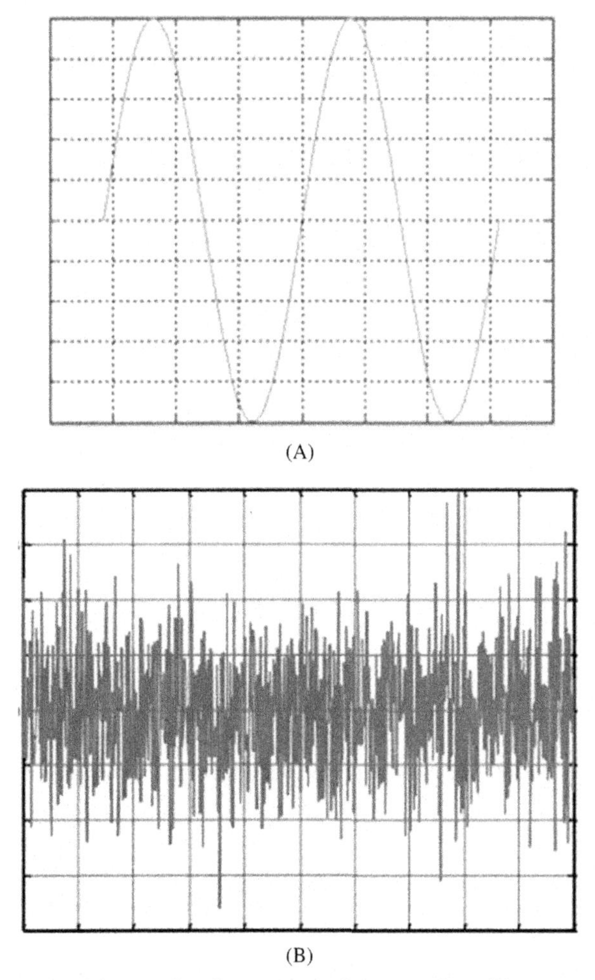

Figure 1.11 Stationary variables can be deterministic (A) or random (B).

1.2.2.2 Linear ordinary time invariant system

In a continuous system, the dynamic inputs are related to the dynamic outputs by differential and integral equations. To study the dynamic characteristics of the transducers used in biomedical applications, linear behavior is assumed. Most electronic instruments and physical systems can be described by linear ordinary differential equations up to second order with constant coefficients. The relationship between the input and output of a linear dynamic system can be represented in the time domain by

$$a_n \frac{d^n y_n}{dt^n} + \cdots + a_1 \frac{dy}{dt} + a_0 y(t) = b_m \frac{d^m x}{dt^m} + \cdots + b_1 \frac{dx}{dt} + b_0 x(t) \tag{1.5}$$

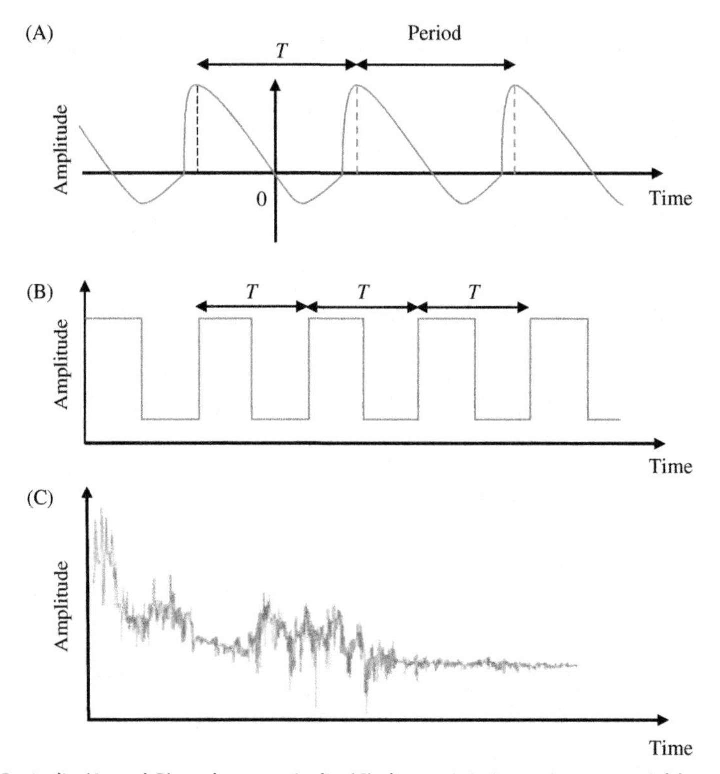

Figure 1.12 Periodic (A and B) and nonperiodic (C) deterministic stationary variables.

where

a_i ($i = 0, 1, 2, \ldots, n$) and b_j ($j = 0, 1, \ldots, m$) are constant coefficients,
$x(t)$ is the input variable,
$y(t)$ is the transducer output,
$f(t)$ is the transfer function of the system.

Equation (1.5) is linear differential because a_i and b_j coefficients are constant and they are not time or input dependent. In addition, the following linearity relationships are valid (k is constant):

$$x_1(t) \rightarrow y_1(t)$$
$$x_2(t) \rightarrow y_2(t)$$
$$kx_1(t) \rightarrow ky_1(t)$$
$$x_1(t) + x_2(t) \rightarrow y_1(t) + y_2(t)$$

Equation (1.5) is ordinary because there is only one independent variable, the transducer output, $y(t)$.

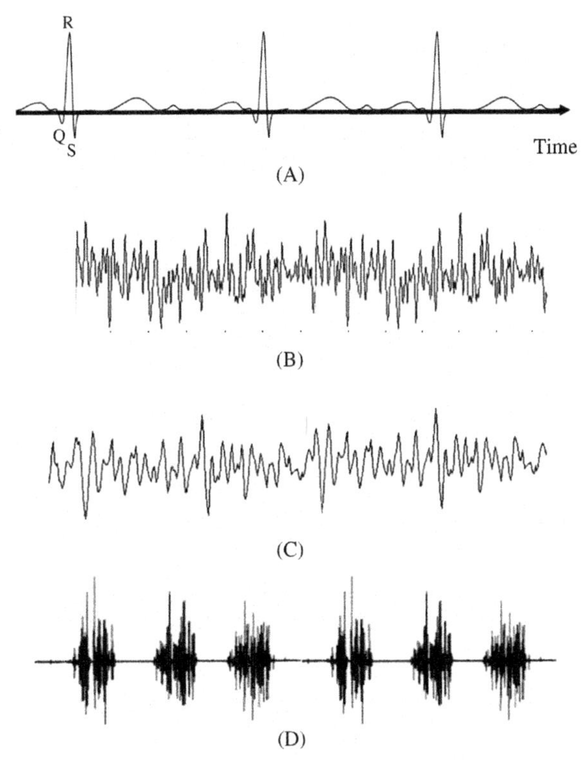

Figure 1.13 Examples of biomedical variable signals. (A) Electrocardiogram (ECG), a periodic signal. (B) Electroencephalogram (EEG), a random signal. (C) Surface electromyogram (SEMG), a random signal. (D) Electromyogram of isolated or single fiber muscle (SFEMG) contraction, a transient signal.

Equation (1.5) is used in time domain analysis of a linear ordinary time invariant system. The Laplace transform allows to represent the relationship between the input and output of Eq. (1.5), in the frequency domain (Eq. 1.6):

$$a_n Y(s)s^n + \cdots + a_1 Y(s)s + a_0 Y(s) = b_m X(s)s^m + \cdots + b_1 X(s)s + b_0 X(s) \qquad (1.6)$$

where

$X(s)$ is the Laplace transform of $x(t)$,

$Y(s)$ is the Laplace transform of $y(t)$,

$s^k = (\mathrm{d}^k/\mathrm{d}t^k)$ is the k-order derivative with respect to time.

The properties of this transform (linear, translation, and scaling the time derivative, etc.) facilitate analysis of linear dynamic systems. The most interesting advantage of this transform is that integration and derivation become multiplications and divisions. It allows to solve differential equations as polynomial equations, which are much simpler to solve. The Laplace transform has its name in honor of the French mathematician Pierre Simon Laplace.

1.2.2.3 Zero-order, first-order and second-order systems

The performance of most transducers can be described by linear ordinary time invariant systems of zero, first, and second order, which allows to deal with simplified forms of Eqs. (1.5) and (1.6). Mathematical description of these systems is presented below.

Zero-order system is mathematically described in Eq. (1.7):

$$a_0 y(t) = b_0 x(t) \tag{1.7}$$

The equation of a zero-order system has all coefficients null, except a_0 and b_0. It does not undergo transitory because it has no element to store energy (capacitor or inductor) and needs just one parameter to characterize it (static sensitivity). Output is frequency independent; its value is proportional to input value at any frequency and does not present phase or amplitude distortion. Any transducer which equivalent circuit has only resistive elements behaves like a zero-order system. For example, displacement transducers constructed with linear or angular potentiometers. Figure 1.14 shows an angular potentiometer used as displacement transducer, as well as output when an unit step is applied in its input.

The variable resistor is powered by an external voltage source V_S. The output voltage V_{out} is attenuated relative to V_S by a voltage drop proportional to the angular deflection θ_i.

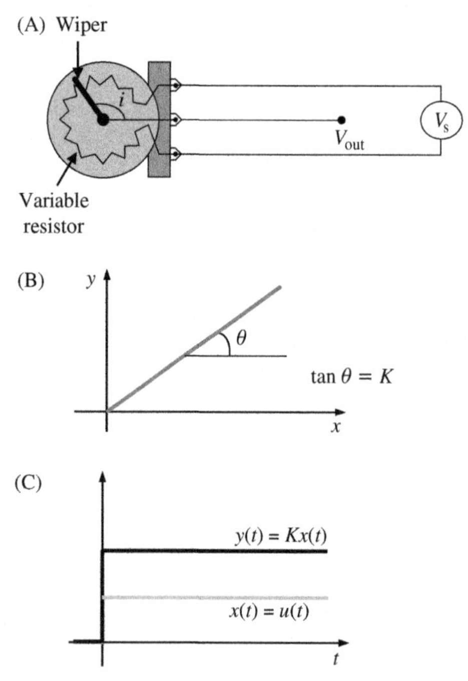

Figure 1.14 Example of zero-order system: angular potentiometer-based displacement transducer (A), output versus input characteristic (B), unit step ($u(t)$) input and transducer output $y(t)$ (C).

This transducer is considered as a zero-order system if the changes in the angle θ_i are sufficiently slow so that the inductive and capacitive effects associated with the operation of the potentiometer (mainly due to inertia and friction) can be disregarded.

Figure 1.15 shows another example of transducer that can be represented by zero-order system, a thermocouple-based thermometer.

If a unit step voltage $x(t) = u(t)$ is applied to the input of a zero-order system, the output is $y(t) = K\,x(t)$.

The transfer function of a zero-order system, in frequency domain, is:

$$F(s) = \frac{Y(s)}{X(s)} = \frac{b_0}{a_0} = K \tag{1.8}$$

where K is the static sensitivity of the system.

The modulus of the transfer function (K) versus frequency for a first-order system is a straight line parallel to the abscissa, that is, the static stability of the zero-order system is constant, equal to k does not vary with frequency. The phase versus frequency corresponds to a line parallel to the abscissa at zero, that is, the phase is zero for any frequency value.

Measurement systems are usually represented by equations of order greater than zero, but in most cases, it is possible to make simplifications to turn them into simpler

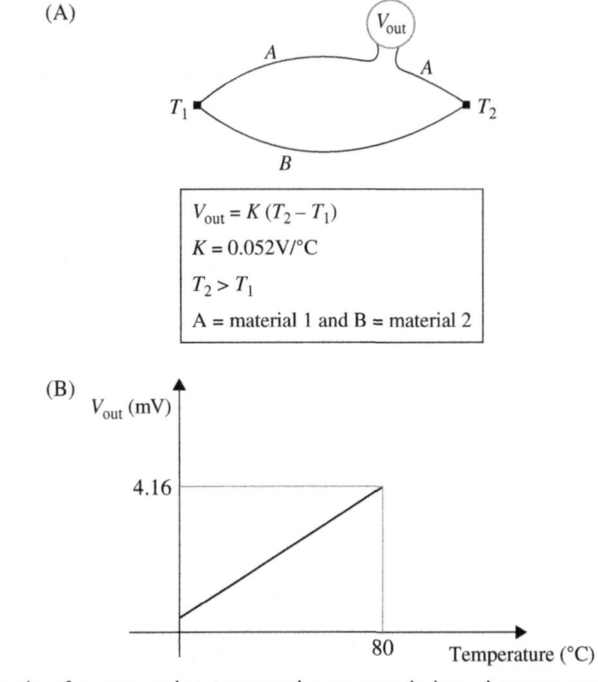

Figure 1.15 Example of a zero-order system: thermocouple-based temperature transducer (A) and thermocouple output voltage *versus* temperature (B).

systems. Many measuring elements or systems can be represented by a first-order differential equation in which the highest derivatives are of the first order. A first-order system contains a single energy storage element (capacitor, inductor) and is described mathematically in time domain by Eq. (1.9) and in frequency domain by Eq. (1.10). Equation (1.11) is the canonical form of the transfer function of a first-order system.

$$a_1 \frac{dy}{dt} + a_0\, y(t) = b_0\, x(t) \tag{1.9}$$

$$(a_1 s + a_0) Y(s) = b_0\, X(s) \tag{1.10}$$

$$F(s) = \frac{Y(s)}{X(s)} = \frac{b_0}{a_1 s + a_0} = \frac{(b_0/a_0)}{(a_1/a_0)s + 1} = \frac{K}{\tau s + 1} \tag{1.11}$$

where

$K = b_0/a_0$ is the static sensitivity or gain

$\tau = a_1/a_0$ is the time constant, or the response time of the transducer or system.

K and τ are the only parameters needed to characterize a second-order system.

Substituting $s = j\omega$ in Eq. (1.11), the transfer function is represented by Eq. (1.12):

$$F(j\omega) = \frac{K}{\tau j\omega + 1} \tag{1.12}$$

Equation (1.12) has a modulus and a phase, which can be plotted against frequency (Figure 1.12).

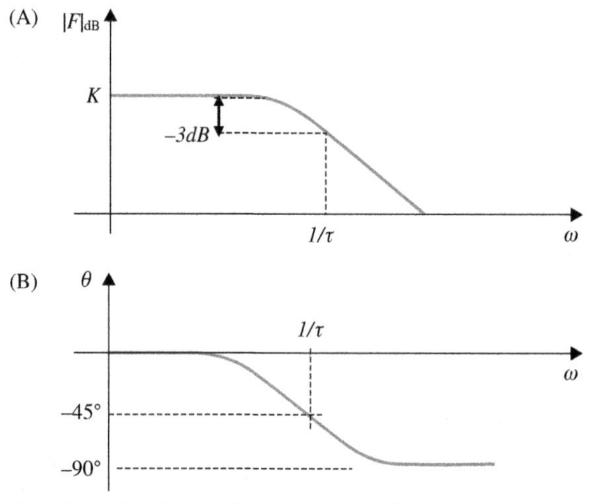

Figure 1.16 Transfer function of a first-order system: modulus versus angular frequency (A) and phase versus angular frequency (B).

$$F(j\omega) = \frac{K}{1 + \tau j\omega} = \frac{K}{\sqrt{1 + \omega^2\tau^2}} \angle\theta = \arctan(-\omega\tau) \tag{1.13}$$

Resonance frequency is equal to $1/\tau$. Computing the transfer function modulus at resonance frequency results that the modulus is 3 dB below the maximum value (Figure 1.16A) and phase value is $-45°$ (Figure 1.16B). If a sinusoidal input of the form

$$x(t) = a \sin \omega t \tag{1.14}$$

is applied into a first-order system, the response will be also sinusoidal. The steady state output will be of the form

$$y(t) = b \sin(\omega t - \theta) \tag{1.15}$$

where θ is the phase lag between input and output. The frequencies are the same but the output signal will lag behind the input.

Any transducer which equivalent circuit has one charge-storage element, capacitor or inductor, has a transfer function like Eq. (1.11). Figure 1.17 shows a series RL circuit. For an unit step input, $v_{in}(t) = u(t)$, $V_{in}(s) = U(s) = 1$ and the current (output variable) in time domain through the circuit and transfer function in frequency domain are (for initial conditions null):

$$L\frac{di(t)}{dt} + R\, i(t) = v_{in}(t) \tag{1.16}$$

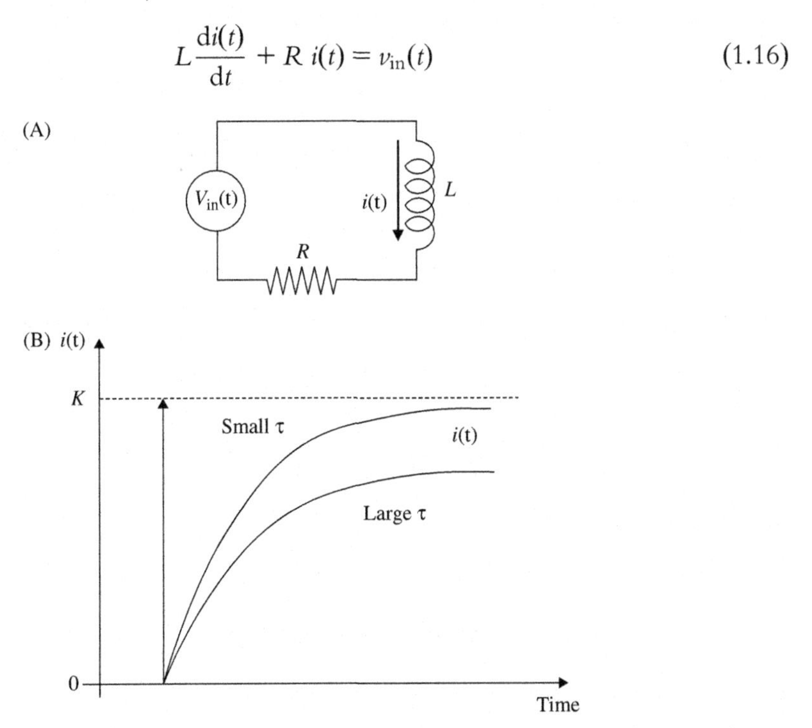

Figure 1.17 Series RL circuit (A) and output current against time and the influence of time constant τ (B).

$$F(s) = \frac{1/R}{1 + sL/R} \tag{1.17}$$

where $\tau = L/R$ and $K = 1/R$.

The current across the series RL circuit, in frequency domain, is:

$$I(s) = F(s) \cdot V_{\text{in}}(s) \tag{1.18}$$

$$I(s) = \frac{K}{1 + \tau s} U(s) \tag{1.19}$$

And in time domain:

$$i(t) = v_{\text{in}}(t) \otimes f(t) \tag{1.20}$$

or

$$i(t) = L^{-1}\left\{\frac{K}{\tau s + 1}\right\} \tag{1.21}$$

Solution comes from resolving Eq. (1.20) or using well-known equation of the Laplace anti-transform:

$$i(t) = K(1 - e^{-t/\tau}) \tag{1.22}$$

Equation (1.22) shows output current in the RL circuit as unit step input voltage. Current across R and L increases toward maximum value (K), rapidly or slowly, according to τ value. If time constant is large, output current takes a longer time to reach maximum value (Figure 1.17B).

Several types of transducers are described as a second-order system, particularly those with a moving element associated to a spring and some damping device, for example, pressure, force, velocity, and acceleration transducers. Equivalent circuits of these transducers are similar to a dumped mass-spring system and are represented by a second-order differential equation where the highest derivative is of the form d^2x/dt^2.

A second-order system has two charge-storage elements (e.g., two capacitors, two inductors, or one of each). Its dynamic performance is described by a second-order differential equation (a simplified version of Eq. (1.5)):

$$a_2 \frac{d^2y}{dt^2} + a_1 \frac{dy}{dt} + a_0 y(t) = b_0 x(t) \tag{1.23}$$

Or in frequency domain:

$$(a_2 s^2 + a_1 s + a_0) Y(s) = b_0 X(s) \tag{1.24}$$

And the transfer function is

$$F(s) = \frac{Y(s)}{X(s)} = \frac{b_0}{a_2 s^2 + a_1 s + a_0} = \frac{b_0/a_0}{(a_2/a_0)s^2 + (a_1/a_0)s + 1}$$
$$= \frac{K}{(s/\omega_n)^2 + 2\xi(s/\omega_n) + 1} \tag{1.25}$$

where

$$\begin{cases} K = \dfrac{b_0}{a_0} \leftarrow \text{Static sensivity(gain)} \\ \xi = \dfrac{a_1}{2\sqrt{a_0 a_2}} \leftarrow \text{Damping ratio} \\ \omega_n = \sqrt{\dfrac{a_0}{a_2}} \leftarrow \text{Natural oscillation frequency without damping} \end{cases}$$

The module and phase of the transfer function of a second-order system are

$$|F(j\omega)| = \frac{k}{\sqrt{1 - (\omega/\omega_n)^2 + 4\xi^2(\omega/\omega_n)^2}} \tag{1.26}$$

$$\phi = \arctan\left(\frac{2\xi}{(\omega/\omega_n) - (\omega_n/\omega)}\right) \tag{1.27}$$

The shape of the dynamic solution of Eq. (1.25) to a step input depends on the type of damping (Figure 1.18). The magnitude of the damping ratio affects the transient response of the system to a step input change, as shown below:

$$\xi \begin{cases} >1\text{: over-damped, output does not oscillate} \\ =1\text{: critically damped, does not oscillate} \\ <1\text{: under-dumped, oscillates} \end{cases}$$

A second-order system is said to be critically damped ($\xi = 1$) when a step input is applied and there is no overshoot and hence no resulting oscillation. If $\xi > 1$, the system is said over-damped, and its output does not oscillate. When $\xi = 1$, the system is said to be critically damped, and its output oscillates.

Consider a damped mass-spring system and an external force $f(t)$ displacing a mass M, initially at rest, against a spring and a fixed structure. The friction between mass and the structure is considered viscous. According to Hooke's law, if the spring is stretched (or compressed) y units of length, then it exerts a restoring force

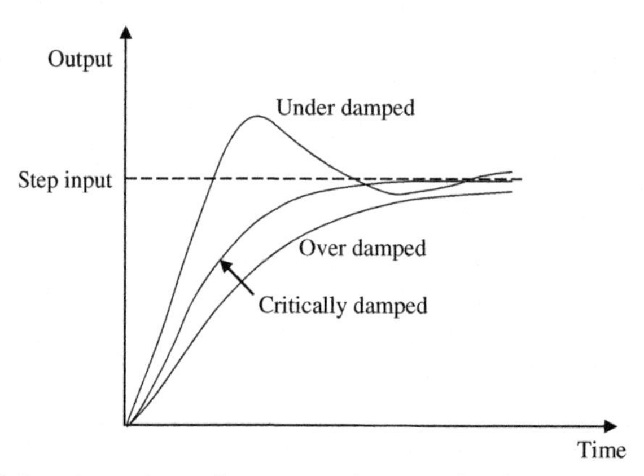

Figure 1.18 Effect of damping ratio on the output of a second-order system.

proportional to y (Eq. (1.28)). The friction between the mass M and the fixed part is considered perfect and viscous with coefficient B and is proportional to the mass velocity (Eq. (1.29)). The sum of force is equal to the product between mass and acceleration (Eq. (1.30)).

$$F_{\mathrm{spr}} = -K_{\mathrm{m}} y(t) \tag{1.28}$$

where K_{m} is the spring positive constant (linear).

$$F_{\mathrm{fric}} = -B\frac{\mathrm{d}y(t)}{\mathrm{d}t} \tag{1.29}$$

$$x(t) - B\frac{\mathrm{d}y(t)}{\mathrm{d}t} - K_{\mathrm{m}} y(t) = \frac{\mathrm{d}^2 y(t)}{\mathrm{d}t^2} M \tag{1.30}$$

or

$$\mathrm{M}\frac{\mathrm{d}^2 y(t)}{\mathrm{d}t^2} + \mathrm{B}\frac{\mathrm{d}y(t)}{\mathrm{d}t} + K_{\mathrm{m}} y(t) = x(t) \tag{1.31}$$

Suppose that the input force is x_1, a harmonic (sinusoidal) input, that is,

$$x_1 = x_{\mathrm{o}} \sin \omega t \tag{1.32}$$

where x_{o} is the amplitude of the input displacement and ω is its angular (or radial) frequency. The steady state output is

$$y(t) = X \sin(\omega t - \theta) \tag{1.33}$$

When a sinusoidal input is applied to a second-order system, the response of the system is rather more complex than when applied to the first-order system and depends

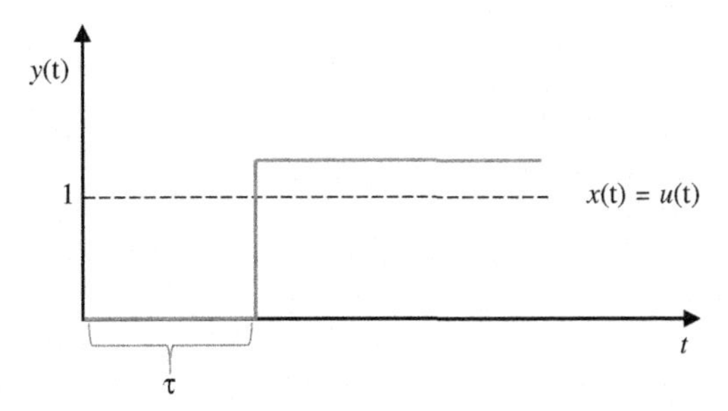

Figure 1.19 Effect of time delay in the output of a zero-order measuring system.

upon the relationship between the frequency of the applied sinusoid and the natural frequency of the system and the amount of damping present (Eq. (1.26) and (1.27)). The phase shift characteristic depends strongly on the damping ratio for all frequencies.

1.2.2.4 Time delay

An important factor in the performance of a measuring system is that the full effect of an input signal (i.e., change in measured quantity) is not immediately shown at the output but is almost inevitably subject to some lag or delay in response. This is a delay between cause and effect due to the natural inertia of the system and is known as time delay. Mathematically, for a zero-order system it is described as

$$y(t) = Kx(t - \tau_d) \tag{1.34}$$

where

x(t) is the input signal (a unit step, u(t) in the example shown in Figure 1.19)
y(t) is the output signal of the zero-order system
τ_d is the time delay
K is the static sensitivity and $t > \tau_d$.

Figure 1.19 shows a representation of the effect of time delay in the output of a zero-order measuring system. The output is identical to the input, unless the temporal delay. Time delay can cause oscillations if there is feedback in the system. It is usually present in electrical, hydraulic (vessels), mechanical (respiratory pneumatic tubing) transmission systems. It is also called dead time or transport delay.

RECOMMENDED READINGS

Beckwith, T. G., Marangoni, R. D., & Lienhard, J. H. (2007). *Mechanical measurements* (6th ed.). Pearson: Prentice-Hall, Cloth.

Chan, A. Y. K. (2008). *Biomedical device technology: Principles and design*. Charles C. Thomas.

Cobbold, R. S. C. (1974). *Transducers for biomedical measurements: Principles and applications*. John Wiley & Sons.

Dally, J. W., Riley, W. F., & McConnell, K. G. (1993). *Instrumentation for engineering measurements* (2nd ed.). John Wiley & Sons.

Doebelin, E. O. (Ed.), (1995). *Engineering experimentation, planning, execution, reporting.* McGraw-Hill.

Doebelin, E. O. (Ed.), (2004). *Measurements systems—Application and design* (5th ed.). McGraw Hill.

Gueddes, L. A., & Baker, L. E. (1968). *Principles of applied biomedical instrumentation.* John Wiley & Sons.

Khandpur, R. S. (2005). *Biomedical instrumentation: Technology and applications.* McGraw-Hill.

Morris, A. S., & Langari, R. (2012). *Measurement and intrumentation: Theory and application.* Elsevier.

Neuman, M. R., Fleming, D. G., Cheung, P. W., & Ko, W. H. (1977). *Physical sensors for biomedical applications.* CRC Press.

Ogata, K. (1997). *Modern control engineering* (3rd ed.). Prentice-Hall.

Webster, J. (Ed.), (2010). *Medical instrumentation: Application and design* (4th ed.). Wiley & Sons, Inc.

CHAPTER 2

Electrodes for Biopotential Recording and Tissue Stimulation

Contents

2.1 INTRODUCTION

Biopotential electrodes act as an interface between the biological tissue and the electronic measuring circuit, performing the transduction of ion current into electronic current. They are generally made of noble metal (silver, steel, gold) in different shapes

Principles of Measurement and Transduction of Biomedical Variables.
DOI: http://dx.doi.org/10.1016/B978-0-12-800774-7.00002-7

(circular, rectangular, needle-shaped, etc.) and are coated with a salt, such as silver chloride, or polymers, such as Nafion® (fluoropolymer—copolymer based on the sulfonated tetrafluoroethylene discovered in the late 1960s by Walther Grot de Du Pont). The surface of a metal electrode is coupled to the skin through electrolyte gel. The salt and the electrolyte gel help transducing the flow of ionic charges into an electronic current.

This chapter presents the main concepts for understanding how biopotentials are registered, the functioning of the electrode/electrolyte and electrolyte/skin interfaces, the electrical characteristics of biopotential electrodes and the different types of electrodes used to register biopotential. At the end of chapter, it will be possible to understand how the transduction of a biopotential occurs, that is, how the events which begin with the exchange of ions across the cell membrane can be represented by an electrical signal captured with a metal electrode placed over the body surface or inserted into the biological tissue.

2.2 BIOPOTENTIALS

The dynamic equilibrium that maintains the human body functioning involves chemical reactions to break the bonds of ingested nutrients, the construction of biopolymers such as proteins, nucleic acids, lipids, and carbohydrates and the disposal of metabolic wastes like urea and water. Although chemical reactions are always in the origin of energy distribution and synthesis of molecular constituents in living organisms, other types of energy are also needed, such as electric (biopotentials), mechanical (motion), thermal (especially in endothermic vertebrates), and even light (bioluminescence).

Electrical activity in biological tissues is dependent on the cells membrane state. Usually a difference in electrical potential is detected between the inside (cytoplasm) and the outside of the living cells. In membrane resting state, the value of this potential difference varies, according to cell type, between 5 and 100 mV, often with the interior of the cell with negative polarity relative to the outside. Figure 2.1 shows the record of the resting potential of a cell made with a microelectrode inserted through the membrane and a table with typical values of the resting potential of some biological tissues.

In biological tissue, there is no availability of free electrons and holes moving in an analogous way to what occurs in conduction and valence bands of conductive and semiconductive materials. Electric charges correspond to ions of dissociated compounds in intra- and extracellular aqueous media. Thus, the intra- and extracellular environments are conductive solutions containing charged atoms or ions, and the main are potassium (K^+), sodium (Na^+), and chloride (Cl^-). Mechanisms of ions selective transport across the cell membrane regulate the ionic concentration in the intra- and extracellular environments. Among other factors, the cell's transmembrane

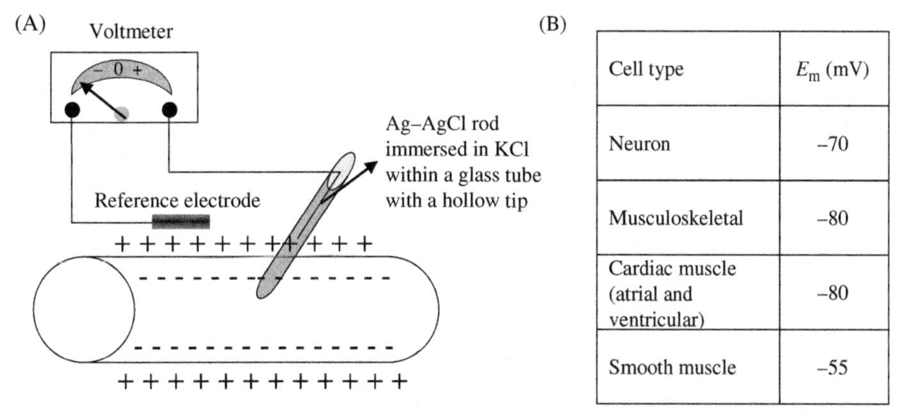

Cell type	E_m (mV)
Neuron	–70
Musculoskeletal	–80
Cardiac muscle (atrial and ventricular)	–80
Smooth muscle	–55

Figure 2.1 (A) Schematic diagram of the measurement of the difference in electrical potential between the interior and exterior of the resting membrane of a living cell (E_m). (B) Membrane potential values of different biological tissues cells.

Table 2.1 Ionic equilibrium potential (E_{eq})

Ionic concentration	K^+	Na^+	Cl^-
Intracellular (mM)	120	25	10
Extracellular (mM)	4	145	110
E_{eq} (mV)	−90	+60	−60

resting potential is due to the unequal concentration of ions on both sides of the membrane, active or passively partitioned by selective mechanisms of transmembrane ion transport. The effect of intra- and extracellular concentrations of potassium, sodium, and chloride ions at the ionic equilibrium potential is illustrated in Table 2.1.

The cell membrane acts as a capacitor, storing spatial distribution energy of the electrically charged ions in the intra- and extracellular environments. This potential energy is available to be quickly used and stabilizes the membrane, preventing this system to be disturbed, for example, by a subthreshold excitation.

Excitable cells, which are neurons, myocytes, and endocrine cells, can be activated when some form of energy (ionic current flow, temperature variation, pulse ultrasound, electric current, etc.) is applied to their membranes. Figure 2.2 shows a typical waveform of an action potential triggered by any stimulus, provided that it is suprathreshold. The characteristics of the active membrane change:

- sodium ions enter the cell (sodium channels open initiating depolarization or rising phase);
- the membrane potential leaves the "resting," its value rises and can even reverse its polarity (for a few miliseconds), that is, the inner side of the cell becomes more positive than the outside;

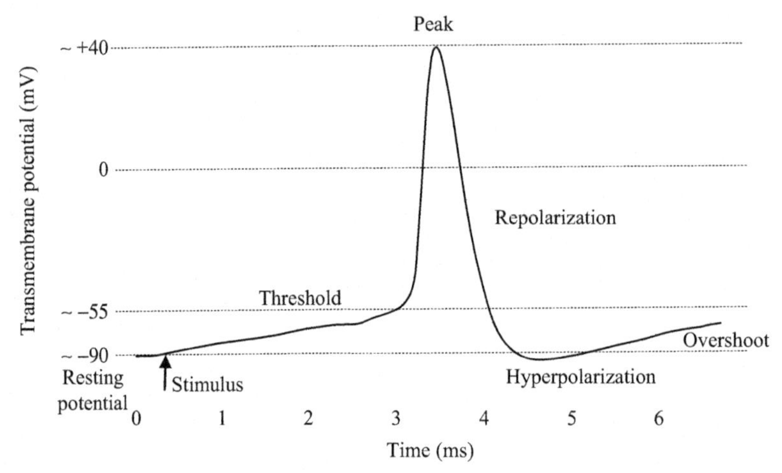

Figure 2.2 A typical action potential waveform.

- potassium channels open (take longer than sodium) and potassium ions leave the cell;
- at the same time the sodium channels begin to close, reversing the depolarization (descent or repolarization phase);
- potassium channels are slow to close and membrane hyperpolarization can occur reaching lower values than the resting potential;
- the nonexcited condition of the membrane permeability is reversed and the resting potential is restored;
- after the restoration of the resting potential, the cell goes through a refractory period (there are exceptions) and is not able to respond to a new stimulus.

The propagation of the action potential across the membrane of an excitable cell occurs by the succession of depolarization and repolarization phases caused by the flow of transmembrane ionic currents, with ions flowing in and out of the cell. Figure 2.3 shows the schematic diagram of the propagation of the action potential in excitable cell.

Biopotentials are ionic potentials, produced by ionic currents and have to be converted into electric potentials before being measured by conventional methods. Ideally free of noise and stable devices, metal electrodes convert ionic current into electrical current, and thus play the role of transducers. Therefore, a transducer that converts ionic current into electrical current can measure the ionic displacement that generates the action potential. A single action potential can be detected in some types of cells, but involves the use of an electrode of very small dimensions, and its placement within the cell. The measurement of the cell transmembrane potential can be made with an Ag–AgCl microelectrode placed in the intracellular environment and a metal electrode placed outside the cell as shown in Figure 2.1.

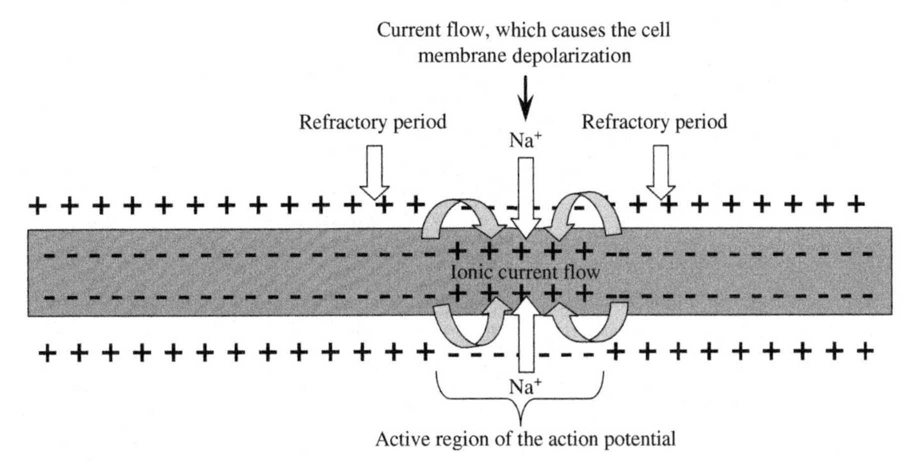

Figure 2.3 Propagation of the action potential along the membrane of an excitable cell.

The ionic currents run through small physical distances, but the electric field variations produced can be detected at a considerable distance. The most common way to register a biopotential is to measure the combined effect of many action potentials that reach the surface of the body. The tissues crossed by the electric field variations of the cell membrane activations act as a volume conductor allowing that these variations, which occur inside the body, to be transmitted to the surface and captured with electrodes placed over the skin. A biopotential source, such as the heart, generates electrical field gradients that can be detected any place over the body surface. The most common way to measure cardiac potentials is to place the electrodes on the chest. Augustus Waller registered, for the first time, the electric field on the surface of the thorax, produced by the electrical activity of the human heart, in 1887 (Waller, 1887). He recorded the isopotential lines over the thorax, that is, the electric field lines generated by ionic currents from depolarization of heart cell membranes, spreading through the conductor volume (tissues of the thorax) and found that the cardiac electric generator had a dipolar nature; he determined the correspondent dipolar source and suggested the current flow lines that would generate such an electric field. Waller even suggested that the electrocardiogram (ECG) should be registered using 10 bipolar leads defined by 5 measurement points, both hands, both legs, and the mouth.

2.3 ELECTRODE–ELECTROLYTE INTERFACE

Figure 2.4A shows an electrode formed by atoms of a metal M immersed in electrolyte, an aqueous solution containing cations of the metal (M^+) and anions A^-. Figure 2.4B represents the interface between the metal and the electrolyte. When the metal is exposed to the solution, the reactions represented by Eqs. (2.1) and (2.2)

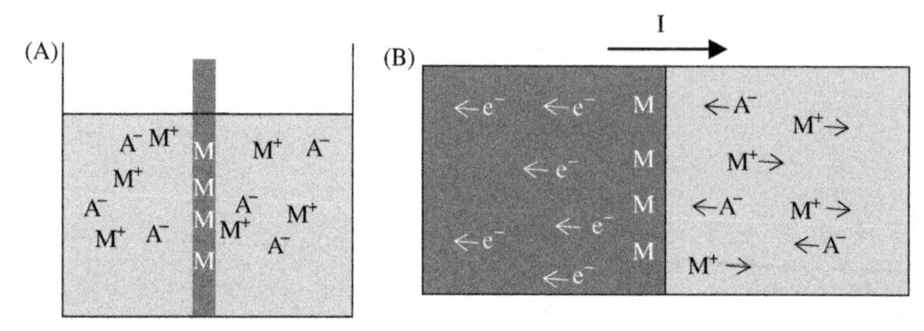

Figure 2.4 (A) Metal electrode immersed in an electrolyte solution and (B) electrode–electrolyte interface.

begin to occur, predominantly in one direction, depending on the cations concentration in the solution and the equilibrium conditions for each of these reactions.

The atoms of the metal M in the electrode–electrolyte interface can be oxidized to form cations and one or more free electrons (Eq. (2.1)). The cations are discharged into the electrolyte and the electrons are transported through the electrode.

$$M \leftrightarrow M^{n+} + ne^{-} \tag{2.1}$$

where n is the valence of M, the metal electrode.

Any anion that comes from the electrode–electrolyte interface can be oxidized into a neutral atom transfering one or more free electrons to the electrode (Eq. (2.2)).

$$A^{m-} \leftrightarrow A + me^{-} \tag{2.2}$$

where m is the valence of the component A from the electrolyte.

Both oxidation reactions in Eqs. (2.1) and (2.2) can be reversed with a reduction process. The displacements of electronic and ionic charges are the result of oxidation and reduction chemical reactions occurring at the interface between the metal electrode and the electrolyte.

The net current I through the electrode–electrolyte interface, shown in Figure 2.5B, flows from the electrode to the electrolyte. It is the result of the electrons displacement in the opposite direction through the electrode, the cations (M^{+}) displacement in the same direction, and anions (A^{-}) displacement moving in the opposite direction, through the electrolyte. When the resulting current flows from the electrode to the electrolyte, the oxidation reactions are dominant. When current flows through the electrolyte to the electrode, the reduction reactions are dominant. In addition, when the frequency of the oxidation reactions is equal to the rate of reduction reactions, the net charge transfer, that is, the current through the interface, is null. It is important to note that no electronic or ionic charge crosses the interface, but there is electronic charge displacement through the metal electrode and there is ionic charge displacement through the electrolyte (Geddes & Baker, 1968; Webster, 2010).

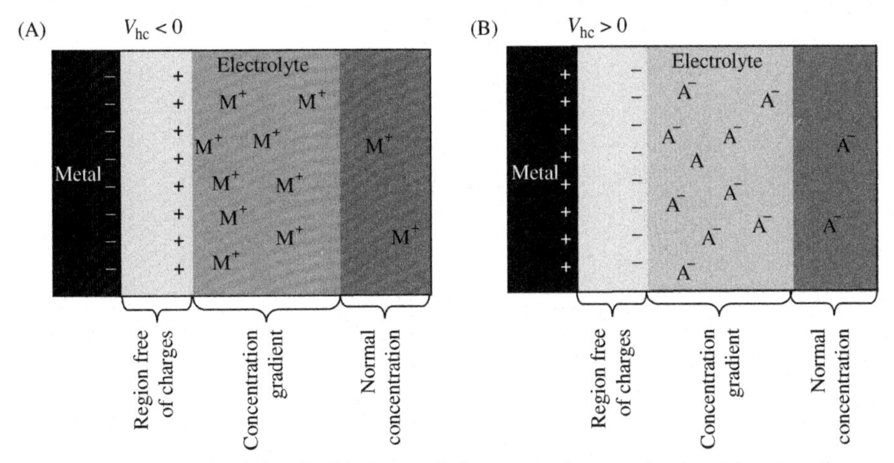

Figure 2.5 Representation of the double layer of charges in the metal–electrolyte interface to positive and negative valence metals, or $V_{hc} < 0$ (A) and $V_{hc} > 0$ (B), respectively.

2.3.1 Half-cell potential (V_{hc})

The spatial separation of opposite charges in the electrode–electrolyte interface establishes a "double layer" of charges: one type of charge is dominant in the metal surface and the opposite charge distributes in the electrolyte adjacent to the electrode. The electrolyte concentration of cations and ions near to the interface changes: a charge gradient arises in the electrolyte immediately adjacent to the metal. Therefore, the electrolyte near the interface region presents an electrical potential that is different from the rest of the solution. Figure 2.5 shows the representation of the charge distribution which results in a difference in electrical potential between the metal and the electrolyte. This potential difference is determined by the metal of the electrode, the ions concentrations in the electrolyte solution and the temperature, and is called "half-cell potential" (V_{hc}).

It is not possible to measure the V_{hc} of a metal electrode without using a second electrode as reference. Because the second electrode also has a V_{hc}, it is only feasible to measure the electric potencial difference between the V_{hc} of the first electrode and the V_{hc} of the second electrode. There could be numerous combinations of pairs of electrodes and a standard convention adopted a particular electrode, of hydrogen, as having a null V_{hc}, under specific conditions reproducible in the laboratory. One can then measure the half-cell potential of any electrode material in relation to the hydrogen electrode called the reference electrode. In addition to the hydrogen electrode, the Ag–AgCl and calomel electrodes, operating under certain conditions, are defined as constant electrode potentials too, although not null, and they also are called reference electrodes.

The operation of each of the three types of electrodes that are commonly used as reference, hydrogen, Ag–AgCl, and calomel, is explained below (Chan, 2008; Cobbold, 1974; Geddes & Baker, 1968).

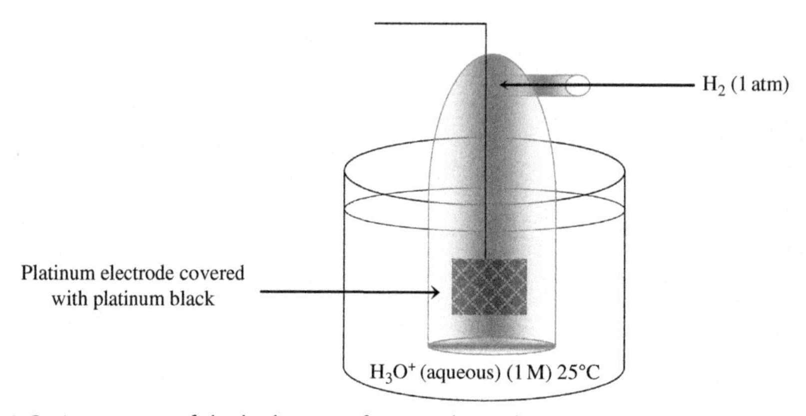

Figure 2.6 Basic structure of the hydrogen reference electrode.

2.3.1.1 Hydrogen reference electrode

Figure 2.6 shows the basic structure of the hydrogen reference electrode.

The hydrogen electrode comprises a platinum wire or sheet in which black platinum (platinum salt) is electroplated to form a fine mesh layer of metallic platinum on which the H_2 is bubbled; the gas molecules are adsorbed in the platinum mesh layer forming a "hydrogen electrode" and increasing the available surface for chemical reactions. The light is absorbed in platinum mesh surface, giving it a darkened appearance. The hydrogen electrode is the only metallic electrode that does not consist of a solid metal in equilibrium with its ion. The black platinum, covered with H_2 molecules, is immersed in acidic solution (H_3O^+). H_2 electrode operation is based on the reversible reactions represented by Eqs. (2.3) and (2.4).

$$H_2 \leftrightarrow 2H \tag{2.3}$$

$$2H \leftrightarrow 2H^+ + 2e^- \tag{2.4}$$

If the activity of the hydrogen ion is 1 mol/l (pH = 0) and hydrogen gas is bubbled into the solution so that partial pressure of hydrogen is 1 atm, the electrode potential is defined as zero volts at any temperature: $E_0 = 0.000$ V.

Figure 2.7 shows an electrochemical cell used to determine the half-cell potential (V_{hc}) of an electrode (X). The hydrogen electrode is the reference. The electrolyte, an acid solution with a concentration 1 mol of H_3O^+, also contains cations of the X material. A voltmeter, connected between the two electrodes, measures the potential difference between them. As the V_{hc} of the hydrogen electrode is set to zero, the reading value will correspond to the V_{hc} of the X material electrode.

Table 2.2 shows some common metal electrodes and their respective half-cell potentials measured under standard conditions (25°C, 1 atm pressure and 1.0 mol dm^{-3} concentration) and referenced to the standard hydrogen electrode (Haynes, 2013).

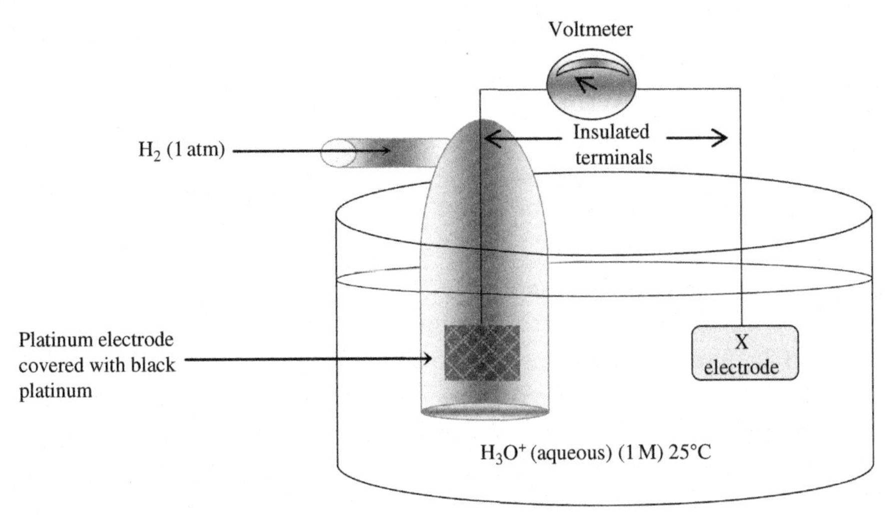

Figure 2.7 Electrochemical cell used to determine the half-cell potential (V_{hc}) of any metal, for instance, *X*.

Table 2.2 Half-cell potential (V_{hc}) of electrodes

Electrode	Reduction half reactions	Half-cell potential V_{hc} (*V*)
Lithium	$Li^+ + e^- \rightarrow Li$	−3.04
Potassium	$K \rightarrow K^+ + e^-$	−2.92
Calcium	$Ca^{2+} + 2e^- \rightarrow Ca$	−2.84
Sodium	$Na^+ + e^- \rightarrow Na$	−2.71
Aluminum	$Al^{3+} + 3e \rightarrow Al$	−1.71
Zinc	$Zn^{2+} + 2e^- \rightarrow Zn$	−0.74
Chromium	$Cr^{3+} + 3e^- \rightarrow Cr$	−0.74
Iron	$Fe^{2+} + 2e^- \rightarrow Fe$	−0.41
Cadmium	$Cd^{2+} + 2e^- \rightarrow Cd$	−0.40
Nickel	$Ni^{2+} + 2e^- \rightarrow Ni$	−0.23
Lead	$Pb \rightarrow Pb^{2+} + 2e^-$	−0.13
Hydrogen	$2H^+ + 2e^- \rightarrow H$	(by definition) 0.00
Silver chloride	$AgCl + e^- \rightarrow Ag + Cl^-$	+0.23
Mercuric chloride	$Hg_2Cl_2 + 2e^- \rightarrow 2Hg + 2Cl^-$	+0.27
Copper	$Cu^{2+} + 2e^- \rightarrow Cu$	+0.34
Copper	$Cu^+ + e^- \rightarrow Cu$	+0.52
Silver	$Ag^+ + e^- \rightarrow Ag$	+0.80
Gold	$Au^{3+} + 3e^- \rightarrow Au$	+1.42
Gold	$Au^+ + e^- \rightarrow Au$	+1.68
Fluorine	$F_2 + 2e^- \rightarrow 2F^-$	+2.87

The hydrogen electrode has high reproducibility and low offset voltage (a pair of hydrogen electrodes immersed in the same acid solution presents a DC voltage difference of 10 mV). When subjected to the action of oxidizing agents, the hydrogen concentration near the electrode reduces, changing the electrode potential. In adittion, its use requires high purity hydrogen gas. It is mainly used in calibrations and rarely in routine procedures (Chan, 2008; Cobbold, 1974; Geddes & Baker, 1968).

2.3.1.2 Ag–AgCl reference electrode

Another widely used reference electrode is the silver electrode coated with silver chloride, Ag–AgCl. Figure 2.8A illustrates this type of electrode, which consists of a silver wire or plate coated with a thin layer of soluble ionic compound of the metal (Ag^+) with a suitable anion (Cl^-). This electrode is generally used with KCl electrolyte solution (x mol/l), saturated with silver chloride, which ensures that the solution in the electrode vicinity is saturated with Ag^+ and Cl^- ions. When the Ag–AgCl electrode

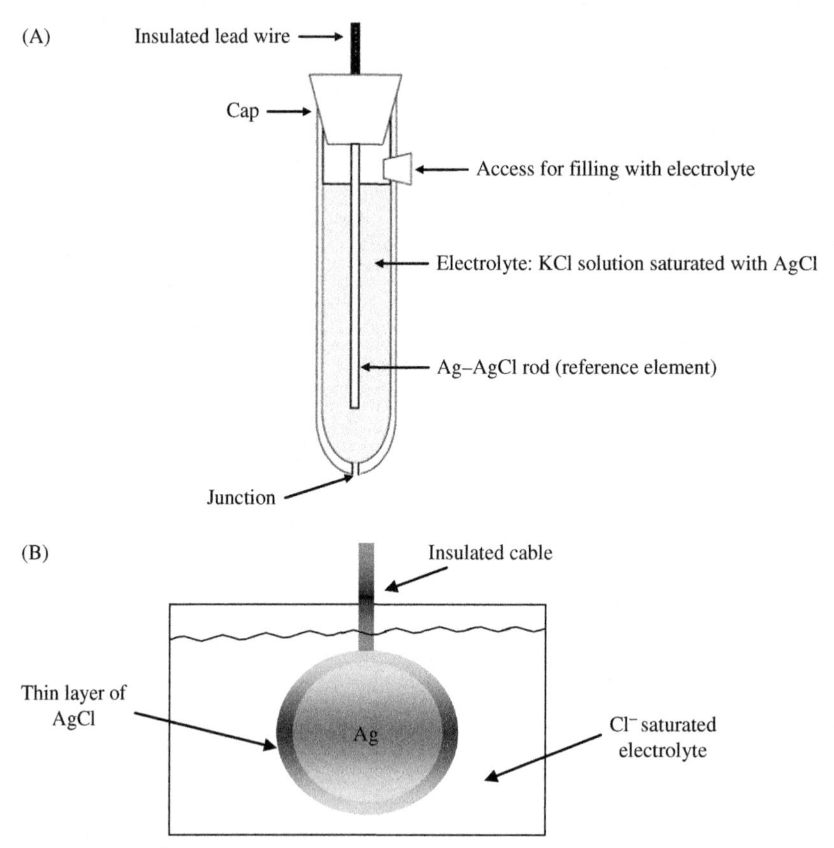

Figure 2.8 (A) Ag–AgCl reference electrode and (B) disc electrode, shown in section, immersed in electrolyte.

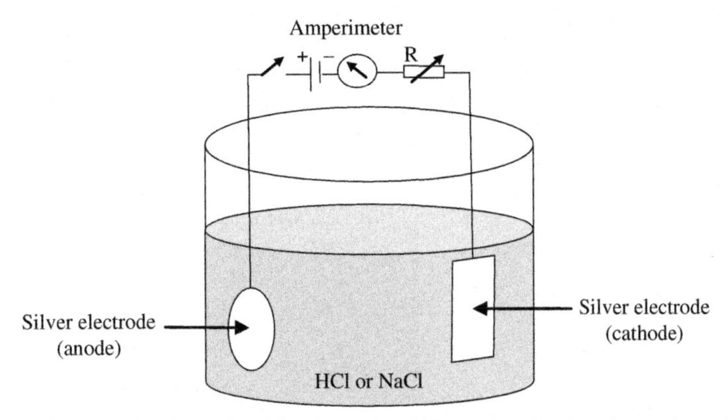

Figure 2.9 Electrochemical cell used to deposit an AgCl layer on the Ag electrode surface.

is immersed in this solution, oxidation reactions of the silver atoms (Eq. (2.5)) occur at the electrode surface, releasing silver cations in the solution and free electrons in the metal interface. These silver cations react with the electrolyte Cl^- anions (Eq. (2.6)), forming AgCl, which is soluble in water and precipitates in the silver electrode surface, contributing to enhance the silver chloride layer. Figure 2.9B also represents an Ag–AgCl electrode, but in format of disc, similar to the electrode used in biopotential recording.

$$\text{On the electrode surface: } \mathrm{Ag(solid)} \leftrightarrow \mathrm{Ag^+} + \mathrm{e^-} \tag{2.5}$$

$$\text{In the electrolyte: } \mathrm{Ag^+} + \mathrm{Cl^-} \leftrightarrow \mathrm{AgCl\ (solid)} \downarrow \tag{2.6}$$

The V_{hc} of the Ag–AgCl electrode is stable when the electrolyte contains Cl^-. Biological tissues have high concentration of Cl^- and this type of transducer is relatively stable in invasive biological applications. The equilibrium potential of the silver–silver chloride electrode is given by the Nernst equation:

$$V_{Ag} = V^0_{Ag/Ag^+} + \frac{RT}{nF} \ln(\alpha_{Ag^+}) \tag{2.7}$$

where

V^0_{Ag/Ag^+}, standard potential of the silver–silver chloride electrode
R, molar gas constant ($8.3144621\ \mathrm{J\ mol^{-1}\ K^{-1}}$) (*source*: NIST Reference on Constants, Units, and Uncertainty)
T, temperature in Kelvin ($25°C = 298$ K)
n, atom valence, in this case, $+1$
F, Faraday's constant ($96{,}485.3365\ \mathrm{C\ mol^{-1}}$) (*source*: NIST Reference on Constants, Units, and Uncertainty)
α_{Ag^+}, silver solubility.

The silver chloride solubility at 25°C is:

$$Ks = \alpha_{Ag^+} \cdot \alpha_{Cl^-} \approx 1.78 \cdot 10^{-10} \tag{2.8}$$

Substituting Ks in Nernst equation results:

$$V_{Ag} = V^0_{Ag/Ag^+} + \frac{RT}{nF}\ln\left(\frac{Ks}{\alpha_{Cl^-}}\right) \tag{2.9}$$

$$V_{Ag} = V^0_{Ag/Ag^+} + \frac{RT}{nF}\ln\left(\frac{Ks}{\alpha_{Cl^-}}\right) - \frac{RT}{nF}\ln(\alpha_{Cl^-}) \tag{2.10}$$

$$V_{Ag} = V^0_{Ag/Ag^+} + \frac{RT}{F}\ln(1.78 \cdot 10^{-10}) - \frac{RT}{F}\ln(\alpha_{Cl^-}) \tag{2.11}$$

Making use of tabulated values:

$$V_{Ag} = V^0_{Ag/Ag^+} - 0.0256\ \ln(\alpha_{Cl^-}) \tag{2.12}$$

$$V_{Ag} = 0.224 - 0.0256\ \ln(\alpha_{Cl^-}) \tag{2.13}$$

The Ag–AgCl electrode obeys the Nernst equation for a wide range of values of Cl^- activity and its potential depends on the temperature and concentration of the electrolyte. When the reference electrode is filled with saturated KCl:

$$Ag-AgCl/_{KCl\ Sat.} = 197.0\ mV\ (at\ 25°C)\ \ or\ \ = 191.9\ mV\ (at\ 30°C)$$

Using 3 mol/l KCl solution, the equilibrium potential is:

$$Ag-AgCl/_{KCl\ 3\ mol/l} = 207.0\ mV\ (at\ 25°C)\ \ or\ \ = 203.4\ mV\ (at\ 30°C)$$

The presaturation of the KCl electrolyte prevents the erosion of the electrode surface silver chloride layer. The silver chloride electrode has reproducibility and reliability comparable to that of the hydrogen electrode and offset potential $<50\ \mu V$. It can be built in various formats and sizes: sheet, wire, or as microelectrode (for intracellular measurements). Equation (2.11) indicates that a modification in the electrolyte concentration modifies the electrode potential and also that the silver chloride electrode is a function of temperature.

The electrolytic process to form an Ag–AgCl electrode with wire or sheet format uses an electrochemical cell such as that shown in Figure 2.9: a silver electrode in which the AgCl layer will be deposited is the anode and another silver electrode, with a larger surface, is the cathode. A DC voltage source feeds the chemical cell (typically 1.5 V); a variable resistor R limits the peak current controlling the chemical reactions velocity; an amperimeter indicates the current intensity which value is proportional to the reactions velocity. When the switch closes, the reactions rate (Eqs. (2.5) and (2.6)) increases causing the current to achieve a maximum value. The thickness of the AgCl layer deposited increases, until the reaction rate begins to fall due to lack of anions (Cl^-) in the electrolyte, decreasing the current to values near zero (Chan, 2008; Cobbold, 1974; Geddes & Baker, 1968; Webster, 2010).

2.3.1.3 Calomel reference electrode

Figure 2.10 shows the schematic diagram of calomel electrode. This electrode has two glass tubes with porous plugs in the bases. The inner tube contains a platinum wire connected to the output wire lead and is filled with mercury (Hg metalic) and a paste with Hg_2Cl_2, or calomel, which is slightly soluble in water, Hg and KCl. The calomel comes into contact with the solution of potassium chloride (also soluble in water) that fills the second tube, through the pores of the plug in the base of the first tube. The pores of the plug in the base of the second glass tube close the ionic circuit in the electrochemical cell, for example.

The calomel dissociates (reversibly) in ions Hg_2^{2+} and Cl^- according to Eq. (2.14).

$$Hg_2Cl_2(sol) \leftrightarrow Hg_2^{2+}(liq) + 2Cl^- \quad (2.14)$$

The presence of Cl^- ion in the solution reduces the activity of the Hg_2^{2+} to a value inversely proportional to the Cl^- ion activity. At equilibrium, in the interface mercury–mercury chloride, oxidation and reduction reactions occur according to

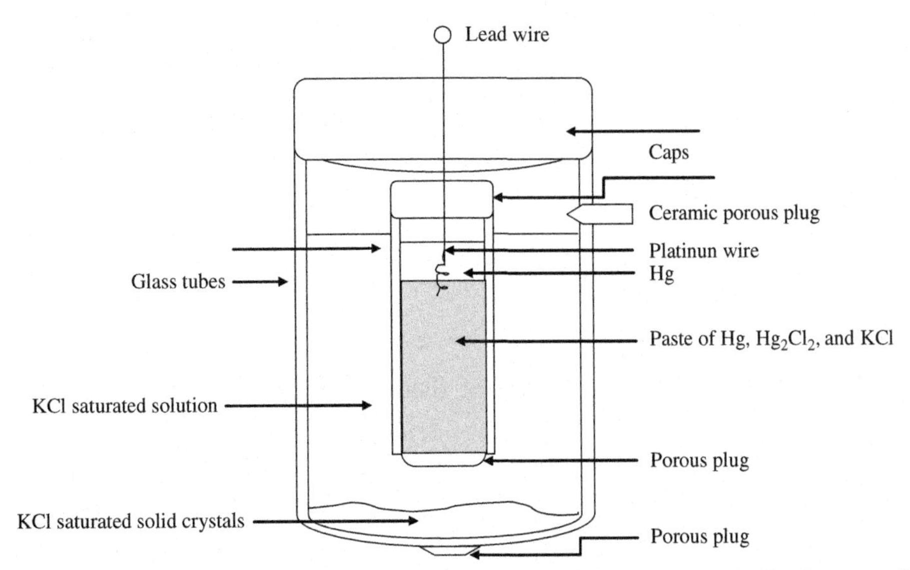

Figure 2.10 Calomel electrode used as reference electrode for determining half-cell potentials of metal electrodes.

Eq. (2.15). The Hg metal atoms are oxidized to form mercury cations and free electrons, which are transported through the platinum wire.

$$2\text{Hg} \leftrightarrow \text{Hg}_2^{2+}(\text{liq}) + 2\text{e}^- \tag{2.15}$$

The contact of mercury (metal) with calomel paste results in a half-cell potential that depends on the concentration of the KCl solution. The activities of Cl^- and Hg_2^{2+} ions define the potential of the calomel electrode. The solubility of the calomel electrode at 25°C is

$$Ks = (\alpha\text{Cl}^-)^2 \cdot \alpha\text{Hg}_2^+ \approx 1 \cdot 10^{-18}$$

The Nernst equation for the calomel electrode is

$$V_{\text{Hg}} = V^0_{\text{Hg/Hg}_2^{2+}} + \frac{RT}{F}\ln(\alpha_{\text{Hg}_2^{2+}}) \tag{2.16}$$

Replacing $\alpha_{\text{Hg}_2^+}$ in Eq. (2.16) with Ks, results:

$$V_{\text{Hg}} = V^0_{\text{Hg/Hg}_2^{2+}} + \frac{RT}{F}\ln(Ks) - \frac{RT}{F}\ln(\alpha_{\text{Cl}^-}) \tag{2.17}$$

Using tabulated values $E^0_{\text{Hg/Hg}_2^{2+}} = 0.797$ V and $Ks = 1.10 - 18$ at 25°C:

$$V_{\text{Hg}} = 0.797 + \frac{RT}{F}\ln(1 \cdot 10^{-18}) - \frac{RT}{F}\ln(\alpha_{\text{Cl}-}) \tag{2.18}$$

The KCl solution in calomel electrode is used at concentrations of 0.1, 1 N, or saturated, corresponding to half-cell potentials equal to −0.334, −0.281, and −0.242 V, respectively, at 25°C. The saturated KCl solution is the most used resulting in a very stable reference electrode and producing a very good reference at constant temperature. The calomel electrode exhibits less stability with temperature changes than the silver–silver chloride and hydrogen electrodes. At high temperatures (above 60°C), thermal decomposition of mercury chloride (calomel) occurs. Its use is indicated for pH measurement in clinical laboratories, in solutions with proteins and with heavy metals which react with Ag–AgCl (Chan, 2008; Cobbold, 1974; Geddes & Baker, 1968; Webster, 2010).

2.3.2 Equivalent electronic circuit of the electrode/electrolyte interface

The equivalent circuit that represents the interface between the metal electrode and the electrolyte, shown in Figure 2.11, includes resistive and capacitive components which values are determined by the electrode material and by the composition and concentration of the electrolyte. The capacitance C_{dl} is in the model because V_{hc} is due to ionic charges distribution, represented as two layers of charges with opposite polarities separated by a region free of charges, which behaves as a capacitor. Thus, C_{dl}

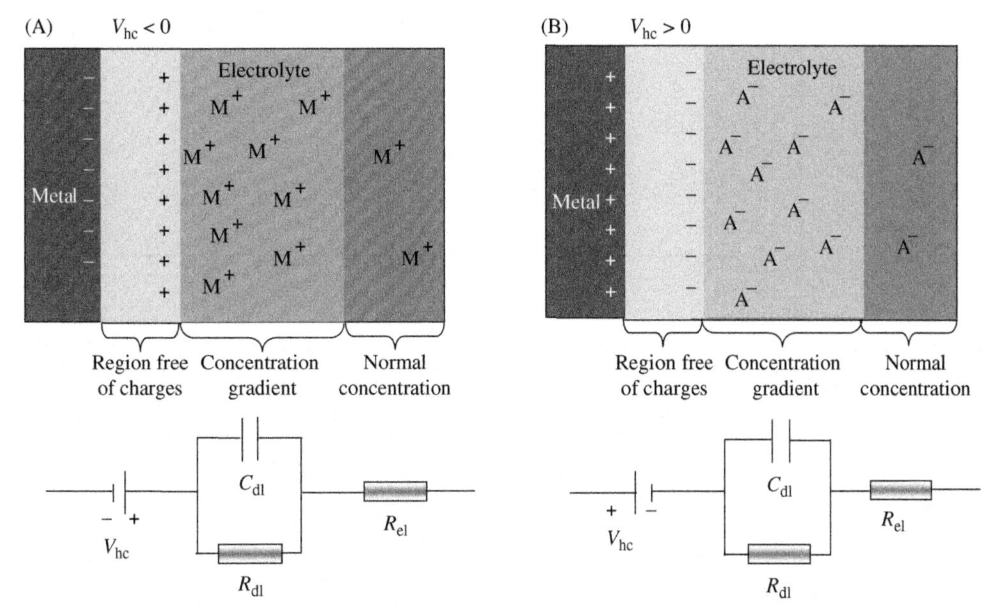

Figure 2.11 Equivalent circuit of a biopotential electrode in contact with an electrolyte: (A) negative valence metal and (B) positive valence metal.

corresponds to the double layer capacitance in the electrode–electrolyte interface. The typical range values of this capacitance are between 0.1 and 10 μF. The parallel resistance R_{dl} is the resistance across this double layer (typical values are above 2 kΩ). The series resistance R_{el} represents the variation of the ion concentration in the electrolyte from the interface with the metal. A DC voltage source represents the metal half-cell voltage and completes the electrical equivalent circuit of a biopotential electrode coupled to the electrolyte. The polarity of this DC voltage source depends on the valence of the metal used in the electrode (Chan, 2008; Cobbold, 1974; Geddes & Baker, 1968; Webster, 2010).

The electrode–electrolyte equivalent circuit (Figure 2.11), at high frequencies, has capacitive reactance much smaller than the resistance of the double layer, that is, $1/\omega C_{dl} \ll R_{dl}$ (ω = angular frequêncy). Thus, the parallel arrangement of R_{dl} and C_{dl} has an equivalent resistance even smaller than the capacitive reactance of C_{dl}. In conclusion, at high frequencies, the interface impedance is approximately constant and equal to R_{el} (electrolyte resistance). At lower frequencies, $1/\omega C_{dc} \gg R_{dl}$, and the interface impedance is also approximately constant, but its value is greater and equal to $(R_{dl} + R_{el})$.

The impedance frequency dependance of a 0.25 cm^2 surface area silver electrode is shown in Figure 2.12(1). Figure 2.12(2–5) shows the curves of the impedance frequency dependance of Ag–AgCl electrodes, equal areas, and different AgCl layer

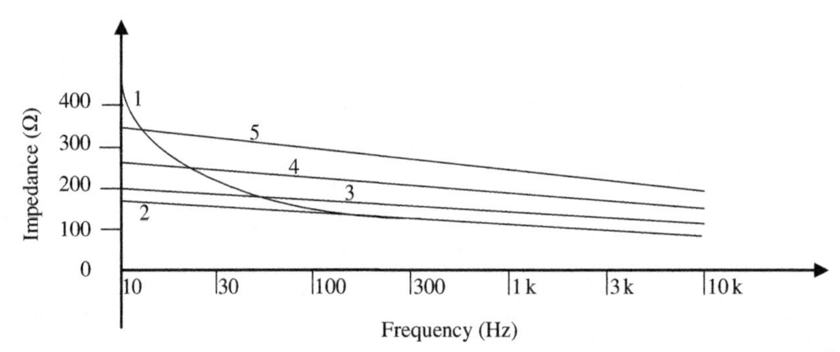

Figure 2.12 Impedance as a function of frequency for electrodes with an area of 0.25 cm^2 made of pure silver (1) and silver coated with AgCl layer deposited electrolytically with (2) 7.5 mA · s; (3) 125 mA · s; (4) 275 mA · s; and (5) 425 mA · s.

thicknesses. The impedance of the Ag—AgCl electrode differs greatly from the silver electrode at frequencies lower than 100 Hz. At 10 Hz the silver electrode impedance is almost three times its value at 300 Hz, showing the influence of the reactive component in the equivalent circuit. The electrolytic deposition of AgCl layer reduces electrode impedance at low frequencies; for both, pure silver electrode and Ag—AgCl electrode, impedance decreases with increasing frequency. The impedance of the Ag—AgCl electrode exhibits a linear and decreasing behavior with frequency. The thicker the AgCl layer, higher is the impedance, regardless of frequency (Cobbold, 1974; Geddes & Baker, 1968; Webster, 2010).

2.4 ELECTROLYTE—SKIN INTERFACE

The skin—electrolyte interface can also be included in the equivalent circuit that represents the biopotential measurement over the body surface. The layers organization of the skin is shown in Figure 2.13. The skin, an organ in constant renovation, is divided into three layers: epidermis, dermis, and subcutaneous layer. Epidermis has five layers and the outer one is the *stratum corneum*, formed mainly of dead cutaneous cells, which acts like a protection barrier against water loss, microorganisms, and sun, for instance. *Stratum corneum*, considered like an ion semipermeable, has high electrical resistance compared to other layers and its effect is minimized through partial removal (cleaning or abrasion).

Figure 2.14A shows a representation of the interfaces electrolytic gel—electrode—skin and Figure 2.14B shows the electrical equivalent circuit for these interfaces. Note that *stratum corneum* is modeled in Figure 2.14B as a DC potential V_{sc}.

A parallel RC circuit represents the effect of the epidermis, and therefore its impedance changes with frequency: the impedance of 1 cm^2 of skin is equal to approximately 200 kΩ at 1 Hz and 200 Ω at 1 MHz. The effect of the sweat glands and ducts

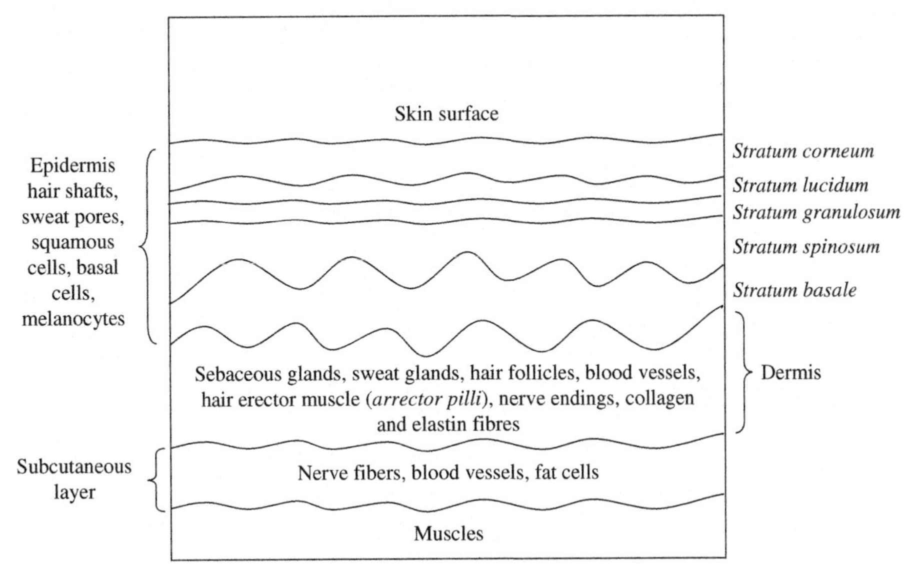

Figure 2.13 Representation of the layers of the skin, epidermis subdivision, and main components of the layers.

is omitted in the absence of thermal stimulus (dashed lines). The effect of the deeper layers produces negligible DC potential (voltage drop across R_{dsl}) (Chan, 2008; Cobbold, 1974; Geddes & Baker, 1968; Webster, 2010).

2.5 ARTIFACTS OF MEASUREMENT

Figure 2.15A shows the representation of a biopotential (electromyogram, EMG) measurement with two metallic surface electrodes, coupled to the skin through electrolytic gel. Figure 2.15B shows the equivalent circuit, where the left and right branches represent the surface electrodes. The ideal situation requires identical electrodes, that is, equal resistives and capacitives components and half-cell voltages for both electrodes. Any situation that breaks the symmetry of values of the elements of the equivalent circuit gives rise to measurement artifacts. Some of these situations discussed in sequence are offset voltage, motion artifact, electrode polarization, and liquid junction potential.

2.5.1 Offset voltage

The half-cell potential, ideally stable and constant for identical metal electrodes, can constitute a source of artifact in the measurement. Even using two electrodes made by the same manufacturer and with the same characteristics, they may have different V_{hc}, what can result in current flow between the electrodes, giving rise to an undesired

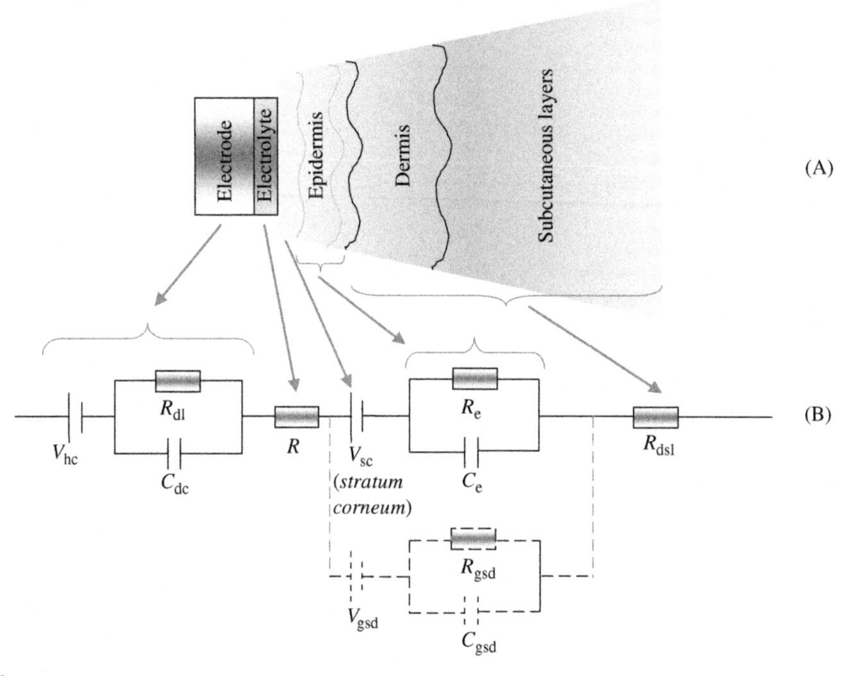

where:

C_{dl} = Capacitance of the double layer in the metal/electrolyte interface
V_{hc} = Half-cell potential of the metal electrode
R_{dl} = Resistance of the double layer in the metal/electrolyte interface
R = Resistance of the electrolyte
V_{sc} = Potential drop, defined by Nernst equation, that results from the difference of ionic concentration between the *stratum corneum* (semipermeable membrane) and the electrolyte
C_e and R_e = Capacitance and resistance of the epidermis impedance
R_{dsl} = Resistance that represents dermis and subcutaneous layers (nerves, blood vessels, glands, and sweat ducts and hair follicles)
V_{gsd}, C_{gsd}, and R_{gsd} = Elements that represent glands and sweat ducts in the presence of thermal stimulus

Figure 2.14 (A) Interfaces electrode–electrolyte–skin. The skin is represented by its layers: epidermis, dermis, and subcutaneous layers. (B) Equivalent simplified electric circuit.

voltage, called offset voltage. This voltage is added to the voltage drop across R_{tissue} (biopotential to be measured) and can be mistakenly interpreted as a physiological event.

2.5.2 Motion artifact

When a nonpolarized electrode is in contact to the electrolyte, a double layer of charges is formed in the interface. Any event that modifies the charges distribution in the metal/electrolyte interface modifies the electrode V_{hc}. When measuring a biopotential with two equal electrodes and one of them moves, for example, due to an excessive amount of electrolyte under the electrode, while the other stays stationary, a DC

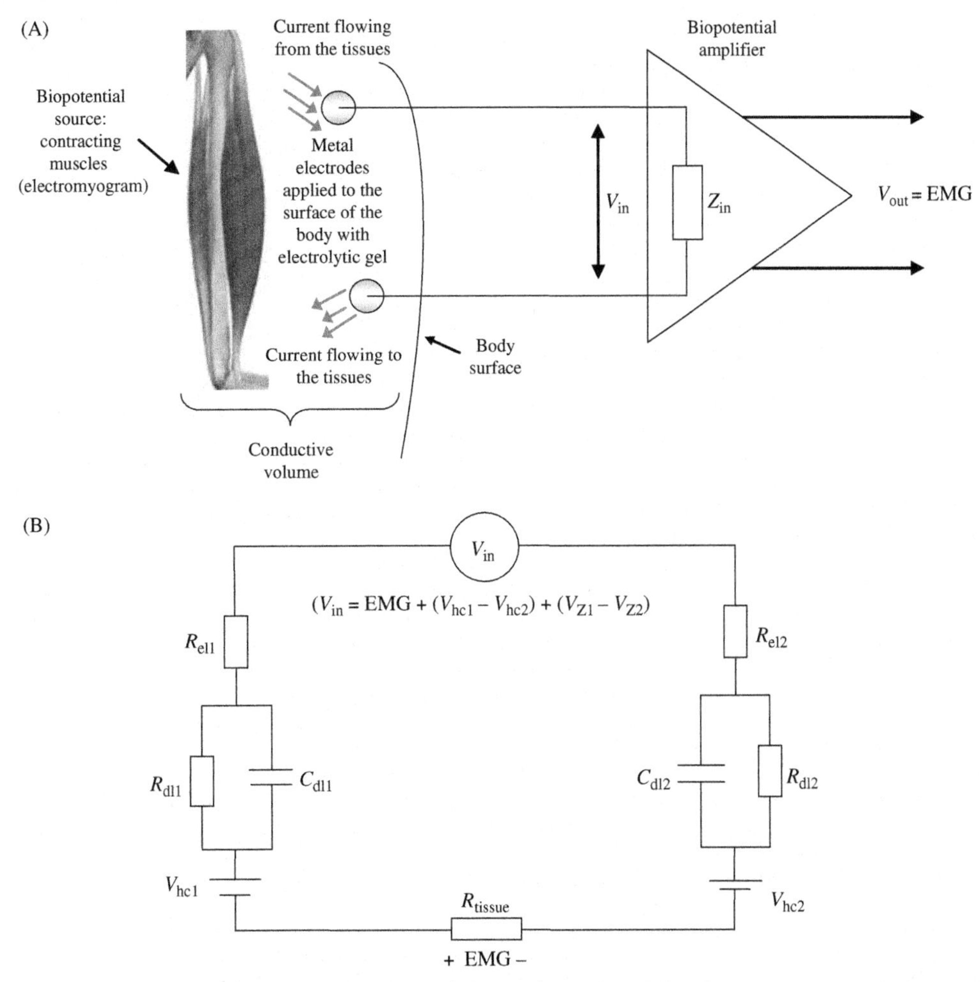

Figure 2.15 Biopotential measurement with two electrodes: (A) schematic representation and (B) equivalent circuit. Z_{in} is the input impedance of the amplifier; V_{in} is the voltage difference effectively amplified; V_{hc1} and V_{hc2} are half-cell potentials of electrodes; V_{Z1} and V_{Z2} are the potential drops across the double layers of the interfaces; and R_{el1} and R_{el2} are the impedances of the electrolytes under the electrodes.

potential will arise due to the difference in their V_{hc}. The DC potential is called motion artifact; it is added to biopotential signal, amplified and may be misinterpreted as a physiological event. The electrode movement may also be due to patient's respiration. When the electrodes are applied to the patient's thorax, for ECG recording, and the skin under the metallic electrodes stretches during the inspiration phase, the charges distribution is modified creating a potential difference between the electrodes V_{hc}.

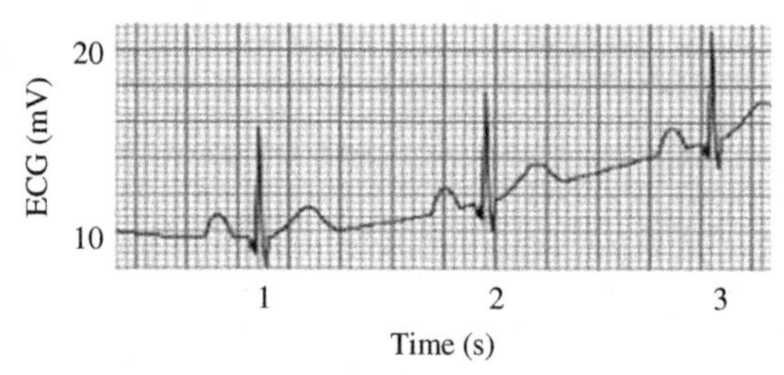

Figure 2.16 Motion artifact in ECG recording with Ag–AgCl electrodes. Motion artifact is identified as a tracing deviation from the baseline.

Figure 2.16 shows an example of motion artifact caused by the relative displacement between electrolyte and electrode of a pair of Ag–AgCl electrodes used in ECG recording. The baseline of the biopotential floats due to a variable DC level that is added to the signal captured by the pair of electrodes.

2.5.3 Electrode polarization

The equilibrium or half-cell potential of a metallic electrode is defined under conditions in which no current flows between the electrode and the electrolyte. In an ideally polarizable electrode no stationary net current flows through the electrical double layer. There is no real current between the electrode surface and the electrolyte: what happens is the displacement of charges (electrons in the electrode and ions in the electrolyte) and the interface behaves like a capacitor. No real electrode behaves exactly as ideally polarizable or nonpolarizable. Electrodes made with noble metals, such as gold, platinum, and titanium, behave approximately as ideally polarizable. In an ideally nonpolarizable electrode, in contrast, current flows freely without polarization and no overpotential is generated. Silver–silver chloride and mercury–mercury chloride electrodes behave approximately like ideally nonpolarizable electrodes.

Temperature and ion activity changings in the electrolyte are the main causes of electrode V_{hc} modification. If current flows through the electrode/electrolyte interface, concentration and ion activity change, modifying V_{hc} according to Nernst equation (specific application for Eq. (2.1) reaction):

$$V_{hc} = V_{hc^0} + \frac{RT}{nF}\ln(\alpha_c^{n+}) \tag{2.19}$$

where

V_{hc}, half-cell potential

V_{hc^0}, equilibrium or standard half-cell potential

α_c^{n+}, activity of cation C^{n+} (valence $+n$).

The generic equation for a redox reaction can be written as in Eq. (2.20):

$$\alpha A + \beta B \leftrightarrow \gamma C + \delta D + ne^- \tag{2.20}$$

where n electrons are transferred. Nernst equation can be written as in Eq. (2.21):

$$V_{hc} = V_{hc^0} + \frac{RT}{nF} \ln \left(\frac{\alpha_C^\gamma \cdot \alpha_D^\delta}{\alpha_A^\alpha \cdot \alpha_B^\beta} \right) \tag{2.21}$$

where αs represent the activities of the ions participating in the reactions.

When current flows through a real electrode, its V_{hc} changes due to electrode polarization. The difference between the observed V_{hc} and the expected equilibrium V_{hc} is known as polarization or overpotential. Some mechanisms that contribute to electrode polarization are resistance or ohmic overpotential, concentration overpotential, and activation overpotential (Webster, 2010). These distinct types of electrode polarization are additive and represent a deviation of the V_{hc} from equilibrium:

$$V_{Pol} = V_R + V_C + V_A \tag{2.22}$$

where

V_{Pol}, electrode polarization or overpotential
V_{Ohm}, resistence or ohmic overpotential
V_{Conc}, concentration overpotential
V_{Act}, activation overpotential.

2.5.3.1 Ohmic overpotential

In Figure 2.15B, R_{el1} and R_{el2} represent the resistances of the eletrolyte applied to the electrode surfaces during EMG register. When a current flows through these electrodes, there are voltage drops across the electrolytes due to their resistances. The voltage drops are proportional to the current and to the electrolyte conductivity (electronic and ionic). The electronic conductivity is often higher than the ionic conductivity, which conductivity depends on the ionic concentration of the electrolyte. Ideally, in the circuit of Figure 2.15B, the voltage drops across R_{el1} and R_{el2} are equal, cancel each other and do not contribute to the biopotential measurement. If a concentration profile develops and becomes different under each electrode, the magnitudes of the ohmic drops may change, resulting in a DC potential difference that is added to the biopotential.

2.5.3.2 Concentration overpotential

The equilibrium V_{hc} results from ionic distribution near the electrode–electrolyte interface, when no current flows between the electrode and the electrolyte. Under these conditions, the reactions represented by Eqs. (2.1) and (2.2) reach equilibrium, and oxidation and reduction occur at the same rate. When current flows through the interface, ion concentration changes and gives rise to a concentration gradient, which in turn, will lead to a voltage drop. The concentration polarization of an electrode results from the buildup of ion concentration gradient near the interface, which modifies the equilibrium V_{hc}. The difference between this new potential and the equilibrium V_{hc} is the concentration overpotential.

2.5.3.3 Activation overpotential

The oxireduction reactions represented by Eq. (2.1) are not exactly reversible. The oxidation of the metal atom results in charge transference to the metal (e^-) and to the electrolyte (metal cation), which requires the atom to overcome an energy barrier or activation energy. The reverse reaction, reduction of a metallic cation, also involves activation energy, but it is not necessarily the same as that involved in the oxidation reaction. When current flows through the interface, oxidation or reduction predominates and the activation energy changes according to the current flow direction. The activation energy difference, required for overcoming the barrier, modifies the electrode half-cell potential.

2.5.4 Liquid junction potential

If two eletrolytes with distinct concentrations are in contact, for instance, through a porous membrane, there is a tendency of the more concentrated solution to give ions to the other, giving rise to a potential difference, called liquid junction potential, V_{lj}.

The Ag–AgCl electrode shown in Figure 2.8A has a porous plug separating the electrode filling solution from the external test electrolyte of the measuring cell. If there is difference of ion concentration between these two solutions, there is a liquid junction potential. The standard voltage given by a reference electrode is correct only if there is no additional voltage like the one supplied by the liquid junction potential at the porous plug of the Ag–AgCl electrode. The liquid junction potential is another component that modifies the V_{hc} of an electrode. When the Ag–AgCl reference electrode is used in an electrochemical cell, the liquid junction potential formed at its porous plug may represent an offset voltage of units to hundreds of milivolts of the standard half-cell potential of the second metal electrode.

Liquid junction potential appears whenever two dissimilar electrolytes come into contact. At this junction, a potential difference will develop because of the tendency of the smaller and faster ions to move across the boundary more quickly than those of lower mobility. When a semipermeable membrane (like the porous plug) separates two aqueous ion solutions with different concentrations, there is a potential difference through the membrane described by Nernst equation:

$$E = \frac{RT}{nF} \ln\left(\frac{\alpha_1}{\alpha_2}\right) \tag{2.23}$$

where α_1 and α_2 are ion activities on both sides of the membrane.

The ion activity in a solution coincides with its availability to react. In a diluted solution, the ion activity is equal to the ion concentration. At higher concentrations, the ion activity is lower due to intermolecular effects (the intermolecular forces holding the liquid or solid together must be broken up by the solvent in order to form a solution). The V_{hc} values in Table 2.1 are standard half-cell potentials determined under controlled conditions. If the electrode–electrolyte system deviates from the standard condition, the observed V_{hc} differs from standard V_{hc}.

In electrolytic solutions with similar compositions, but distinct concentrations, the ion mobilities are different; the liquid junction potential is calculated by Eq. (2.24):

$$V_{lj} = \left(\frac{\mu_+ - \mu_-}{\mu_+ - \mu_-}\right)\frac{RT}{nF}\ln\left(\frac{\alpha'}{\alpha''}\right) \tag{2.24}$$

where μ_+ and μ_- are the mobilities of positive and negative ions of the solutions.

Concluding, the half-cell potential is dependent on overpotentials, ions activities, and ions mobilities (Chan, 2008; Cobbold, 1974; Webster, 2010).

2.6 ELECTRODES CLASSIFICATION

There is more than one classification of electrodes for biopotential measurement or biological tissue stimulation. Recording or monitoring electrode is used to measure biopotential, a tissue activity, while stimulating electrode delivers electrical stimulus to the tissue. Macroelectrode has contact area larger than a cell, while microlectrode has contact area of cell dimension. Surface or noninvasive electrode measures biopotentials or stimulates tissue through the body surface, without cutting the skin, while invasive recording or stimulating electrode is applied inside the biological tissue. Here electrodes are classified as noninvasive, invasive, and stimulation electrodes (Chan, 2008; Cobbold, 1974; Geddes & Baker, 1968; Khandpur, 2005; Webster, 2010).

2.6.1 Noninvasive electrodes

Noninvasive electrodes are used to register biopotentials without invading the biological tissue, that is, without disrupting cell membrane. They are classified as metal and flexible.

2.6.1.1 Metal electrodes

Metal electrodes, applied to the skin through electrolytic gel, register biopotentials as ECG, eletromyogram (EMG), and electroencephalogram (EEG). To avoid chemical reactions with electrolyte or sweat, that may cause skin irritation, the electrodes are made, preferably, of inert or almost inert metals and metal alloys such as gold, platinum, silver, titanium, and stainless steel. The metal electrodes class can be classified as limb, suction, disc, EEG, floating (top-hat and disposable), and dry electrodes.

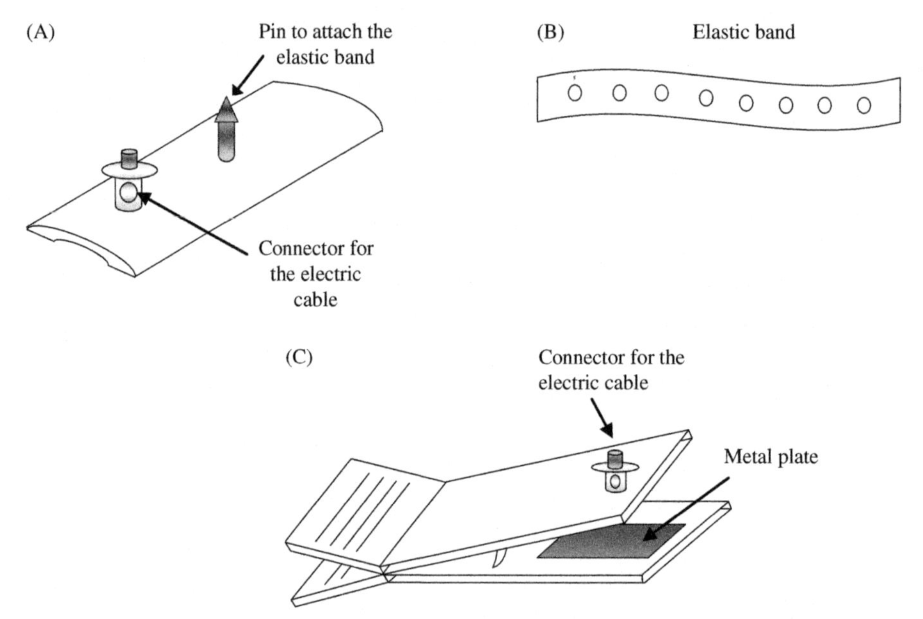

Figure 2.17 Limb electrodes: (A) curved plate, (B) fixation elastic bands and (C) plate electrode mounted in clip support.

2.6.1.1.1 Limb electrodes

This type of electrode usually has rectangular format and plane contact area. Its surface can also be curved to a better adjustment to the format of arms and legs (Figure 2.17A). They are used, for instance, as return plate in electrosurgery and right leg electrode in ECG recording. The inner side of the electrode receives a layer of electrolytic gel and it is fixed with the help of elastic bands. Smaller sizes of plates are also mounted in clip supports (Figure 2.17B), eliminating the need of the bands. In addition to gold, silver, and stainless steel, they can be made of a metallic alloy of copper, zinc, and nickel, known as German silver or alpaca. German silver is extensively used because of its hardness, toughness, resistance to oxidation, and high electrical resistance; the percentage of the three elements varies, ranging for copper from 50% to 61.6%; for zinc from 17.2% to 19%; and for nickel from 21.1% to 30%.

2.6.1.1.2 Suction electrodes

The suction electrode has a metallic dome shape with a connector to the electric cable, and a suction rubber bulb (Figure 2.18A and B). Different metal and alloys can be used in the dome: gold, silver, Ag–AgCl, Ni–Cu, and german silver (an alloy of copper, nickel, and zinc; for instance, 60% copper, 20% nickel, and 20% zinc). The main use of suction electrodes is in precordial ECG recording. The rubber bulb is squeezed and then the electrode is connected to the chest through suction, which

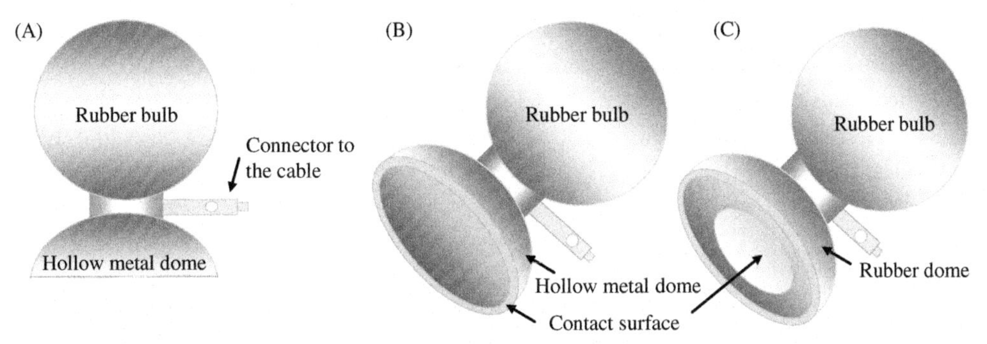

Figure 2.18 Suction electrodes: (A and B) components of a suction electrode and (C) variation of suction electrode with a recessed Ag–AgCl disc and rubber dome.

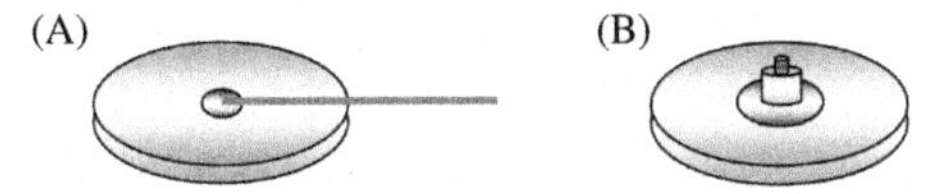

Figure 2.19 Metal disc electrodes with (A) lead wire and (B) cable connector soldered in the center of the top face.

removes the air between the electrode and the skin, keeping the electrode in place without the need of elastic bands or adhesives. An electrolyte layer is applied in the edge of the dome before the electrode is adjusted to the skin surface. The suction can cause skin irritation and this type of electrode should be used for short periods of time; moreover, it also causes discomfort to the patient since its use can be painful. It is manufactured in different diameters to child and adult use (15, 24, and 30 mm). Among the metal electrodes, the suction electrode is the one with the higher impedance due to the small contact area (edge of the dome).

Figure 2.18C shows a suction electrode that has the dome made of rubber with a recessed metal disc inside (Ag–AgCl), which contributes to decrease the electrode impedance (larger contact surface) and to reduce the discomfort (rubber, instead of metal suctions the patient skin). The electrolytic gel layer is applied on the disc surface. One example of this version of suction electrode, also used in chest wall for ECG recording, is the H5 1800 fabricated by Servoprax®.

2.6.1.1.3 Metal Disc Electrodes

This type of electrode is formed by a metal disc with a wire or a cable connector welded to the center of one of the disc faces (Figure 2.19). A layer of gel is applied to the bottom side of the electrode before it is placed on the skin. These electrodes are used in precordial ECG and surface electromyography (EMG) recording. Various diameter values are available to suit the age of the patient and the body region under examination. They are made of Ag–AgCl, stainless steel, gold, or platinum, to minimize chemical reactions occurrences due to gel or sweat during the exams. Elastic bands or adhesive tape are used to attach the electrodes on the skin.

Other types of recording electrodes also use metal discs, like the top-hat electrode, that will be discussed in floating electrodes, or formats similar to a disc like EEG electrodes.

2.6.1.1.4 EEG electrodes

EEG electrodes are manufactured as stamped, cast, or sintered electrodes. The stamped EEG electrodes, used in routine examinations, are made from a thin plate of silver, gold, or Ag–AgCl. They are also named stamped cup electrodes due to their format. They have a wide edge (Figure 2.20A and C) where a layer of colloidal paste is applied to fix the electrodes in the scalp skin; a hole in the top of the electrode (Figure 2.20B) allows easy filling of the electrolytic gel after adhesion of the cup to scalp (and also any excess gel to get out during the positioning of the electrode); and a lateral connector, usually stamped together with the disc, where the lead wire is welded (Figure 2.20A–C). EEG stamped discs are sold as individual electrodes or mounted in colored flat cable, which facilitates their application on the scalp with the 10–20 system. The discs are fabricated with different external diameter (6 and 10 mm), central hole diameter (1.5 and 2 mm), and cable lengths (100, 150, and 200 mm) to suit to adult and infant utilization. Cast disc EEG electrodes made of gold usually are cast of pure silver with heavy gold plating. EEG cups are also manufactured as disposable electrodes and in this case they are usually made of Ag–AgCl.

Stamped electrodes made of silver and coated with silver chloride may loose the AgCl layer during biopotential recording and cleaning process and need rechloriding

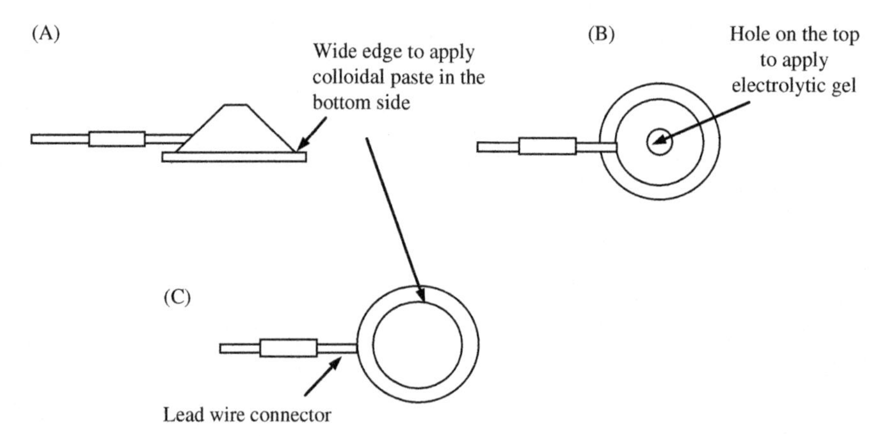

Figure 2.20 EEG electrodes: (A) lateral view and (C) bottom view of the hollow cup showing the wide edge where the colloidal paste is applied to fix the electrode on the scalp. (B) Top view showing the hole to apply the electrolytic gel.

(deposition of a new layer of AgCl). The EEG electrodes are also fabricated by sintering process. In this process, a homogeneous mixture of fine powders of Ag and AgCl is compressed by a special technique, without the use of binders. As a result, these electrodes are homogeneous across the thickness, do not bend, have high mechanical strength and do not require rechloriding. They have wide contact area and present as further characteristics, very low offset voltage, polarization, rate of drift and noise level and are less susceptible to artifacts than the conventional electrodes (Tallgren, Vanhatalo, Kailaa, & Voipio, 2005). Figure 2.21 shows some examples of sintered EEG electrodes. Figure 2.21A shows sintered fixed wired electrode without housing and Figure 2.22B shows the electrode with plastic cover. Sintered discs are manufactured with and without a central hole (Figure 2.21C), in different disc diameters (4–12 mm) to suit to infant and adult use; they are coupled to the scalp skin with electrolytic gel and are fixed using collodion like the conventional electrodes. They are widely used with caps for brain mapping and long-term brain activity monitoring.

The noninvasive EEG recording routines include some types of nonscalp electrodes, like the earlobe clips, used as reference, and nasopharyngeal electrodes, used in investigation of the origin from specific epilepsy activities.

The earlobe electrode has two EEG sensors made of gold, silver, or Ag–AgCl, mounted on a clip type plastic holder showed in Figure 2.22A. The electrical connection is made by soldering the lead wire to the metal sensor (Figure 2.22A) or by a

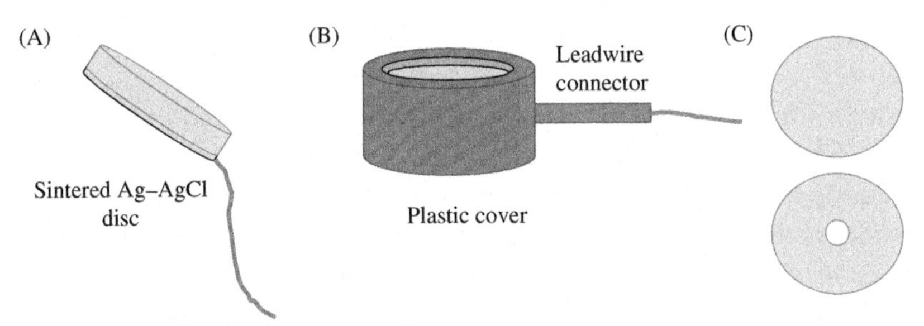

Figure 2.21 Sintered EEG electrodes. (A) Ag–AgCl sintered fixed wired electrode without housing. (B) Ag–AgCl disc with housing (plastic cover); the disc face is recessed to apply the electrolytic gel. (C) Top view of Ag–AgCl discs with and without a central hole.

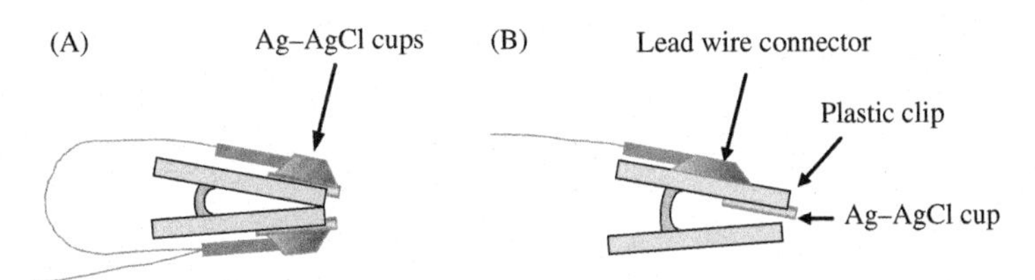

Figure 2.22 Earlobe electrodes (A) with soldered lead wire and (B) with lead wire connector (the plastic clip has a top hole coinciding to the electrode central hole to apply the electrolyte gel).

conector (Figure 2.22B). The metallic sensor is manufactured with different disc and hole diameters and cable lengths (same as EEG electodes) to suit to infant and adult patients. The discs must be made from the same material of the scalp electrodes to avoid measurement artifacts caused by dissimilar electrodes.

Nasopharyngeal electrodes are rigid and have a format similar to the letter *z* with the first and central (10–15 cm) parts made of insulated lead wire (usually silver) and the third part (tip, 2–3 cm) coated with gold ending in a ball (active region) with 2–5 mm diameter. They are inserted through the nostrils until the balls reach the region of the nasopharynx roof near the temporal lobe. Rarely used nowadays, decades ago they were considered as standard to improve the recording of frontal and inferior temporal responses.

2.6.1.1.5 Floating electrodes

The floating classification is related to the electrodes contact design made through a thick electrolytic gel layer. Floating electrodes are less susceptible to motion artifact because the metal sensor is recessed, placed inside a casing and do not enter em contact with the skin. The casing fixed to the skin is filled with the electrolyte, in a way that the metal sensor "floats" in the electrolytic gel and prevents the double layer of charges to be disturbed. This classification includes reusable top-hat and disposable electrodes.

2.6.1.1.5.1 Top-hat electrodes Figure 2.23 shows a schematic diagram of a reusable metal disc top-hat electrode for biopotential recording. The Ag–AgCl disc is placed inside a hollow insulating casing and do not touch the skin. The inner part of the casing is filled with electrolyte and a double-sided adhesive tape promotes fixation of the electrode to the skin face. The embedded electrolyte does not move relative to the electrode, assuring that there is no relative movement between the skin and the double layer of charges in the metal/electrolyte interface. If the metallic element is sintered rather than stamped, these electrodes become even more stable.

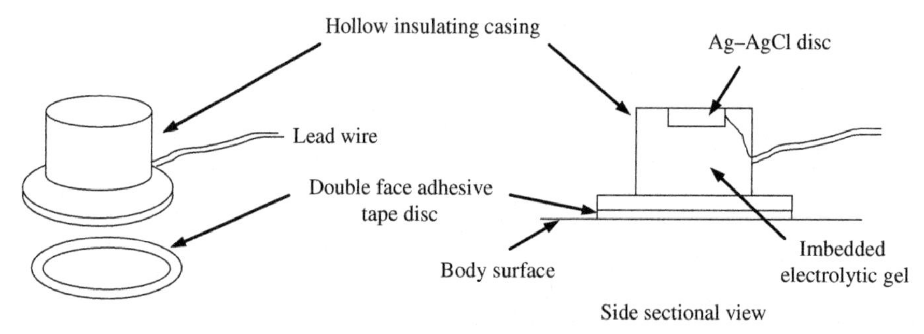

Figure 2.23 Schematic diagram of a reusable metal disc top-hat electrode.

2.6.1.1.5.2 Disposable electrodes The disposable metal disc electrode is the most commonly used type of macroelectrode. Similar to reusable top-hat electrode, the disposable electrode also has a recessed metal sensor, but instead of electrolyte gel, it uses a dense foam (polyethylene, 60 kg m^{-3}) soaked in electrolytic paste (KCl solid gel) to provide contact with the skin. The foam placed between the electrode and the skin generates mechanical stability and minimizes motion artifact. Figure 2.24A shows a side sectional view of a disposable electrode: the Ag–AgCl disc is mounted between dense foam, which is embedded with an electrolyte, and the plastic casing. The top side of the Ag–AgCl disc is insulated and has a metal snap, usually made of stainless steel or Ag–AgCl, to connect the cable, or the cable itself is welded on the disc face (Figure 2.24C). The bottom side of the outer foam pad is coated with hypoallergenic adhesive that fixates the electrode to the skin. They are manufactered in many sizes and formats and are suitable for long-term monitoring; should be used only once and discarded.

2.6.1.1.6 Dry Electrodes

Dry surface electrodes, applied directly on the skin, can record biopotentials without the need of removing fat and sweat or even applying electrolytic gel. This type of electrode has very high input impedance encapsulated with the metal sensor, and it is also named active electrode. The input impedance, electronically enhanced, ensures lower sensitivity to the impedance of the electrode/skin interface.

The electrode impedance is primarily resistive though having capacitive component originated from contact of the electrode with the skin. The first layer of skin, the *stratum corneum*, has a high electrical resistance compared to the deeper regions of the skin (dermis). It is possible to define a capacitor where one of the conducting plates is the metal electrode, the other plate is the dermis and the dielectric is the *stratum corneum*. Another difference compared to the use of conventional electrode with electrolyte is that the *stratum corneum* represents a larger dielectric (the spacing between the plates is larger) than the double layer of charges at the electrode–electrolyte interface, resulting in a lower capacitance. Amplifier input impedance must be at least a few gigaohms to get good quality output signals. Dry electrodes manufactured with

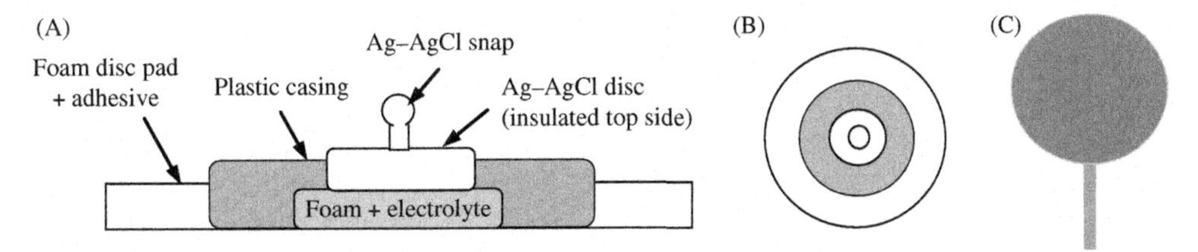

Figure 2.24 Schematic diagram of a disposable electrode with lead wire connector: (A) side section, (B) top view, and (C) electrode with soldered lead wire.

JFET (junction field effect transistor) amplifiers have input impedance equal or higher than 10 TΩ and capacitance lower than 5 pF.

Dry electrodes are fabricated in disposable and reusable models. The use of disposable dry electrodes allows long-term ambulatorial ECG recording. Usually this type of electrode has microstructures in its bottom face to enlarge the contact area with the skin; it is affixed to the skin with adhesive tape (Orbital Research Inc.). Reusable dry electrodes are used for EEG and evoked potentials (visual—VEP and somatosensorial—SEP) recording. This type of electrode is frequently fabricated from gold alloy and is connected to a especial casing that is fixed in the scalp or in a cap adjusted in the patient's head. These dry electrodes allow to capture the whole EEG frequency spectrum (0.1−40 Hz) and are sold in different sizes to fit adequately to the occipital, parietal, central, and frontal regions in infant and adult patients (Guger Technologies).

The use of disposable dry electrodes allows long-term ambulatorial ECG recording. Usually the electrode has microstructures in its bottom face that enlarge the contact area with the skin; is affixed to the skin with adhesive tape (Orbital Research Inc.).

One disadvantage of using dry electrode is its susceptibility to interference caused by nearby electric fields (e.g., the power grid) that affects the functioning of the electrode preamplifier. During a long monitoring process a layer of fat or sweat can arise on the skin, which can lead to a lower capacitance than expected, and affect the capacitive reactance ($Xc = 1/2\pi fC$) of the electrode, compromising its response at low frequencies.

The absence of any electrolyte in contact with the skin eliminates the motion artifact and prevents undesirable chemical effects and skin irritation that may occur during long-term monitoring.

2.6.1.2 Flexible electrodes

A flexible electrode is fabricated depositing a metallic film, for example, Ag−AgCl, on a flexible substrate (polymeric); usually the substrate side receives a layer of conductive adhesive to fix the electrode to the skin, and the metallic face, which is connected to a lead wire, receives a layer of insulating material. The electrode must be thin, flexible, and easy to adjust to the contours of the body and stay at the place for long periods. They are used primarily for monitoring children and premature newborns because they are light, thin, and adapt to body contours, avoiding motion artifact and ulceration in the contact region, which may occur in the case of rigid electrodes applied with electrolyte and adhesive tapes. The electrode shown in Figure 2.25A was developed in the 70s for use in newborns. The substrate is made from a very thin Mylar® film (13 μm thickness) coated by an Ag layer (1 μm thickness); then a thin layer of AgCl is deposited electrolytically giving the electrode an appearance of mesh. The flexible electrode fabricated with Mylar® substrate, a polyester film invented in the early 1950s (DuPont, Mylar®), is also transparent to X-rays, and this means that the patient may be subjected to X-ray examination without removing the electrode from

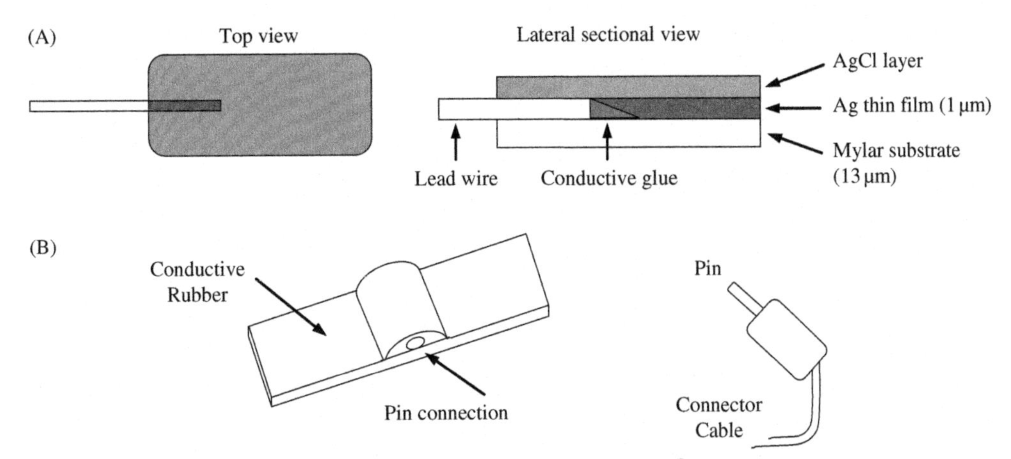

Figure 2.25 Flexible electrodes (A) with Mylar film (DuPont, Mylar®) and (B) of conductive rubber.

the skin, which minimizes skin irritation, mainly in babies. Other polymeric materials used as flexible electrode substrate are PDMS (polydimethylsiloxane), Parylene, and Polyimide (Baek, An, Choi, Park, & Lee, 2008; Ochoa, Wei, Wolley, Otto, & Ziaie, 2013; SCS Specialty Coating Systems).

Figure 2.25B shows another type of flexible electrode, the conductive rubber electrode, made from silicone rubber with embedded carbon particles. This electrode is often used as stimulation electrode, for instance, in the application of transcutaneous electrical nervous stimulation or TENS.

The fixation of flexible electrode is made with a thin, also flexible layer, the same size of the contact surface of the electrode, of a gelatinous material, called electrolytic hydrogel. It is adhesive (minimizes the motion artifact) and conductive and its electrical impedance is higher than that of the conventional electrolytic gel. The large electrical impedance is not a problem because biopotential is usually amplified in very high input impedance buffered differential amplifier stage of instrumentation amplifiers (e.g., the AD624 (Analog Devices, AD624 Precision Instrumentation Amplifier tag) differential impedance with $R_{in} = 10^9\ \Omega$ and $C_{in} = 10$ pF, a high precision, low noise, instrumentation amplifier from Analog Devices designed primarily for use with low level transducers). The electrolytic gel used with the conductive rubber must have the right composition, that is, must have the C^+ cation available to the oxireduction reactions develop correctly in the electrode/electrolyte interface.

2.6.2 Invasive electrodes

The invasive capture of biopotentials requires transcutaneous electrodes, which means cutting the skin and other biological tissues with the electrodes. The patient skin/electrolyte no longer exists and in the metal electrode/electrolyte interface, extra- and intracellular fluids of the patient body replace the electrolyte. Invasive electrodes are classified as needle, wire, and microelectrodes, according to their diameter. The diameter itself is chosen according to the biological tissue being examined. For a transmembrane measurement, the diameter of the electrode tip is determined through the cell size and its membrane resistance to avoid the cell destruction. The diameters of the cells of biological tissues are usually in the range between 50 and 500 μm (Cobbold, 1974; Geddes & Baker, 1968; Webster, 2010).

2.6.2.1 Needle and wire electrodes

Needle and wire electrodes are used to register biopotentials, such as EMG, ECG, and EEG and in invasive monitoring during surgical proceedures. Although biopotentials can be recorded with surface electrodes, invasive recording allows registering the electrical signals with less loss of frequency content. The EMG invasive recording is the golden pattern to measure muscle activity and allows obtaining the electrical activation of a few muscle fibers, with needle electrodes, and even motoneuron unit action potential trains (MUAPT), with very thin wire electrodes.

Figure 2.26 shows needle and wire invasive electrodes used to capture ECG and EMG biopotentials. The picture in Figure 2.26A is a representation of a needle electrode, usually made from a stainless steel needle, isolated throughout its shank by a coating, having only its sharpened tip exposed. The other end of the needle is connected to the lead wire. The insulation coating of the needles shank is made from nylon or Teflon, which also provides mechanical stiffness. In the EMG recording, the electrode is placed within the muscle or group of muscles under examination. In the

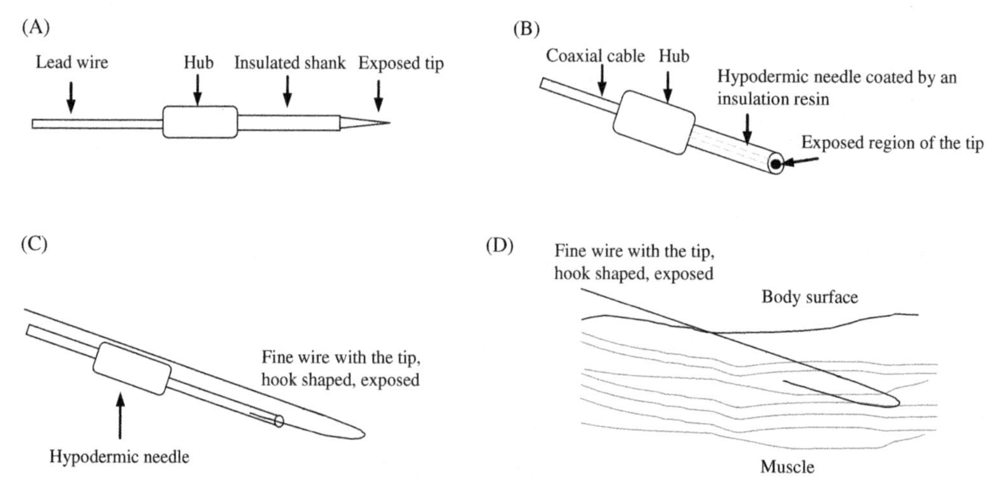

Figure 2.26 Invasive electrodes for biopotential recording: (A) needle electrode; (B) shielded needle electrode; (C) wire electrode with hook shaped tip; and (D) wire electrode inserted in the tissue.

ECG invasive recording, the electrodes are inserted, for instance, in the muscles of arms and legs, according to the derivation used.

Figure 2.26B ilustrates a shielded needle electrode. This type of electrode is obtained placing a fine wire inside a hypodermic needle and filling its lumen with an isolating material (e.g., epoxy resin). One side of the needle is connected to the ground and the other extremity is obliquely cut, leaving only the tip of the wire exposed; this tip will be the active electrode in a monopolar configuration. This type of needle electrode is used in EEG invasive monitoring; the needle in transcuneously inserted in the scalp skin. A second insulated wire can be inserted in the needle leaving only its tip exposed to obtain a bipolar electrode, that is, a needle electrode with two sensing surfaces (areas from tens to hundreds of microns). With a similar procedure, it is possible to introduce several wires in the hollow needle, to obtain multiple active electrodes, used in EMG recording to investigate the action potential of isolated muscle fibers.

Figure 2.26C shows an invasive electrode made from insulated fine wire (25–125 μm) having only its tip exposed. The wire, with its tip, bent into a hook shape, is placed in the hypodermic needle lumen. The set is percutaneously inserted into the region to be examined and the needle is removed, leaving the wire electrode at the right place (Figure 2.26D). The hook-shaped tip of the wire prevents it from moving. If the fine wire is helically wound, it becomes more resistant to any movement or muscle contraction, preventing ruptures during the exam. To remove the electrode, the wire should be pulled, in order to unfold and release its tip.

The wire electrodes are made from metallic alloys usually of platinum, silver, nickel, iridium, and chromium, for example, 90% platinum and 10% iridium. These alloys have an appropriate combination of strength, stiffness, and chemical inertness.

2.6.2.2 Microelectrodes

The microelectrodes are used to study cell electrophysiology by intra- and extracellular measurements. For example, microelectrode arrays implanted intracortically monitor neuronal activity and locate the cortical area responsible for epileptic seizures (disturbed neuronal activity in the brain). As showed in Figure 2.1, a glass microelectrode inserted in the cell (*in vivo* or *in vitro*) measures potential differences across the cell membrane. These electrodes have cell dimensions (diameter ranging from 0.05 to 10 μm) to avoid damage that would compromise the normal functioning of the cell. Although small, these electrodes must have sufficient resistance to be inserted through the tissue and stay in the place for measuring extra- and intracellular potentials. There are several ways to classify microelectrodes; basically they are made of metal, glass, or from techniques used in microelectronics to fabricate integrated circuits. These three types of microelectrodes are presented below: glass microelectrodes (glass micropipettes); metal microelectrodes; and microelectrodes fabricated using microelectronic technology.

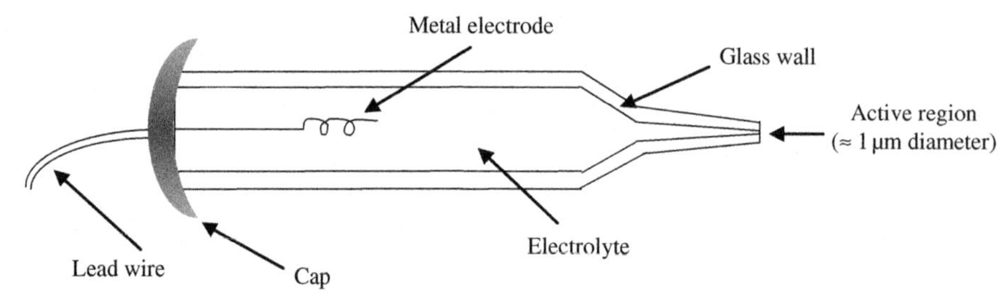

Figure 2.27 Components of a glass micropipette.

2.6.2.2.1 Glass microelectrodes (glass micropipettes)

This electrode is fabricated from a glass capillary tube that is heated and pulled through its extremities forming a very narrow constriction in its center region (≈ 1 μm diameter). Then the tube is cut in the constriction forming two glass micropipettes. Each micropipette is filled with electrolyte (KCl 3 M) and receives a cap with a metal electrode rod or wire (Ag–AgCl) coupled; this metal electrode is inserted in the electrolyte (Figure 2.27). The opening at the tip of the micropipette is the active region of the microelectrode and is large enough to allow ions exchange between the electrolyte and the outer environment (intra- or extracellular fluids).

The glass capillary tube can be pulled and stretched manually (by very skilled people) but this is not recommended because of lack of reproducibility. Vertical and horizontal pullers with a platinum or nichrome heating element, preheat selectable times and one or two pull stages, allow to achieve good reproducibility, although setting them up correctly is time consuming. Pullers are good to obtain fine tip micropipettes with short shanks and resistance up to 300–500 MΩ, and with long shanks and resistance value in the range 30–300 MΩ. The outer diameter of the tip is typically of the order of 50–500 nm (Cobbold, 1974; Geddes & Baker, 1968; Montenegro, Queirós, & Daschbach, 1991; Webster, 2010).

Micropipettes are made from high quality glass (borosilicate, aluminosilicate, or quartz). Borosilicate (for instance, Premium Corning Type 7740 composition: 81% SiO_2, 13% B_2O_3, 4% Na_2O, 2% Al_2O_3—Pyrex, Warner Instruments Inc.) is the most commonly used glass in electrode fabrication because of its mechanical strength, chemical durability, electrical resistivity, and its ability to withstand thermal stress.

It is also possible to use a glass fiber-containing capillary to pull electrodes. When the micropipette is pulled, the lumen shape is preserved up to the tip, which makes easier to fill the micropipette with the electrolyte. The solution tracks down the channels formed either side of the fiber right down to the tip. If bubbles form, they usually will not occlude the lumen completely.

The simplified equivalent electrical circuit showed in Figure 2.28 explains the measurement of the transmembrane potential V_{cell} with a micropipette and a metal in

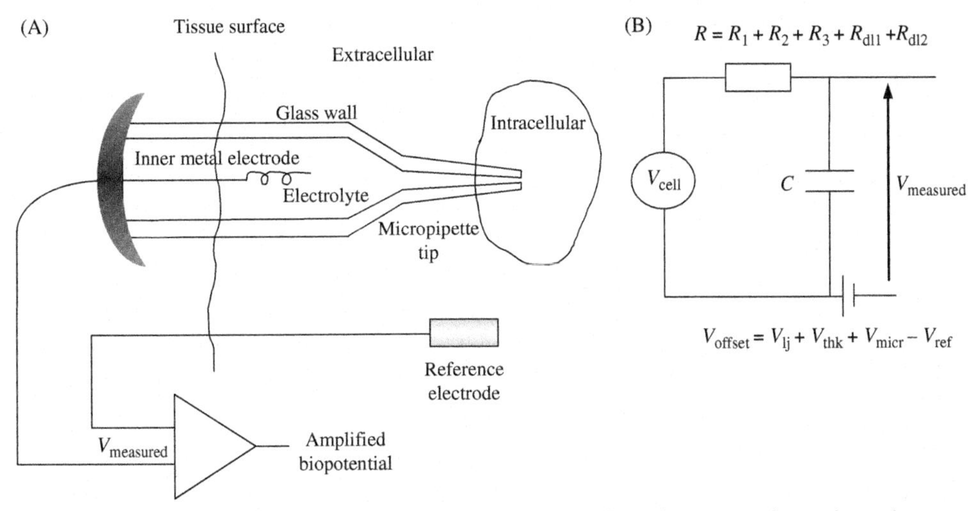

Figure 2.28 (A) Transmembrane potential measurement with a glass microelectrode and a metal reference electrode and (B) simplified equivalent circuit.

different or reference electrode. The cell membrane is modeled as an AC voltage source V_{cell}. The desired V_{cell} value is modified by resistive and capacitive components, which represent the micropipette, the reference electrode and surrounding liquids, and an offset voltage, which is the sum of the half-cell potential of the microelectrode V_{micr}, the half-cell potential of the reference electrode V_{ref}, and the micropipette tip potential V_{tip}. Ideally, if the metal of both electrodes, inside the glass pipette and the reference, are equal, their half-cell potentials cancel. The tip potential results from the liquid junction potential V_{lj}, between the electrolyte in the pipette tip and the intracellular fluid, and the potential of the wall thickness of the micropipette V_{thk}. V_{lj} is a Nernst potential-like voltage, defined by the ionic composition of electrolyte inside the micropipette and the intracellular fluid. The thin glass wall of the pipette tip inside the cell behaves like a membrane that separates two solutions of different ionic concentration; V_{thk} depends on the tip size and shape and can represent a negative offset voltage as large as 100 mV. Offset voltage adjustment in the amplification stage can compensate the DC level that represents all potential contributions.

The resistor R of the equivalent circuit (Figure 2.28B) represents the series arrangement of resistive components of the reference electrode/extracellular fluid (R_{dl1}) and metal electrode/electrolyte (R_{dl2}) interfaces, the electrolyte inside the pipette (R_1) and the intra- (R_2) and extracellular fluids (R_3). The capacitor C (Figure 2.28B) is due to the capacitive contributions of the metal/fluid interfaces of both electrodes, one coaxial capacitor, which represents the extracellular fluid and the electrolyte separated by the thin glass wall of the micropipette shank, and a second coaxial capacitor, formed by the intracellular fluid and the electrolyte, separated by the glass wall of the micropipette tip. The thin glass wall behaves like dielectric. The coaxial (distributed) capacitance values are dependent of the length of the micropipette inserted in the biological tissue. The resultant C is high enough (in the range of units of pF) to define, with the resistance R (in the range of units to tens of megaohms), a large time constant for the electrode $\zeta = RC$. The resistance R and the capacitance C form together a low-pass filter that responds slowly ($\zeta \sim$ tens of microseconds) to rapid changes in cell membrane potential, due to the high series resistance and distributed capacitance. A proper capacitance compensation circuit in the recording amplifier reduces the time constant and enhances the microelectrode response to low frequency spectral components (Cobbold, 1974; Geddes & Baker, 1968; Webster, 2010).

2.6.2.2.2 Metal microelectrodes

An American physiologist, Ida Henrietta Hyde (1857–1945), invented the intracellular microelectrode in 1921. The utilization of glass micropipettes led to a golden age of neurophysiological discoveries from 1930 to 1950. Since the 1960s, nonglass microelectrodes, less fragile, like glass-insulated platinum or silver electrodes, used for many years in extracellular recordings with isolated cells, became the main choice in neurophysiological recordings made in intact animals (Israel & Schulder, 2004).

Metal microelectrode fabrication begins with a very fine metal needle, insulated by a film of polymeric material, except at one end (Figure 2.29A). Then the needle is mounted in an electrochemical cell to slowly erode the noninsulated end, while, at the same time, it is withdrawn from the electrolyte bath to form a sharpened thin tip (Figure 2.29B). The most used needle materials are stainless steel, tungsten, and platinum iridium. An external metal case, connected to the ground, gives mechanical strength to the electrode. The metal needle is connected to the lead wire and an insulating material, leaving only the tip exposed, coats the set (Cobbold, 1974; Geddes & Baker, 1968; Webster, 2010).

A variation of the metal microelectrode is obtained from a glass capillary tube, which is filled with molten metal (melting point close to, but lower than the glass). Then, the whole set is heated to a temperature higher than the melting point of the glass and its ends are pulled until the center of the capillar becomes very narrow. In this region, the set is cut forming two glass metal filled micropipettes. The glass acts as an insulator and the active tip is the exposed metal area where the capillary tube was

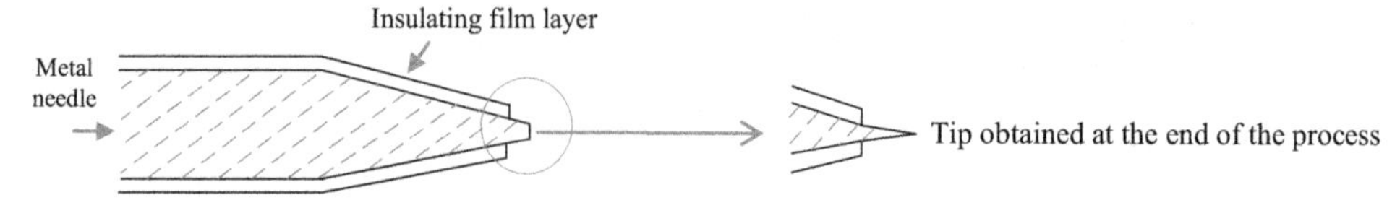

Figure 2.29 Metal microelectrode fabrication begins with an insulated needle to obtain a sharpened tip through electrolysis.

divided. At the opposite end to the tip, the lead wire is connected to the metal inside of the glass capillar (Cobbold, 1974; Geddes & Baker, 1968; Webster, 2010).

Another type of metal electrode is fabricated starting with a (borosillicate) glass capillary rod that is heated beyond the melting point of the glass and then pulled, forming a constriction in its central region; the rod is cut in the constriction, giving rise to two solid micropipettes. Each micropipette receives a thin metal film, only a few tenths of microns thickness, using metal etching. This technology, used in microelectronics to fabricate semiconductors integrated circuits, allows forming a very thin and uniform layer on the surface of the micropipette. The final steps are to connect the lead wire and to coat the micropipette with an insulating polymer material, leaving just the metal tip exposed (active microelectrode region) (Cobbold, 1974; Montenegro et al, 1991; Webster, 2010).

Electrical characteristics of metal microelectrodes are described below from the simplified equivalent electric circuit of a transmembrane potential recording showed in Figure 2.30 (Cobbold, 1974; Geddes & Baker, 1968; Webster, 2010). When the microelectrode penetrates the biological tissue, the amplifier receives an input voltage, the potential captured between the microelectrode and the reference electrode. This input voltage is the combination of different contributions: the transmembrane potential V_{cell}; the microelectrode half-cell potential V_{micr}; the half-cell potential of the reference electrode V_{ref}; and the voltage drop across the metal/liquid interfaces. Ideally, if the metal of both electrodes, metal microelectrode and reference, are the same, their half-cell potentials are equal and cancel.

The cell membrane is modeled as a variable voltage source V_{cell} in Figure 2.30B. The resistance of the metal microelectrode shank is in the range of hundreds of ohms; the reference electrode/extracelular fluid interface also contributes with a resistive

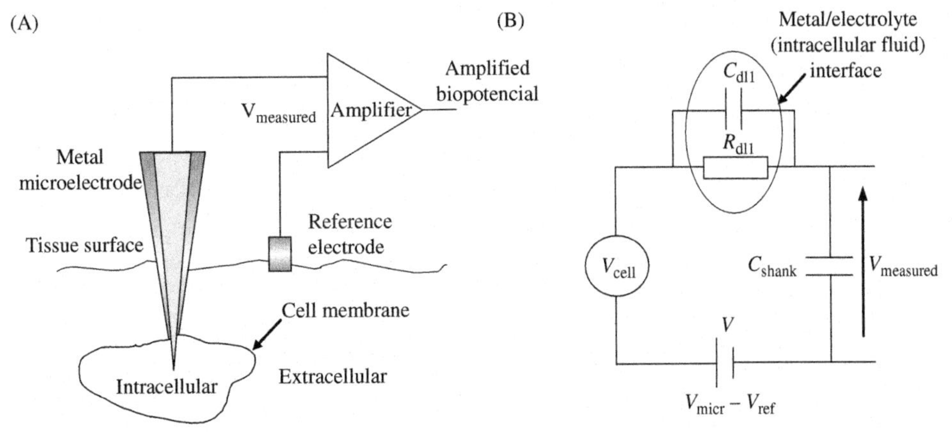

Figure 2.30 (A) Transmembrane potential recording with a metal microelectrode and (B) simplified equivalent electric circuit.

component; and there are the series resistances of the intra- and extracellular fluids. These resistive contributions may be negligible, when compared to the resistive component of the impedance of microelectrode/electrolyte interface R_{dl1}, whose value is in the range of hundreds of megaohms (to areas of the order of tens of square micrometers). The deposition of black platinum in the tip of the metal electrode increases its effective area and reduces the electrode impedance, avoiding the attenuation of the captured transmembrane potential.

In Figure 2.30B, C_{dl1} represents the effect of the double layer charge distribution in the metal electrode tip/intracellular fluid interface. Its capacitance is dependent on the length of the metal tip inserted through the cell membrane.

The insulated (dieletric) shank of the metal microelectrode, in contact with the extracellular fluid, defines a coaxial capacitor C_{shank}, which value depends on the permitivity and thickness of the insulating material and the shank length immersed in biological tissue:

$$\frac{C_{shank}}{L} = \frac{2\pi\varepsilon_r\varepsilon_0}{\ln(D/d)} \tag{2.25}$$

where

ε_r, dielectric constant of free space

ε_o, relative dielectric constant of the insulating material

D, diameter of the shank (metal electrode + insulating, approximately cylindrical)

d, diameter of the metal shank (microelectrode)

L, length of the shank.

The impedance of the microelectrode is frequency dependent and using a high input impedance amplifier helps compensating the attenuation of the spectral components in low frequency of the transmembrane potential, mainly to a small area deeply immersed microelectrode (large C_{shank}).

2.6.2.2.3 Silicon-based microelectrodes

The first implantable arrays were microwire arrays developed in the 1950s. In the 1970s, a planar 2×15 array of gold electrodes plated with platinum black, each spaced 100 μm apart from each other was used to record from cultured cells. In the 1990s, the use of the technology employed in the manufacture of transistors and integrated circuits allowed producing microelectrodes with multiple active areas with high reproducibility and accuracy.

Silicon-based microelectrodes are frequently fabricated as 1D, 2D, and 3D arrays. Microelectrode arrays are devices that contain multiple plates or shanks through which biological, mostly neural signals, are obtained, essentially serving as interfaces that connect cells to electronic circuitry. The same structure is also used to deliver electrical stimulation to tissues. Microelectrode arrays are widely used in fundamental

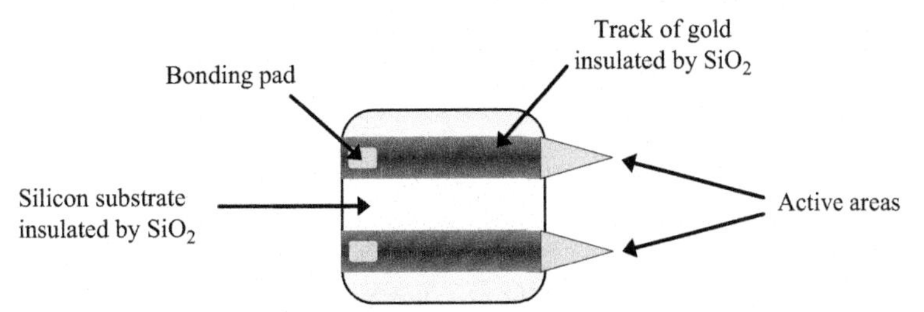

Figure 2.31 Microelectrodes of gold in SiO_2 insulated silicon substrate.

electrophysiological research areas for recording and stimulating neurological, muscular, and cardiac tissues, *in vitro* and *in vivo* (or implantable). The action potential, an all-or-nothing phenomenon, initiates with the cell membrane depolarization and generates a sharp change in voltage in the extracellular environment, which is what the microelectrode array electrodes ultimately detect. Typical electrode sizes are in the order of tens of *micra* with interelectrode distances down to 30 μm.

Figure 2.31 shows an example of microelectrode manufactured from a silicon substrate. An insulating film of SiO_2 is deposited on the substrate top face and two (or more) tracks of gold are deposited over the oxide. Then the set gets a new layer of insulating oxide (SiO_2). The etching technique is used to remove excess material, adjusting size and thickness of the set to suitable dimensions, and to expose only the gold active and bonding pad areas of the microelectrode.

Figure 2.32A shows a 1D array of microelectrodes. To construct this array, a thin film of metal (e.g., gold) is deposited on the top face of a silicon substrate. A layer of insulating oxide (SiO_2) is deposited over the metal film, defining the areas and formats of the tracks, bonding pads, and active areas. The gold layer area, which is not covered by SiO_2, is etched away. Then, the remaining insulating layer is removed partially to expose only the active areas and bonding pads. This type of microelectrode can record biopotentials from different depths of biological tissue reached by its active areas. For example, the 1D array can be inserted in the cortex to capture potentials from its distinct layer structure. Figure 2.32B shows a 2D microelectrode with active areas of different sizes and integrated electronic to preprocess the signals recorded.

A research group of University of Utah and Cybernetics Incorporation created in 1991 the monolithic 3D array with a hundred active areas (tips of the needles) distributed in a 16-mm^2 region (Hatsopoulos & Donoghue, 2009). Based on sawing and isotropic wet etching techniques, the 3D pattern of needles was created from a thick silicon substrate; the substrate base was filled with glass for electrical passivation and the needle shanks were coated with an insulating material (polyimide). Titanium, tungsten, and platinum layers were deposited in each tip forming the active areas. This array microelectrode can be implanted in areas of the brain responsible for limb movements or other functions, to sense neuro activity (or to deliver electrical

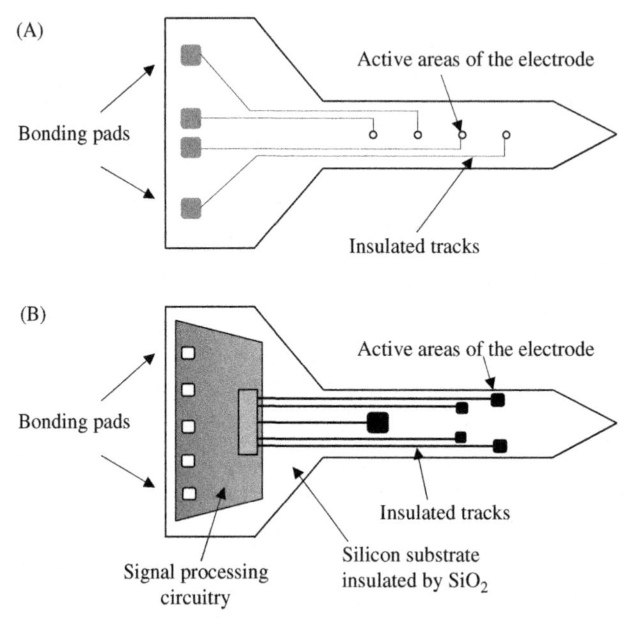

Figure 2.32 Arrays of multiple microelectrodes (A) 1D with four active areas at different depths and (B) 2D with five active areas at different depths and integrated electronic.

stimulus) of many individual cells, but all at the same depth; this array is functionally 2D instead of 3D. With needles of different lengths, the array becomes 3D and thus, its tips will access different depths of neuronal tissue.

A research group of Twente University (Netherlands), in 1996, developed an array applying the LIGA (german acronym for Lithographie Galvanoformung, Abformung) process, which uses, among other techniques, an aligned deep X-ray lithography to format the silicon substrate. It was a 3D array with 200 μm tall columns of square section from bottom to the top. Each column was coated by Si_3N_4 and iridium oxide was electrodeposited in its top (Bielen, Schmidt, Weiel, & Rutten, 1996).

To overcome the construction and performance problems (e.g., lack of reproducibility, electrical interconnection of needles) of the Utah and Twente array microelectrodes, other designs and techniques of construction were employed to obtain 3D arrays. A research group of Michigan University developed a practical microassembly process for 3D microelectrode arrays for recording and stimulation in the central nervous system (Bai, Wise, & Anderson, 2000). An overall idea of the structure of this microassembled 3D array is explained below. It is formed by a micromachined silicon platform with an integrated ribbon cable and slots where 2D planar probes with four shanks each are inserted and held orthogonal to the platform by spacers. Gold plated electrobeams are responsible for the lead transfer between the probes and the cable of the platform. This construction process allows the numbers of 2D planar probes to be increased to obtain

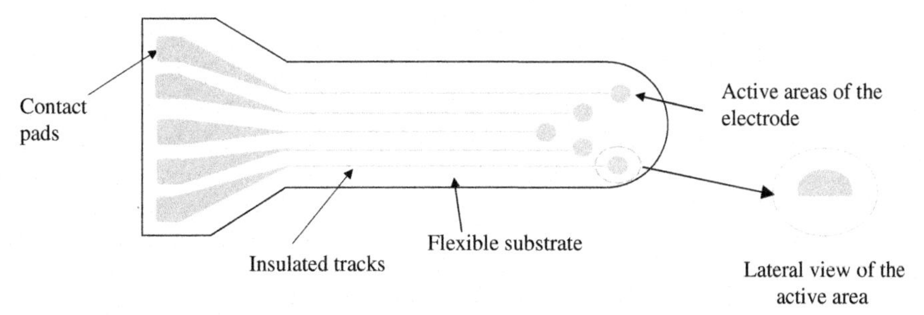

Figure 2.33 Schematic diagram of a flexible implantable 3D array microelectrode with enlarged active areas to reduce the electrical impedance.

high-density 3D arrays, even in multilayer configurations, and the incorporation of electronic platform with signal processing CMOS circuitry (Bai et al., 2000). The use of integrated circuits of CMOS technology allows on-chip dedicated circuitry (filters, amplifiers), which means that low amplitude signal, conditioned at the electrode, are faithfully recorded. CMOS technology is also used to fabricate a large number (tens of thousands) of electrodes on a small chip and to measure the cells electrical activity without disrupting their membrane, using extracellular techniques.

During *in vivo* extracellular measuring process, as in long time monitoring of the central nervous system activity, the implantable microelectrode must make good contact but should not damage the living tissue. Flexible microelectrodes, fabricated by the process of microelectrical mechanical system (MEMS), adjust their formats to accommodate the tissue shape. Flexible biocompatible implants have one or more layers of flexible thin polymer substrate, as for instance, polyimide and parylene, which works also as insulator between thin layers of metal used to make electrodes, interconnection tracks and cables, contact pads and electronic components with standard micromachining technologies, such as photolithography and etching.

Some microelectrode characteristics, as small contact area, and thus high selectivity, high number of electrode sites for good spatial selectivity and low impedance, are desired when recording electrical activity or stimulating biological tissue, to quality warranty of the signal acquired or the charge transfer, respectively. One solution to enlarge the effective active areas of the electrode sites is to produce 3D contact. Figure 2.33 shows the schematic diagram of a flexible implantable 3D array microelectrode that has five black platinum-coated hemispherical low impedance active areas. Rui, Liu, Wang, and Yang (2011) developed a similar array and showed that the interface impedance (between the biological tissue and the array) decreased by about 34% compared with conventional planar microelectrodes, and significantly decreased by 84% with Pt-black coatings on electrode sites compared with those uncoated microelectrodes.

High-density deformable arrays (tens to hundreds sites) obtained from thin polymer substrate (thickness of the order of a few tens of micrometers) can be implanted directly on the surface of specific brain areas, like the cortex, to monitor neural activity and help diagnose and locate diseased areas in neurological conditions such as epileptic seizures. These microelectrodes still have the advantage of having integrated electronic circuitry that make the active preprocessing of the recorded signals (Viventi et al., 2011).

2.6.3 Electrodes for tissue stimulation

Stimulation electrodes have similar materials and construction techniques of biopotential recording electrodes. The main difference between them is in the magnitude order of the current through the electrode/electrolyte interface. While during biopotential recording current does not exceed the order of microamperes, stimulation currents are of the order of miliamperes.

Stimulating microelectrodes are used *in vitro* to study the electrophysiology of isolated cells or slices of different tissues. Stimulation electrodes are used *in vivo* in many applications, noninvasively, such as somatosensory evoked potential (SSEP) (Hu et al., 2011; Westerén-Punnonen et al., 2008), transcutaneous electrical nerve stimulation (TENS) for pain relief (Johnson, 2000; Nardone & Schieppati, 1989), functional sensory stimulation (FES) (Hara, 2013; Peckham & Knutson, 2005; Waters, McNeal, Fallon, & Clifford, 1985), electrically eliciting muscle contractions (Chae & Yu, 1999; Ridding, Brouwer, Miles, Pitcher, & Thompson, 2000), or invasively, like in deep brain stimulation (has been effective at treating neurological disorders such as Parkinson's disease and epilepsy) (Bronstein, Tagliati, & Alterman, 2011; Englot, Chang & Auguste, 2011; Rolston, Desai, Laxpati, & Gross, 2011), cochlear implant (to improve hearing by assisting stimulation of the auditory nerve) (Arora, Vandali, Dawson, & Dowell, 2010; Choi & Lee, 2012), retinal implant (to offer prospects of vision restoration for blind patients by eliciting visual percepts of spots of light) (Fried, Hsueh, & Werblin, 2006; Rizzo, Wyatt, Loewenstein, Kelly, & Shire, 2003), etc. Stimulation electrodes are also used in *in vivo* applications, both invasively and noninvasively, as part of medical devices, such as defibrillators, pacemakers, and electrosurgery, among others. Some applications need the electrode to be implanted, permanently or temporarily (pacemakers and defibrillators).

The ideal stimulation electrodes are those that do not change the environment where they are applied, neither their own characteristics during stimulation. Nonpolarizable electrodes made from stainless steel and noble metals are preferred. If the stimulation current oxidizes the electrode, it will be consumed, increasing ionic concentration at the site of application, affecting, for instance, the biological tissue pH, or promoting chemical reactions that will disturb the site equilibrium.

Conventional stimulating metal microelectrodes, for *in vitro* and *in vivo* uses, are fabricated in monopolar, parallel bipolar, and concentric bipolar configurations, of insulated wires of tungsten, iridium, platinum/iridium, and stainless steel (Elgiloy®), in diameters ranging from 2.5 to 150 μm and impedances from 0.1 to 5.0 MΩ.

Tungsten is the most versatile and widely used probe material because of its stiffness, biocompatibility, and cost. It is extensively used for stimulation situations, such as deep brain studies in Parkinson disease and other studies that require a long electrode. Platinum/iridium is extremely inert and biocompatible and is much more resistant to corrosion than either tungsten or stainless steel when used in extensive stimulation protocols; it is an excellent selection for chronic implants. Platinum/iridium also has lower tip impedance than tungsten or stainless steel. Iridium (pure iridium) has by far the lowest tip impedance of any of the noble metals; it is extremely inert and very resistant to corrosion.

Figure 2.34 shows schematic representations of typical microelectrodes in monopolar and bipolar configurations. Generally, the greater the length of the tip, the lower is its impedance, and the greater number of cell potentials will be recorded. Also, the deeper the recording site, the higher electrode impedance is required. Concentric bipolar electrodes are ideal for stimulating and recording from larger cell populations. Typically, concentric electrodes have a preinsulated metal wire or needle inside stainless steel tubing for shielding, and an external insulation layer of polymer coating the microelectrode (WPI World Precision Instruments). Typical diameters are only a few thousandths of an inch unit; small diameter microprobe is important to produce minimal tissue damage, especially with regard to chronic implantation, and to implant a large number of microprobes within a small area. Additional polymer tubing provides stiffness and additional insulation to the electrode shaft and it is recommended when

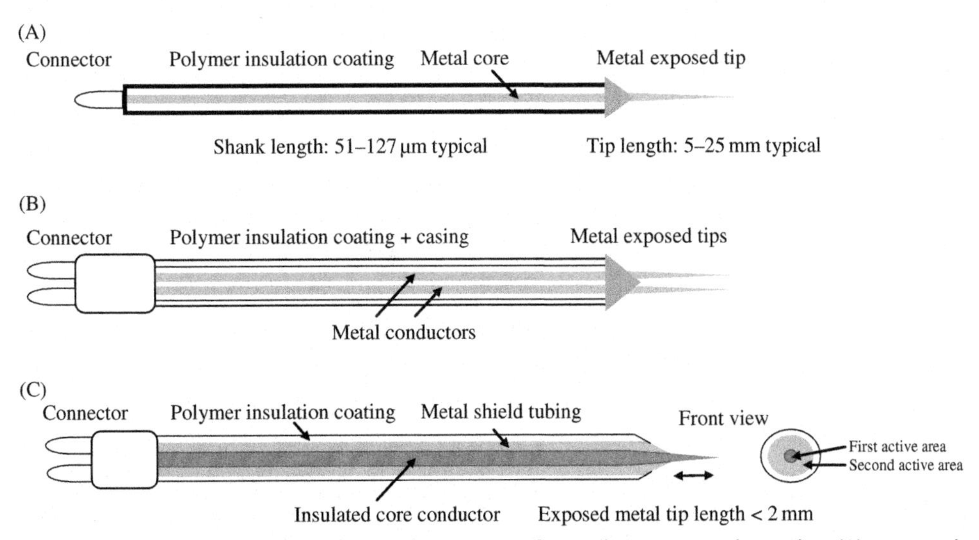

Figure 2.34 Monopolar and bipolar configurations of stimulating microelectrodes: (A) monopolar electrode, (B) parallel bipolar electrode, and (C) concentric bipolar electrode.

the electrode penetrates deep in the tissue. Stimulating electrodes with multiple parallel and concentric active areas can be obtained from similar fabrication techniques.

In bipolar mode of stimulation, the current flows through the two electrodes, that are near each other, resulting in a concentrated current pathway between them, and this stimulates the tissue immediately surrounding the electrodes. When the target is located distant from this current path, or is protected by a high impedance tissue, like the dura mater, a monopolar work electrode and a return electrode can be used to increase the spatial coverage of the stimulus. Some limitations of the parallel bipolar stimulating electrodes are the difficulty in placing the two tips in the desired orientation, for instance, on the tissue slice for optimal tissue activation and the relatively large size of the electrode tips. Concentric bipolar electrodes possess the lowest stimulus artifacts and are easier to orient in the tissue, since they have no directionality.

Figure 2.35A shows an example of surface, noninvasive stimulating electrode: flexible stimulating electrode for TENS. Instead of metal, it is made of silicone rubber

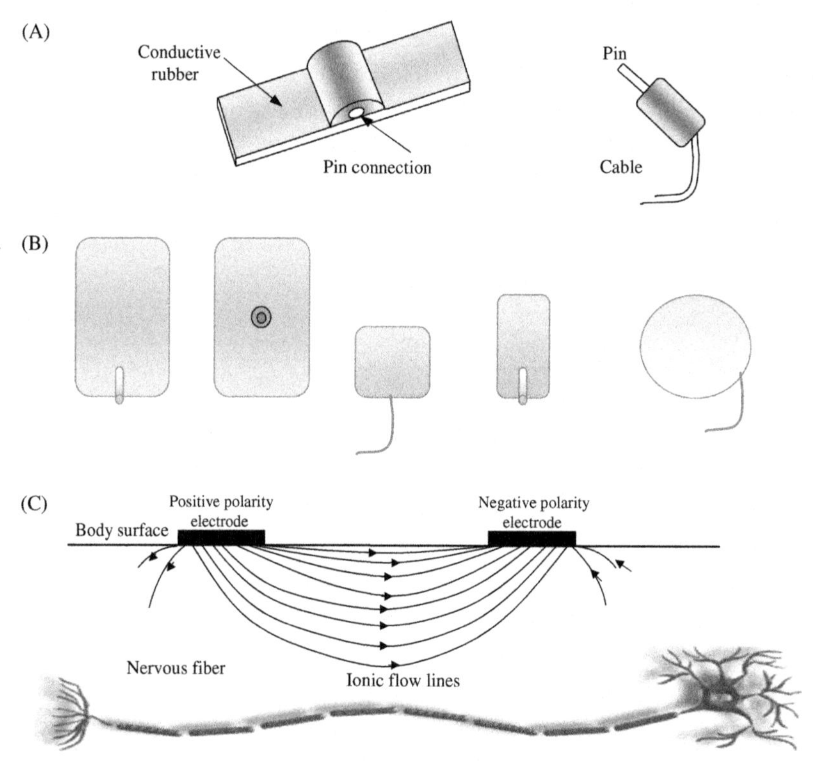

Figure 2.35 (A) Carbon filled rubber electrode for TENS. Rubber pads of different formats, lead wire connections and sizes with adhesive patch for fixing. (C) Schematic diagram of the nerve fiber stimulation with the electric stimulus applied through surface electrodes.

impregnated with carbon particles; it is flexible, which facilitates its adjustment to body shape. The coupling with the skin is made via specific electrolytic gel (hydrogel with C^+) and elastic bands help positioning the electrode in place; alternatively, the bottom surface of the electrode is covered with hypoallergenic adhesive for fixing. Stimulating pads typically are reusable and adhesive, made to stick directly on the skin with the help of a patch (Figure 2.35B). TENS electrodes are available in multiple sizes and features, according to the use. It is important to assure a uniform electrical current distribution over the contact surface to avoid skin burning and other chemical reactions. Figure 2.35C shows a schematic diagram of the functioning of TENS. A pulse of electric current or voltage is applied between the surface electrodes, generating an electric field in the conductor volume formed by the tissues between the skin and the nerve fiber. Ionic current flowing between the two electrodes reaches the fiber membrane; if the current exceeds the threshold of excitability, the cell membrane depolarizes and the action potential is generated. TENS is used in therapeutic treatment of chronic and acute pain (arthritic or muscular) and motor rehabilitation.

Figure 2.36 shows examples of an invasive *in vivo* application of stimulating electrode: implantable electrodes for cardiac stimulation used in pacemakers. These electrodes are intravenously implanted and are insulated with silicone rubber or polyurethan; electrodes should provide low impedance to current flow, and must endure, for several years, the movements of flexion and torsion due to the beating

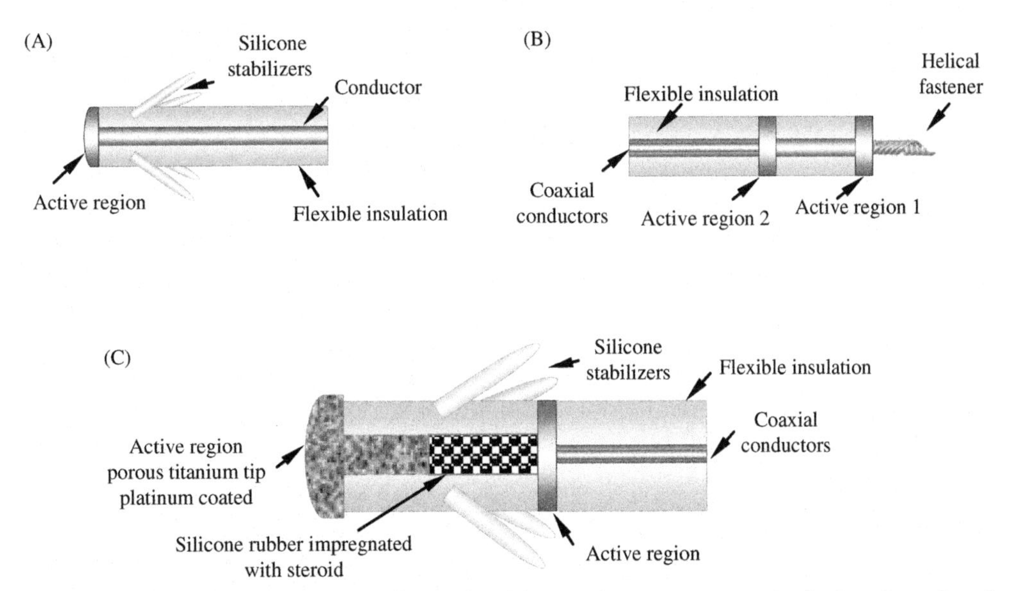

Figure 2.36 Pacemaker stimulating electrodes: (A) unipolar active region with ring-shaped and indented passive fixation; (B) bipolar with active region with ring-shaped and helical active fixation; and (C) cross-sectional view of an intracardiac electrode with release of steroid.

heart. Figure 2.36A and B shows examples of electrodes used with a permanent pacemaker with different ways of attachment to the myocardium. Rings and other forms of active pacing regions are made of metal and biocompatible materials such as platinum, titanium, and alloys such as titanium coated with platinum and iridium, Elgiloy® (iron–cobalt–chromium–nickel–molybdenum–manganese) and MP35N (nickel–cobalt–chromium–molibdenium) or glassy carbon (pyrolytic carbon). The stabilizers in the shape of teeth, claws, and hooks, made from silicone rubber or metal, insulated by silicone rubber, help anchoring the electrode in the trabeculae of the heart muscle. The smaller the active area of the electrode contact, the higher the density of the applied electric field to induce cardiac muscle contraction. Even without increasing the geometric size of the electrode tip is possible to increase the active area and the density of the electric field producing microcavities (pores) on the surface of the electrode tip. Figure 2.36C shows the schematic diagram of the cross-section of an intracardiac electrode with porous tip of titanium coated by platinum, which has an inner plug (monolithic controlled release device) of silicone rubber impregnated with <1 mg DSP steroid (dexamethasone sodium phosphate). The steroid is released into adjacent tissue through the porous tip, thereby reducing the inflammation in the myocardium region where the electrode was fixed. The steroid facilitates tissue healing and stabilization of the electrode, which over time, and ends up being coated by collagen fibers (Medtronic CapSure® Pacing Leads; Ela Medical Implantable Pacing Electrodes; Mond, 1991). Estimulation electrodes used for heart pacing with temporary pacemakers have different ways of fixation on the epicardium, since atraumatic way (just touchs the tissue) to active ways, which involve that the electrode tip be inserted or sewed in the tissue; they are removed, at the end of the temporary stimulation, pulling softly the lead wire end that is outside the body (Osypka AG Medizintechnik in Herten).

2.6.3.1 Constant-current stimulation

When electrical stimulus is applied to biological tissue, the net current between the electrode and the electrolyte should be null, ideally, in order to not accumulate charge at the interface. Even using biphasic stimulation with symmetrical load, there is no warranty that the resulting current magnitude will be the same in each semi cycle of the stimulus, due to the nonlinear tissue/electrolyte/electrode response. The impedances of these interfaces are dynamic, can change under stimulation and depend on the parameters of stimulation, especially the intensity and duration of the stimulus.

Figure 2.37 shows an ideal biphasic, asymmetrical, balanced, and rectangular constant-current pulse (Figure 2.37A), delivered by a metal electrode coupled through electrolyte to a generic tissue, and the resulting typical voltage tissue response (Figure 2.37B). Considering that an equivalent electric circuit, similar to the biopotential recording case (Figure 2.11), represents the stimuling electrode/eletrolyte interface, the voltage response can be explained as follows. Initially the voltage pulse rises

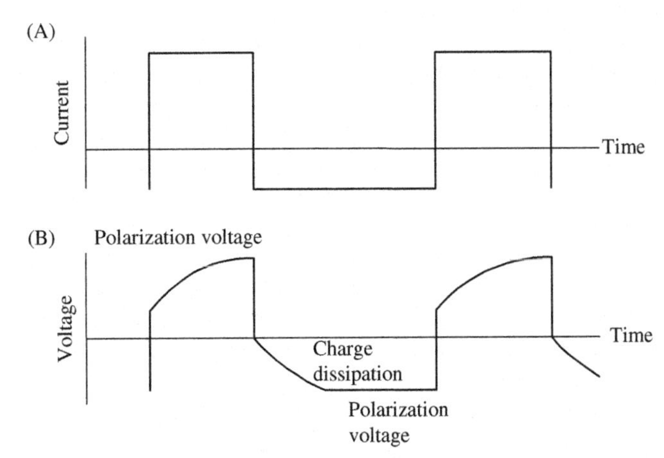

Figure 2.37 Resulting voltage at the interface (stimulation electrode/electrolyte) (B) when a rectangular current pulse (A) is applied.

abruptly due to positive voltage drop across resistive components of the interface. Then, instead of a plateau, the voltage format is typical of a capacitor charging; the unidirectional current flow through the metal/electrolyte interface modifies the charge distribution and consequently, the polarization potential; this polarization effect can be represented by a capacitor, which characteristics depend mainly on current density at the interface. Removing the positive current plateau, there is an abrupt voltage drop, followed by a smoother one, which corresponds to the dissipation of the polarization charge accumulated in the electrode/electrolyte interface. The negative current plateau applied in the second part of the stimulus modifies once more the charge distribution at the interface and the polarization potential polarity (Cobbold, 1974; Webster, 2010).

2.6.3.2 *Constant-voltage stimulation*

Figure 2.38 shows an ideal biphasic, asymmetrical, balanced and rectangular voltage—current pulse (Figure 2.38A), delivered by a metal electrode coupled through electrolyte to a generic tissue, and the resulting typical current tissue response (Figure 2.38B). Again, one considers that stimulating electrode/electrolyte equivalent electric circuit is similar to the biopotential recording case. There is no plateau in the voltage response; instead, its value rises abruptly as the current flows through the resistive elements of the interface, when the positive plateau is applied, and then the voltage decreases slowly as the polarization charge stabilizes. The positive current plateau ends and the voltage drops abruptly, due to the removal of accumulated charge (and even an additional amount of charge) at the interface; then in the second part of the stimulus a negative voltage plateau is applied, the charge distribution changes polarity

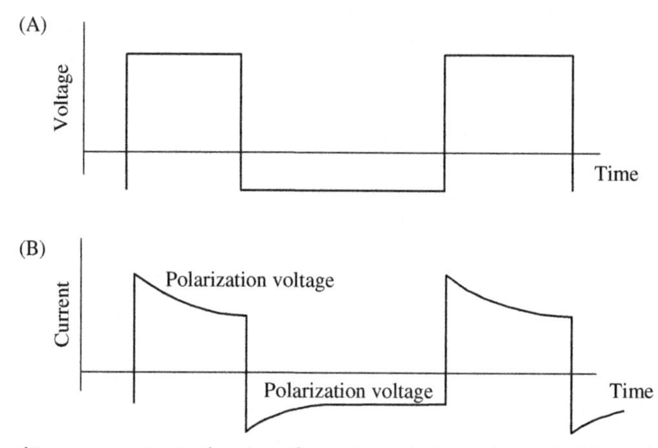

Figure 2.38 Resulting current at the interface (stimulation electrode/electrolyte) (B) when a biphasic, asymmetrical, balanced, and rectangular constant-voltage pulse (A) is applied.

and the polarization voltage stabilizes in a new value proportional to the current applied (Cobbold, 1974; Webster, 2010).

All waveforms are capable of activating the cell membrane. The waveform, intensity, and duration of stimuli vary according to type (*in vivo*, *in vitro*) and objective (cell membrane depolarization, exposed nerve excitation, group of muscles contraction, etc.) of the stimulation. Rectangular, sinusoidal, triangular, trapezoidal, decaying exponential, pulsed, increasing pulsed ramp, burst-square wave modulated, etc., symmetrical, asymmetrical, balanced, unbalanced, monophasic, biphasic, or poliphasic pulses, constant-current or constant-voltage controlled can lead to the desired effect of stimulation (Fisher, 2000; Kuncel & Grill, 2004; Merrill, Bikson, & Jefferys, 2005; Wongsarnpigoon, Woock, & Grill, 2010).

2.7 REVIEW THE LEARNING

1. Explain in your own words what is:
   a. Resting potential of the cell membrane
   b. Action potential
   c. Refractory period
2. Why a metal electrode, used for biopotential recording, is considered a transducer?
3. Why intra- and extracellular ionic component concentrations affect the resting potential of the cell membrane?
4. What chemical reactions occur in the interface between a metal M and an electrolytic solution that contains the cations of this metal?
5. What is half-cell potential of a metallic electrode? How can it be measured?
6. What are the desirable characteristics of a standard electrode?

7. Explain the operation of the standard hydrogen electrode. Complement your explanation with the schematic diagram of the electrode.
8. Show the electrochemical cell used to measure a metal half-cell potential with the standard hydrogen electrode. Identify all components and provide the equations.
9. What are the characteristics of the hydrogen electrode that make it suitable as a reference electrode?
10. Explain the operation of the calomel reference electrode. Complement your explanation with the schematic diagram of the electrode.
11. Show the electrochemical cell used to measure a metal half-cell potential with the standard calomel electrode. Identify all components and provide the equations.
12. What are the characteristics of the calomel electrode that make it suitable as a reference electrode?
13. Explain the operation of the reference Ag–AgCl electrode. Complement your explanation with the schematic diagram of the electrode.
14. Show the electrochemical cell used to measure a metal half-cell potential with the standard Ag–AgCl electrode. Identify all components and provide the equations.
15. What are the characteristics of the Ag–AgCl electrode that make it suitable as a reference electrode?
16. Compare performance and characteristics of hydrogen, calomel, and Ag–AgCl electrodes as reference electrodes. *Tip*: Use a table to organize the data.
17. Explain the operation of the interface metal electrode/electrolyte. Show the circuitry that represents this interface. Explain what represents each component of the circuit.
18. Consider the biopotential measurement with identical electrodes, one for measurement and one for reference.
    a. Show the electrical equivalent circuit and identify each of its components.
    b. How the half-cell potential of these electrodes can influence the biopotential measurement?
19. What is motion artifact? How it affects a biopotential measurement?
20. What components are added to the simplified equivalent electrical circuit to the electrode/electrolyte interface when the skin is included? Show the circuit and describe the new components.
21. How the transduction of ionic current (biopotential) into electronic current occurs at the interfaces electrode/gel/skin during the measurement of a biopotential? What is the importance of the electrolytic gel applied between the metal electrode and the skin?
22. What are perfectly polarizable and perfectly nonpolarizable electrodes? Give examples of electrodes, whose characteristics are close to those definitions, justifying.

23. What are the types of surface electrodes for biopotential recording? Organize a table showing for different types of electrodes, their main features and functions. The table is meant to summarize clearly and concisely your knowledge about the surface electrodes.
24. What are the types of invasive electrodes for biopotential recording? Organize a table showing for different types of electrodes, their main features and functions. The table is meant to summarize clearly and concisely your knowledge about the invasive electrodes.
25. What is the equivalent circuit of the glass microelectrode (micropipette)? Explain the meaning of each component. How the half-cell and liquid junction potential can interfere with the operation of this microelectrode?
26. What is the equivalent circuit of the metal microelectrode? Explain the meaning of each component. What is better to measure an action potential, glass micropipette, or metal microelectrode? Justify your answer.
27. Suppose you are looking for the best measurement system to measure biopotentials using microelectrodes: compare the performance of glass micropipette and metal microelectrode from the simplified equivalent electrical circuits. What do you expect and what will effectively measure if the biopotential waveform:
    a. has spectral content especially at low frequencies?
    b. has spectral content especially at high frequencies?
28. The stimulation electrodes are designed to operate in monopolar or bipolar modes. When one should use one or another?
29. Explain the resulting current waveform when a constant-voltage pulse is applied to the stimulating metal/electrolyte interface.
30. Explain the resulting voltage waveform when a constant-current pulse is applied to the stimulating metal/electrolyte inmterface.

REFERENCES

Analog Devices, *AD624 Precision Instrumentation Amplifier.* http://www.analog.com/static/imported-files/data_sheets/AD624.pdf/> Accessed 15.01.14.

Arora, K., Vandali, A. E., Dawson, P., & Dowell, R. C. (2010). Effects of electrical stimulation rate on modulation detection and speech recognition by cochlear implant users. *International Journal of Audiology, 50*(2), 123–132, 2011.

Bai, Q., Wise, K. D., & Anderson, D. J. (2000). A high-yield microassembly structure for three-dimensional microelectrode arrays. *IEEE Transactions on Biomedical Engineering, 47*(3), 281–289.

Baek, J., An, J., Choi, J., Park, K., & Lee, S. (2008). Flexible polymeric dry electrodes for the long-term monitoring of ECG. *Sensors and Actuators, 143*(A), 423–429.

Bielen, J. A., Schmidt, A. W., Weiel, R., & Rutten, W. L. C. (1996). Fabrication of multi electrode array structures for intra-neural stimulation: Assessment of the LIGA method. In: *Proceedings of the 18th annual international conference of the IEEE Engineering in Medicine and Biology Society,* (pp. 468–469). Amsterdam. <http://doc.utwente.nl/17371/1/00656947.pdf> Accessed 17.02.14.

Bronstein, J. M., Tagliati, M., Alterman, R. L., Lozano, A. M., Volkmann, J., Stefani, A., et al. (2011). Deep brain stimulation for Parkinson disease: an expert consensus and review of key issues. *Archives of Neurology, 68*(2), 165–171.

Chae, J., & Yu, D. (1999). Neuromuscular stimulation for motor relearning in hemiplegia. *Critical Reviews in Rehabilitation Medicine, 11*, 279–297.

Chan, A. Y. K. (2008). *Biomedical device technology: principles and design.* Springfield, Illinois: Charles C. Thomas.

Choi, C. T. M., Lee, Yi-H. (2012). Review of stimulating strategies for cochlear implants. In C. Umat & R. A. Tange (Eds.), *Cochlear implant research updates* (Chapter 5, pp. 77–90, ISBN: 978-953-51-0582-4). <http://www.intechopen.com/books/cochlear-implant-research-updates/stimulating-strategies-for-cochlearimplants> Accessed 15.11.13.

Cobbold, R. S. C. (1974). *Transducers for biomedical measurements: principles and applications.* New York: John Wiley & Sons.

DuPont, *General specifications for Kapton® polyimide films.* <http://www2.dupont.com/Kapton/en_US/assets/downloads/pdf/summaryofprop.pdf/> Accessed 10.01.14.

DuPont, Mylar®, <http://www2.dupont.com/Products/en_RU/Mylar_en.html/> Accessed 10.01.14.

Ela Medical Implantable Pacing Electrodes. <http://www.eletron.gr/en/Leads.html/> Accessed 15.01.14.

Englot, D. J., Chang, E. F., & Auguste, K. I. (2011). Efficacy of vagus nerve stimulation for epilepsy by patient age, epilepsy duration, and seizure type. *Neurosurgery Clinics of North America, 22*(4), 443–448.

Fisher, M. G. (2000). Theoretical predictions of the optimal monophasic and biphasic defibrillation wave shapes. *IEEE Transaction on Biomedical Engineering, 47*(1), 59–67.

Fried, S. I., Hsueh, H. A., & Werblin, F. S. (2006). A method for generating precise temporal patterns of retinal spiking using prosthetic stimulation. *Journal of Neurophysiology, 95*(2), 970–978.

Geddes, L. A., & Baker, L. E. (1968). *Principles of applied biomedical instrumentation.* John Wiley & Sons.

Guger Technologies, *gtec Medical Engineering, gSAHARA Active Dry Electrode System, gtec_ProductCatalogue_gSAHARASys.pdf.* <http://www.gtec.at/Products/Electrodes-and-Sensors/g.SAHARA-Specs-Features> Accessed 22.12.13.

Hara, Y. (2013). Rehabilitation with functional electrical stimulation in stroke patients. *International Journal of Physical Medicine & Rehabilitation, 1*, 147. Available from: http://dx.doi.org/10.4172/2329-9096.1000147.

Hatsopoulos, N. G., & Donoghue, J. P. (2009). The Science of Neural Interface Systems. *Annual Review of Neuroscience, 32*, 249–266.

Haynes, W. H. (Ed.), (2013). *Handbook of chemistry and physics* (94th ed.). CRC Press.

Hu, L., Zhang, Z. G., Hung, Y. S., Ianetti, G. D., & Hu, Y. (2011). Single-trial detection of somatosensory evoked potentials by probabilistic independent component analysis and wavelet filtering. *Clinical Neurophysiology, 122*(7), 1429–1439.

Israel, Z., & Schulder, M. (2004). History of electrophysiological recording for functional neurosurgery. In Z. Israel, & K. Buschiel (Eds.), *Microelectrode recording in movement disorder surgery.* Thieme Medical Publishers Inc.

Johnson, M. I. (2000). The clinical effectiveness of TENS in pain management. *Critical Reviews in Physical Therapy and Rehabilitiation, 12*, 131–149.

Khandpur, R. S. (2005). *Biomedical instrumentation: Technology and applications.* McGraw-Hill.

Kuncel, A. M., & Grill, W. M. (2004). Selection of stimulus parameters for deep brain stimulation. *Clinical Neurophysiology, 115*, 2431–2441.

Medtronic CapSure® Pacing Leads. <http://www.medtronic.com/for-healthcare-professionals/products-therapies/cardiac-rhythm/pacemakers/pacing-leads/#tab3> Accessed 18.02.14.

Merrill, D. R., Bikson, M., & Jefferys, J. G. (2005). Electrical stimulation of excitable tissue: design of efficacious and safe protocols. *Journal of Neuroscience Methods, 141*(2), 171–198.

Mond, H., & Stokes, K. B. (1991). The electrode–tissue interface: the revolutionary role of steroid elution. *PACE, 15*, 95–107.

Montenegro, M. I., Queirós, M. A., & Daschbach, J. L. (Eds.), (1991). *Microelectrodes: theory and applications* (Vol. 197). Springer, NATO ASI Series.

Nardone, A., & Schieppati, M. (1989). Influences of transcutaneous electrical stimulation of cutaneous and mixed nerves on subcortical and cortical somatosensory evoked potentials. *Electroencephalography and Clinical Neurophysiology, 74*, 24–35.

Neuman, M. R., Fleming, D. G., Cheung, P. W., & Ko, W. (1977). *Physical sensors for biomedical applications.* CRC Press.

NIST Reference on Constants, Units and Uncertainty. *CODATA Internationally recommended values of the fundamental physical constants.* <http://physics.nist.gov/cuu/Constants/index.html> Accessed 24.02.14.

Ochoa, M., Wei, P., Wolley, A. J., Otto, K. J., & Ziaie, B. (2013). Published online January 19, *A hybrid PDMS-Parylene subdural multi-electrode array. Biomed microdevices.* New York, NY: Springer Science + Business Media.

Orbital Research Inc. *Silver bumps electrodes.* <http://orbitalresearch.com/PDFs/Orbital_Dry_Electrode_Spec_Sheet.pdf/> Accessed 15.01.14.

Osypka AG. Medizintechnik in Herten, Temporary Myocardial Electrodes (TME). In *Theory and Practice.* <http://osypka.de/media/TME-Booklet_en_2009-06-26.pdf/> Accessed 15.01.14.

Peckham, P. H., & Knutson, J. S. (2005). Functional electrical stimulation for neuromuscular applications. *Annual Review of Biomedical Engineering*, 7, 327–360.

Ridding, M., Brouwer, B., Miles, T., Pitcher, J., & Thompson, P. (2000). Changes in muscle responses to stimulation of the motor cortex induced by peripheral nerve stimulation in human subjects. *Experimental Brain Research, 131*, 135–143.

Rizzo, J. F., Wyatt, J. L., Loewenstein, J., Kelly, S. K., & Shire, D. B. (2003). Methods for acute electrical stimulation of retina with microelectrode arrays and measurement of perceptual thresholds in humans. *Investigative Ophthalmology and Visual Science, 44*(12), 5355–5361.

Rolston, J. D., Desai, S. A., Laxpati, N. G., & Gross, R. E. (2011). Electrical stimulation for epilepsy: experimental approaches. *Neurosurgery Clinics of North America, 22*, 425–442.

Rui, Y., Liu, J., Wang, Y., & Yang, C. (2011). Parylene-based implantable Pt-black coated flexible 3-D hemispherical microelectrode arrays for improved neural interfaces. *Microsystem Technologies*, *17*(3), 437–442.

SCS Specialty Coating Systems. *Parylene properties.* <http://scscoatings.com/docs/brochures/parylene_properties.pdf/> Accessed 15.01.14.

Tallgren, D., Vanhatalo, S., Kailaa, K., & Voipio, J. (2005). Evaluation of commercially available electrodes and gels for recording of slow EEG potentials. *Clinical Neurophysiology, 116*, 799–806.

Viventi, J., Kim, D.-H., Vigeland, L., Frechette, E., Blanco, J., Kim, Y.-S., et al. (2011). Flexible, foldable, actively multiplexed, high-density electrode array for mapping brain activity *in vivo. Nature Neuroscience, 14*(12), 1599–1605.

Waller, A. D. (1887). A demonstration on man of electromotive changes accompanying the heart's beat. *Journal of Physiology (Lond.), 8*, 229–234.

Warner Instruments, a Harvard Apparatus Company. *Electrophysiology tools. Introduction to premium capillary glass.* <www.warneronline.com/product_info.cfm?name=Introduction%20to%20Premium%20Capillary%20Glass&id=992> Accessed 20.02.14.

Waters, R., McNeal, D., Fallon, W., & Clifford, B. (1985). Functional electrical stimulation of the peroneal nerve for hemiplegia. *Journal of Bone and Joint Surgery, 67*(a), 792–793.

Webster, J. (Ed.), (2010). *Medical instrumentation: Application and design* (4th ed.). Wiley & Sons, Inc.

Westerén-Punnonen, S., Yppärilä-Wolters, H., Partanen, J., Nieminen, K., Hyvärinen, A., & Kokki, H. (2008). Somatosensory evoked potentials by median nerve stimulation in children during thiopental/sevoflurane anesthesia and the additive effects of ketoprofen and fentanyl. *Anesthesia & Analgesia, 107* (3), 799–805.

Wongsarnpigoon, A., Woock, J. P., & Grill, W. M. (2010). Efficiency analysis of waveform shape for electrical excitation of nerve fibers. *IEEE Transactions on Neural Systems and Rehabilitation Engineering, 18*(3), 319–328.

WPI World Precision Instruments, Metal Microelectrodes Basics. <http://www.wpiinc.com/blog/2013/04/26/product-information/metal-microelectrodes-basics/> Accessed 15.01.14.

CHAPTER 3

Electrodes for Measurement of Dissolved Gases and Ions Concentration in the Blood Plasma

Contents

3.1 INTRODUCTION

Gasometry is an exam that measures blood component quantities made from a blood sample collected from a vein (venous gasometry) or artery (arterial gasometry). It is a common hospital procedure used to monitor critically ill patients. The blood sample is collected from a central vase, that is, near the heart, using a central catheter like the Swan-Ganz catheter, or from a periphery vase, in the arms or legs.

Principles of Measurement and Transduction of Biomedical Variables.
DOI: http://dx.doi.org/10.1016/B978-0-12-800774-7.00003-9

Blood gasometry is made to evaluate the adequacy of oxygenation and ventilation through the values of the blood partial pressure of dissolved gases, oxygen (pO_2) and carbon dioxide (pCO_2), the oxy-hemoglobin saturation ($SatO_2$), that is, how much hemoglobin is bound to oxygen gas molecules, and acid–base status of the body via the respiratory and nonrespiratory components, such as blood pH (indicates acidity or alkalinity of blood), bicarbonate (HCO_3^-), an important substance in the regulatory system of acidity and alkalinity in our body, and the concentration of inorganic ions dissolved in blood (Na^+, Cl^-, Ca^{2+}, K^+, H^+, etc.), among others (urea, glucose, cholesterol, insulin, etc.).

The partial pressure of oxygen and carbon dioxide gases and pH are always measured with specific electrodes, which provides the most accurate analysis; the levels of bicarbonate, base excess (BE), and oxy-hemoglobin saturation are calculated from the measurements made with electrodes.

3.2 GASOMETRY

Gasometry testing analyzes a blood sample that can be collected from arterial or venous circulation. When the interest is to evaluate pulmonary performance, arterial blood should be used because this sample informs about hematosis (the chemical process of gas exchange that occurs in the pulmonary alveoli) and allows the calculation of oxygen content being offered to tissues. Table 3.1 shows value ranges of gasometry parameters, typically considered normal, of arterial blood. If the test objective is only to assess metabolic parameters, venous blood gasometry can be used. Table 3.2 shows the values considered normal of some gasometry parameters of arterial and venous blood.

Some definitions of important parameters of the gasometry test are presented below, and then, the operation of specific measurement electrodes pO_2, pCO_2, and pH is explained.

Table 3.1 Parameters of arterial blood gasometry

Parameters	Normal range	Electrolytes (mmol/l)		Metabolites (mg/100 ml)	
paO_2	70–100 mmHg	Na^+	135–155	Glucose	70–110
$paCO_2$	35–45 mmHg	K^+	3.6–5.5	Lactate	3–7
pH	7.31–7.45	Ca^{2+}	1.14–1.31	Creatinine	0.9–1.4
Hematocrit	40–54%	Cl^-	98–109	Urea	8–26
Bicarbonate (HCO_3)	22–26 mEq/l				
Hg total	13–18 g/100 ml				
$SatO_2$	95–100%				

Table 3.2 Gasometry parameters of arterial and venous blood

Parameters	Arterial blood	Venous blood
pH	7.35–7.45	0.05 units lower
pCO_2	35–45 mmHg	6 mmHg higher
pO_2	70–100 mmHg	~50% (35–50 mmHg)

3.2.1 Partial pressure of oxygen

The partial pressure of oxygen, pO_2, is measured with electrode and corresponds to the partial pressure exerted on the measuring electrode by molecules of free oxygen dissolved in blood plasma. It does not indicate how much oxygen there is in the blood, just the amount of free oxygen that is dissolved in the plasma.

3.2.1.1 The transport of O_2 in the blood

Approximately 50–60% of the blood volume consists of extracellular fluid called plasma. The remainder of the blood is formed by suspension elements (40–50%) consisting of platelets, leukocytes or white cells and erythrocytes or red blood cells. 90% of plasma is water and acts as a solvent for a wide variety of substances, including dissolved gases (O_2, CO_2, N_2), organic nutrients (glucose, fat), plasma proteins, inorganic ions, nitrogenous remains (urea), and hormones.

Oxygen diffuses from the alveolar air into the blood because the venous blood flowing through the lungs has a $pvO_2 \cong 40$ mmHg (oxygen gas partial pressure), which is lower than the alveolar air ($pAO_2 \cong 102$ mmHg). The diffusion of oxygen to the venous blood turns it into arterial blood where $paO_2 \cong 95$ mmHg. The cellular membrane is a barrier to oxygen diffusion. The oxygen from the blood passing through the lungs does not reach complete equilibrium with the alveolar air and one reason is because the alveolar membrane acts as a barrier to oxygen diffusion.

Oxygen is transported, dissolved in the blood plasma, and in conjunction with the hemoglobin of the erythrocytes (red blood cells). Arterial blood flows through body tissues that have paO_2 lower than that of the blood and, this way, oxygen gas diffuses from blood to tissues. The loss of oxygen with simultaneous gain of carbon dioxide turns the arterial blood into venous blood. Venous blood is collected by veins, conducted to the right side of the heart, and again circulates through the lungs.

The O_2 is not sufficiently soluble in plasma and a carrier of O_2 in the blood is necessary to meet the needs of the body's oxygen: at 38°C, 1 l of plasma dissolves only 2.3 ml of O_2, while the hemoglobin contained in 1 l of blood is capable to transport approximately 87 times more O_2. Figure 3.1 shows the O_2 dissociation curve (at 37°C and $paCO_2 = 40$ mmHg) to pH 7.4. Blood acidosis ($pH < 7.35$) shifts this curve down and alkalosis ($pH > 7.45$) shifts it up (Figure 3.2). The oxygen transport by

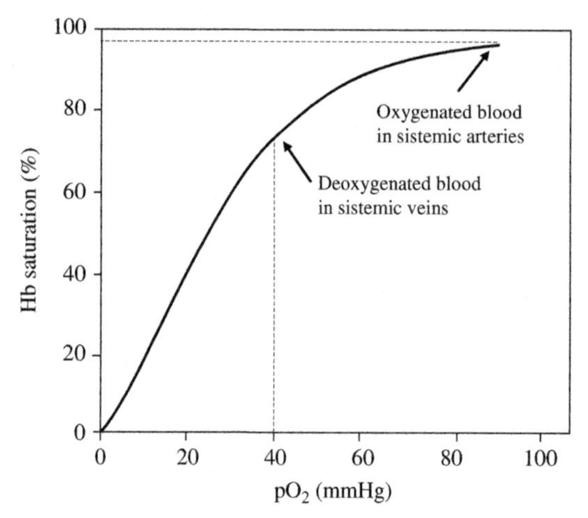

Figure 3.1 Dissociation curve of O_2 at 37°C, for pH 7.4 and paCO_2 40 mmHg.

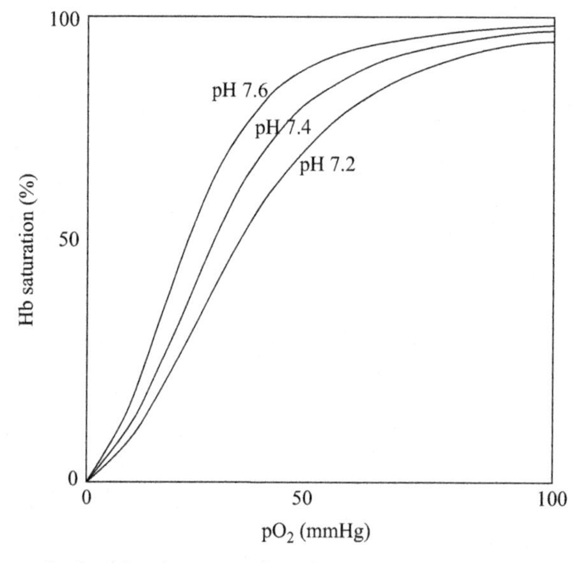

Figure 3.2 pH influence in the blood oxygen dissociation curve.

hemoglobin (one hemoglobin molecule carries four O_2 molecules) depends on the temperature, acid–base balance (pH), and pressure of the gases dissolved in plasma.

3.2.2 Oxy-hemoglobin saturation

During physiological respiration, oxygen binds to the four Fe^{2+} sites (one O_2 to each Fe^{2+}) of the heme component of the protein hemoglobin in erythrocytes; the percentage of red blood cells bound to O_2 molecules (or saturated by O_2) is the oxy-hemoglobin saturation ($SatO_2$), which is calculated by Eq. (3.1)

$$SatO_2 = \frac{[HbO_2]}{[Hb_{total}]} \times 100\% \tag{3.1}$$

where

HbO_2 is the number of oxy-hemoglobin (hemoglobin bound to O_2) and
Hb_{total} is the total quantity of hemoglobin molecules in the blood.

3.2.3 Partial pressure of carbon dioxide

The partial pressure of carbon dioxide, pCO_2, is measured by electrode and corresponds to the pressure that is exerted in the electrode by the dissolved fraction, not combined, of the total CO_2 in the blood. Its value depends basically on the pulmonary ventilation. Venous blood is collected by veins and taken from the right heart to the pulmonary circulation, where it arrives with $pvCO_2$ (venous) in the range 41–51 mmHg and leaves with $paCO_2$ (arterial) between 35 and 45 mmHg; the ideal value is 40 mmHg. To low weight newborn (below 1500 g), under mechanical ventilation, $paCO_2$ until 55 mmHg is allowed (neonatal permissive hypercapnia). $paCO_2$ values below 40 mmHg are associated to chronic lung disease in newborn.

3.2.3.1 The transport of CO_2 in the blood

Carbon dioxide is transported in the blood dissolved in the plasma (it is more soluble than O_2) and bound to hemoglobin as carboxy-hemoglobin and to other blood proteins; the CO_2 binding to hemoglobin molecules enhances 15 times its transport capacity (compared to the amount transported dissolved in the plasma).

The relationship between CO_2 partial pressure and the concentration of hydrogen ions dissolved in blood plasma is approximately described by Handerson–Hasselbach equation. The metabolism produces CO_2 that combines with the water in the blood plasma (reduction of the carbon dioxide) forming carbonic acid, H_2CO_3, which dissociates forming hydrogen ion, H^+, and bicarbonate, HCO_3^- (reversible bonds):

$$CO_2 + H_2O \leftrightarrow H_2CO_3 \leftrightarrow HCO_3^- + H^+ \tag{3.2}$$

There is an intense and constant flow of oxygen, carbon dioxide, and H^+ throughout our body. Despite the large variations in CO_2 production, like the increase during physical activities, for example, blood pH remains practically the same: the concentration of hydrogen ions in the plasma remains in the nanomolar range, 36–43 nmol/l, or pH from 7.35 to 7.45. The pH influence in blood oxy-hemoglobin saturation is shown in Figure 3.2: to the same quantity of oxygen molecules in blood, the lower the pH (acidosis), and the lower the amount of oxygen molecules bound to hemoglobin.

3.2.4 Activity of H^+ ions

The activity of H^+ ions in our body varies from 0.13, in gastric juice (acid), to about 0.00000003 or 3×10^{-8}, in pancreatic juice (alkaline); a practical representation of these concentrations uses the negative base 10 logarithmic scale of the hydrogen ion activity:

$$pH = \log 1/[H^+] \text{ or } -\log[H^+] \quad (3.3)$$

The higher the hydrogen ion concentration, the lower the pH (acidosis); the lower the concentration of H^+ ions, the higher the pH (alkalosis). The pH alone only quantifies the acid–base disturbance, but does not qualify it. The normal concentration of H^+ ions in the extracellular fluid is continuously disturbed by the charge of H^+ ions released by normal metabolism, as shown in Eq. (3.2). This acid load must be neutralized in order to keep the pH in balance and this work is done by the action of buffers in our organism (bicarbonate is one of them), and by respiratory and renal regulation. Table 3.3 shows variation of the values of blood pH, $paCO_2$, and bicarbonate along lifetime.

3.2.5 Bicarbonate

The value of the amount of bicarbonate in the blood is not directly measured, but calculated by the Henderson–Hasselbach equation. Calculating the log on both sides of Eq. (3.2) and rearranging the terms, one comes to Eq. (3.4). Then, using the CO_2 solubility in water and the measured values of pH and partial pressure of carbon dioxide (pCO_2) is possible to determine the bicarbonate value:

$$pH = pk + \log\left[\frac{HCO_3^-}{pCO_2 \times 0.03}\right] \quad (3.4)$$

where

pk is the HCO_3^- (bicarbonate) rate in plasma and

0.03 mmHg or 0.23 kPa is the value of the CO_2 solubility index in water.

Table 3.3 Values of the activity of H^+ ions, arterial partial pressure of carbon dioxide and bicarbonate according to age

Age	pH	$paCO_2$ (mmHg)	HCO_3^- (mEq/l)
1 month	7.39 ± 0.02	31 ± 1.5	20 ± 0.7
3–24 months	7.39 ± 0.03	34 ± 4.0	21 ± 2.0
1.5–3.4 years	7.35 ± 0.05	37 ± 4.0	20 ± 2.5
3.5–5.4 years	7.39 ± 0.04	38 ± 3.0	22 ± 1.5
5.5–12.4 years	7.40 ± 0.03	38 ± 3.0	23 ± 1.0
12.5–17.4 years	7.38 ± 0.03	41 ± 3.0	24 ± 1.0
Adults	7.40 ± 0.02	41 ± 3.5	25 ± 1.0

Metabolic disorders modify the numerator of Eq. (3.4), reducing (acidosis) or increasing (alkalosis) the concentration of bicarbonate. Respiratory disorders interfere with the denominator of Eq. (3.4), increasing (acidosis) or reducing (alkalosis) the $paCO_2$.

3.2.6 Base excess

The BE is the amount of base that must to be added to (negative BE, or base deficit) or subtracted from (positive BE or excess of base) the blood to correct a pH imbalance. BE value is 0 (zero) when pH is 7.4. The normal values range is −2.5 to +2.5 mEq/l. In newborn negative BE levels until −8 mEq/l are acceptable.

3.3 ELECTRODES FOR pO_2, pCO_2, AND pH MEASUREMENT

Next, the operation principle of specific electrodes will be presented for pO_2, pCO_2, and pH measurements. The type of electrode used to measure pO_2 also measures metabolites and the type of electrode used to measure the activity of H^+ ion is also used to measure the concentration of other electrolytes dissolved in the blood plasma. Table 3.4 shows the ranges of expected values of the main parameters measured in gasometry as well as some metabolites and electrolytes.

The activity of hydrogen ions and the partial pressure of CO_2 in a solution are potentiometrically measured. The partial pressure of oxygen in solution is amperometrically measured.

3.3.1 Potentiometric method

Potentiometry is a method used in electroanalytical chemistry, usually to find the concentration of a solute in solution. In potentiometric measurements, a high impedance voltmeter measures the potential between two electrodes. The potentiometric method

Table 3.4 Normal values of arterial gasometry parameters

Dissolved gases in plasma and related parameters		Electrolytes		Metabolites	
pO_2	70−100 mmHg	Na^+	135−155 mmol/l	Glucose	70−110 mg/100 ml
pCO_2	35−45 mmHg	K^+	3.6−5.5 mmol/l	Lactate	3−7 mg/100 ml
pH	7.31−7.45	Ca^{2+}	1.14−1.31 mmol/l	Creatinine	0.9−1.4 mg/100 ml
Hematocrit	40−54%	Cl^-	98−109 mmol/l	Urea	8−26 mg/100 ml
Hg total	13−18 g/100 ml				
$SatO_2$	95−100%				

measures the potential difference between two electrodes immersed in a solution (electrochemical cell). An electrode is the reference and the other the measuring, sensing, or working electrode. The reference electrode has a constant and reproducible potential that is independent of the medium. The potential of the measuring electrode at equilibrium is the potential at the solid/solution interface, where oxidation and reduction reactions occur, and is given by the Nernst law:

$$E = E_0 + \frac{RT}{nF}\ln\frac{[\mathrm{Ox}]}{[\mathrm{Rd}]} \tag{3.5}$$

where

[Ox] and [Rd] are the concentrations of reduced and oxidized forms;
$RT/F = 0.0256$ V (25°C);
F is the Faraday constant;
T is the absolute temperature;
E_0 is the half-cell potential of the metal electrode.

The form of the Nernst law presented in Eq. (3.5) is valid only for very dilute solutions; in other cases, the concentrations should be replaced by the activities of the ions.

3.3.2 Amperometric method

Amperometry is the term indicating a family of electrochemical techniques in which a current is measured as a function of an independent variable that is, typically, time or electrode potential. Voltammetry is a subclass of amperometry, in which the current is measured to different potential levels applied to the electrode. Amperometry is the determination of the current intensity in an electrochemical cell submitted to an electrical potential difference or a constant polarization voltage. At a fixed potential, the current is measured as a function of the analyte concentration, that is, the current intensity is a function of the concentration of the electrochemically active component of the sample. A working electrode performs the oxidation or reduction of the active component during electrolysis and another electrode acts as reference, anode or cathode, depending on the nature of the measurement. The applied potential must be sufficient to cause easy oxidation or reduction of the target analytes. In the measurement of partial pressure of O_2 the working electrode is a platinum electrode polarized by a negative potential, 0.6–0.7 V, which acts as a cathode and the reference electrode is an electrode of Ag–AgCl, which acts as the anode.

3.3.3 pH measurement

The measurement of the activity of H^+ ion in a solution is made potentiometrically. If an unknown solution is separated from a standard solution, which hydrogen ion activity is known, by a selective membrane permeable only to hydrogen ion, the electric potential E through the membrane is given by Eq. (3.6):

$$E = \frac{RT}{nF} \ln \frac{[\mathrm{H}^+]\ \text{known}}{[\mathrm{H}^+]\ \text{unknown}} \tag{3.6}$$

where

R is the constant of gases;
T is the absolute temperature;
n is the valence of ion (in this case one); and
F is the Faraday constant.

The potentiometric measurement of pH requires a working electrode and a reference electrode, each electrode constituting a half-cell (Figure 3.3). The half-cell corresponding to the reference electrode generates a constant voltage that does not depend on the pH. A glass electrode that has an internal reference, usually an Ag–AgCl electrode, immersed in electrolytic solution (HCl) in a glass tube and a sensor element, constitutes the half-cell corresponding to the H+ sensitive electrode. The sensor element of the electrode, located at the bottom of the bulb of the glass tube, consists of a special glass membrane, which has a unique property that distinguishes it from normal glass: the contact with an aqueous solution causes a change in the glass surface structure forming an external gel layer that is selective to hydrogen ion.

The ideal reference electrode follows the Nernst equation, exhibits constant potential over time, returns to its original potential after being subjected to small currents, and has low hysteresis with temperature variations. To hydrogen, calomel and silver coated with silver chloride electrodes, operating under certain conditions, it is

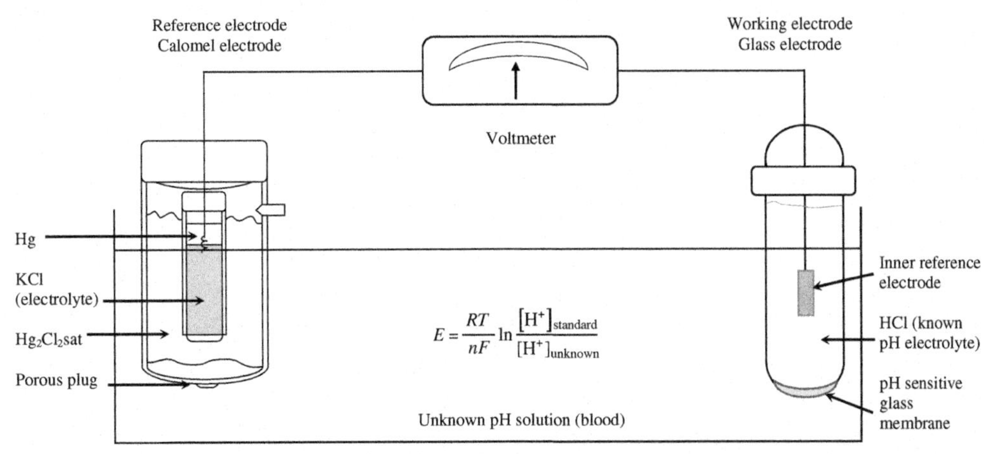

Figure 3.3 Schematic diagram of the electrochemical cell for measuring the pH of a solution, for example, blood. The half-cell corresponding to the reference electrode generates a constant voltage that does not depend on pH.

assigned constant electrode potentials and they are considered nearly ideal reference electrodes. The functioning of these electrodes was explained in Chapter 2.

3.3.3.1 Glass electrode

The potentiometry emerged in the late nineteenth century when the electrometric measurement of the hydrogen ion concentration was discovered by Ostwald in Leipzig, around 1890, and described thermodynamically by Nernst, in 1888. The ion-selective electrodes (ISEs) are a small part of this area of study. The first potentiometric sensor used to measure the acidity of an aqueous solution was the hydrogen electrode, proposed by Nernst in 1897, but due to its complexity had no practical use. Cremer indicated the measurement of the acidity of liquids electrically from his studies in 1906, of liquid interfaces, and found out that it was possible to measure an electric potential in the interface between liquids separated by a thin wall of glass. This idea was taken further by other researchers and Haber and Klemsiewicz discovered in 1909 that a glass bulb (named by him as *glass electrode*) could be used to measure the hydrogen ion activity of a solution, and also, that the electrode response followed a logarithmic function. In the same time, Sorensen, a Danish biochemist, invented the pH scale (Cremer, 1906; Graham, Jaselskis, & Moore, 2013; Haber & Klemsiewicz, 1909; Severinhaus & Astrup, 1985).

For over a century, since the appearance of the glass electrode, controversial theories emerged to explain the mechanism of the functioning of membrane-based ISE. However, the most widespread mechanism is based on the theory of ion exchange between Na^+ ions, in the gel layer of the glass membrane, with H^+ ions in solution (Horovitz, 1923). In the electrochemical cell for pH measurement, the working or indicator electrode is a glass electrode (Figure 3.4), which H^+ sensitive bulb contains:

- electrolyte, a chloride buffer with known concentration (0.1 or 1 M), hydrochloric acid (HCl) or KCl, for example;
- internal reference electrode, for example, Ag–AgCl or platinum, which ensures a constant potential on the interface between the electrolyte and the inner surface of the sensor;
- pH sensor element.

The membrane in the bottom of the glass electrode separates two liquids of different H^+ ion concentrations. A potential difference develops between both sides of the membrane; this potential is proportional to the pH difference of the two liquids (electrolyte and solution under test) and is measured relatively to a reference potential electrode (calomel or Ag–AgCl). Figure 3.4 represents the pH responsive glass electrode immersed in a solution (e.g., blood) which pH value is unknown (Cobbold, 1974; Geddes & Baker, 1968).

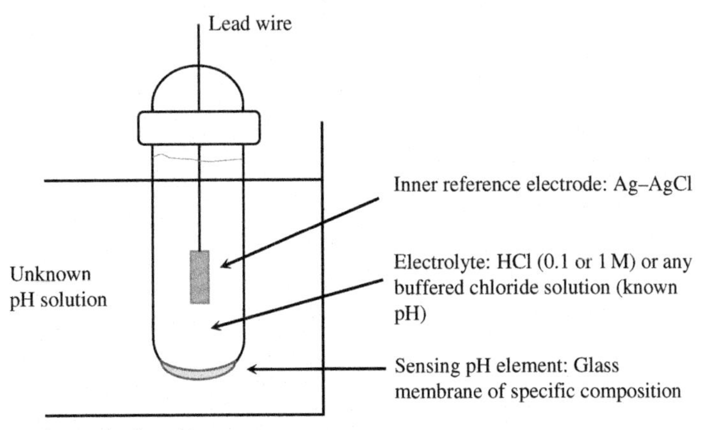

Figure 3.4 Glass electrode for pH measurement.

The membrane is made of a special glass composition (72% SiO_2, 22% Na_2O, and 6% CaO) forming a very thin layer, which is H^+ ion selective (Chan, 2008; Cobbold, 1974). This layer becomes gelatinous in contact with aqueous medium and allows H^+ ions to be changed by sodium ions of the membrane. The ionic changing results in a potential difference that is a linear function of pH and follows Nernst equation. Thus, if a solution with unknown pH ($[H^+]$) is separated from a standard electrolytic solution, which has known hydrogen ion activity ($[H^+_{electr}]$) by a membrane, permeable only to hydrogen ions, the electric potential across the membrane is given by Eq. (3.7)

$$E_{obs} = k + 0.059 \log[H^+_{sol}]/[H^+_{electr}] \tag{3.7}$$

where k is a constant.

Replacing the known values of k and the activity of hydrogen ion in the electrolyte, by a single term K, Eq. (3.7) becomes

$$E_{obs} = K + 0.059 \log[H^+_{sol}] \tag{3.8}$$

or

$$E_{obs} = K - 0.059\ \mathrm{pH} \tag{3.9}$$

The observed potential E_{obs} in the glass electrode depends on the activity of the hydrogen ion in the solution (blood) and the activity of the hydrogen ion in the standard electrolyte. Note that Eq. (3.9) is a term derived from the theoretical Nernst equation. Figure 3.5 shows the influence of temperature on the value of the output voltage of the pH electrode: the graphical representation of output voltage as a function of pH is a straight line, which slope depends on the temperature. At 25°C, the glass electrode generates a voltage of 59 mV (negative) for every pH unit. At 50°C,

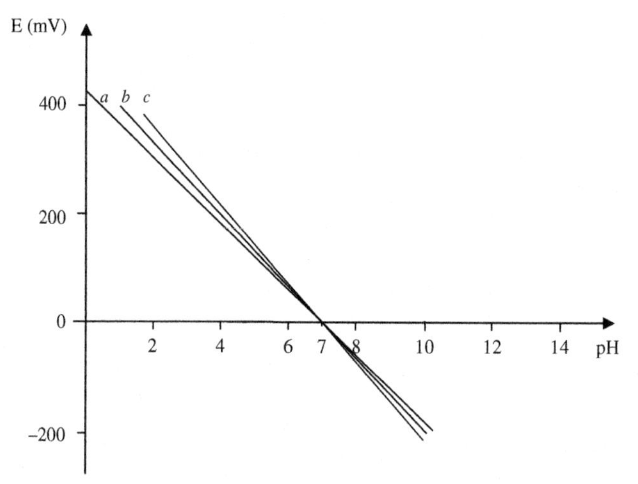

Figure 3.5 Graphical representation of the output voltage of glass electrode as a function of pH value and the influence of (a) 25°C; (b) 50°C; and (c) 100°C.

the output voltage difference is −65 mV and at 100°C, is −74 mV (Chan, 2008; Cobbold, 1974; Webster, 2010).

3.3.3.2 Combined glass electrode

It is necessary to use a pair of electrodes, a working one and another as reference, to determine the concentration of specific ions and pH in viscous solutions and colloidal suspensions. The combined electrode shown in Figure 3.6 is a compact electrode at which the glass electrode is surrounded by the reference electrode (Ag–AgCl or calomel). The lateral aperture is used to electrolyte filling and the junction closes the ionic circuit putting the external electrolyte (inert to pH) in contact with the solution with the unknown pH.

The combined electrode is suitable for most laboratory applications and is easier to handle than a separate pair of electrodes. The most recent ones have an integrated temperature sensor, which is useful for automatic temperature compensation in pH measurements of different samples. Figures 3.6 and 3.7 show the representation of a combined pH electrode used in blood analyzer machine. The pH microelectrode shown in Figure 3.7 has a cuvette shape and a plastic casing and should be discarded after use. At its tip there is an Ag–AgCl wire in a sealed-in buffer, which is separate from the blood sample by the glass membrane. The reference electrode contains a Pt wire immersed in calomel paste surrounded by the electrolyte (KCl solution). Inside the blood analyzer, the sample (1−2 ml) is introduced in such a way that it contacts the tip of the measuring electrode and the KCl solution. The potential difference

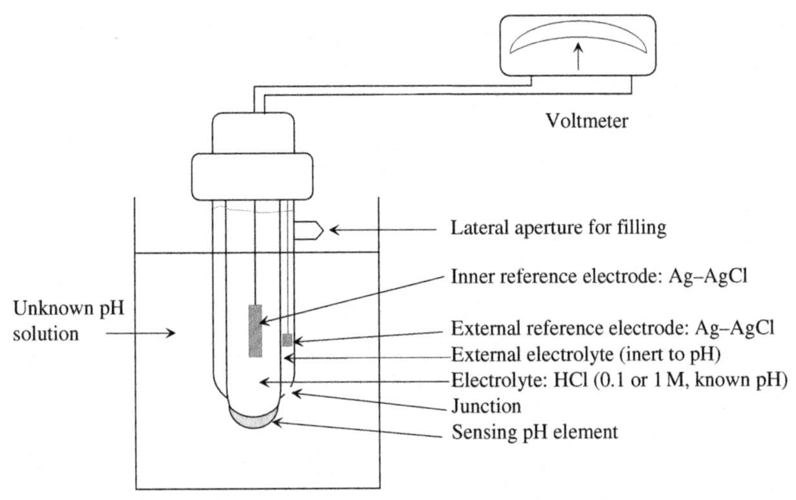

Figure 3.6 Combined glass electrode. Working (sensible to pH) and reference (inert to pH) electrode constructed in the same casing.

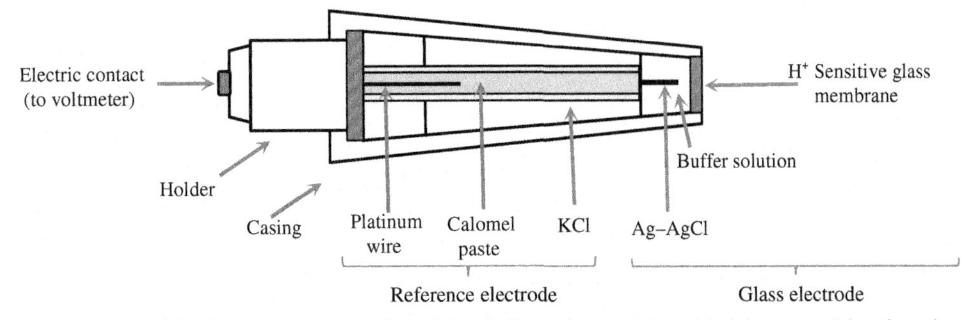

Figure 3.7 Simplified representation of combined glass electrode used in laboratory blood analyzer machine. Working (sensible to pH) and reference (inert to pH) electrodes constructed in the same casing.

output across the sample, which is proportional to the blood pH, goes to the amplifier and voltmeter through the electric contact on the top of the holder.

Due to the elevated resistance of the thin glass wall, typically in the range 10–100 MΩ, the output voltage of the glass electrode could not be accurately measured until adequate electronic devices were developed. The invention of field effect transistors (FETs) and integrated circuits (ICs) with temperature compensation, made it possible to obtain accurate measuring of the glass electrode voltage. Commercial pH meters contain microprocessors that make the necessary corrections for temperature and calibration. Even so, modern pH meters still suffer from drift, which demands frequent calibration.

3.3.3.3 Measurement of electrolyte concentration

The concentration of electrolytes in blood plasma (Na^+, K^+, Li^+, Cu^{2+}, Ca^{2+}, Ag^+, F^-, I^-, Cl^-, NH_4^+, etc.) can be measured with potentiometric-based electrodes which functioning are similar to the pH electrode. According to the ion which concentration is to be measured, the composition of the glass membrane is modified. The membrane becomes permeable to that ion and the electrode will develop a voltage proportional to its concentration. The ideal behavior expected for each glass composition is the membrane to be permeable to only one type of ion, which is impossible in practice, with the exception of the H^+ permeable membrane. Considering that a specific glass composition is permeable to two types of ions, with different sensitivities, the Nernst equation that describes the voltage difference developed through the membrane is:

$$E = E_0 + \frac{RT}{nF}\ln(a_i + k_{ij}a_j) \quad (3.10)$$

where

a_i is the ion i activity
a_j is the ion j activity
k_{ij} is the electrode relative sensitivity to ion j compared to ion i (1 M).

It is possible to produce glass membranes with k_{ij} selectivity that allows effective permeability tens or hundreds times larger to one ion than to other ions present in the glass composition, minimizing the different ions activities interference. The inner electrolytic solution should also be adjusted according to the ion being measured. Additional adjustments (extra measurements, for instance) are required when the measurement is made *in vivo*, directly in living tissue, where there is the additional difficulty of differences in ionic concentration for different tissues, beyond the ion concentration differences between the means intra- and extracellular. Table 3.5 shows the composition of some glass membranes to get selectivity for different ions.

3.3.4 Electrode for paO_2 measurement

The first standard test for dissolved oxygen was reported in 1888 by L.W. Winkler. The Winkler test was a titrimetric method, extremely complex and time consuming (even when automated). *In situ* measurements were practically impossible and no

Table 3.5 Composition of glass membranes permeable to different ions

Ion	Glass composition
H^+	72% SiO_2, 22% Na_2O, 6% CaO
Li^+	60% SiO_2, 25% Al_2O_3, 15% Li_2O
Na^+	71% SiO_2, 18% Al_2O_3, 11% Na_2O
K^+	69% SiO_2, 4% Al_2O_3, 27% Na_2O
Ca^{2+}	3% SiO_2, 6% Al_2O_3, 6% Na_2O, 1% CaO, 16% Fe_2O_3, 67% P_2O_5

real-time monitoring could be done. Some years later, the electrochemical reduction of oxygen was discovered by Danneel and Nernst in 1897. In the decades following, many oxygen detectors were developed using a variety of materials and configurations. The polarography method was discovered in 1922 by Heyrovsky, using dropping mercury, and allowed the first oxygen partial pressure measurement in plasma and blood to be made in the 1940s. His discovery led to the acceptance of electrochemistry as a routine analytical tool. In 1954, Clark constructed the first membrane-covered oxygen electrode having both the anode and cathode separated from the blood sample by a permeable selective membrane. He tested several membranes (cellophane, silastic) until he gets to the polyethylene membrane, which limited permeability to oxygen, reduced depletion of oxygen from the sample, making possible quantitative measurements of oxygen partial pressure in blood, solutions, or gases. Clark's amperometric electrode led to the introduction of present commercial blood gas systems that measure pH, carbon dioxide tension (pCO_2), and pO_2 and calculate many derived variables (Falck, 1997; Severinghaus & Astrup, 1986). By covering cathode and anode with an O_2 selective membrane, Clark changed the polarographic cathode from a sensor of oxygen availability by diffusion, to a measure of oxygen tension (pO_2) in a solution. The term polarography is related to measurement made with the dropping mercury electrode, although much of the literature uses this term to also name voltammetric and amperometric oxygen electrodes.

The Clark electrode makes use of the amperometric method to measure paO_2 and metabolites concentration in the blood. The schematic diagram of the electrode, as its inventor designed it, is shown in Figure 3.8 and the functioning of the Clark electrode is represented in the schematic diagram of Figure 3.9.

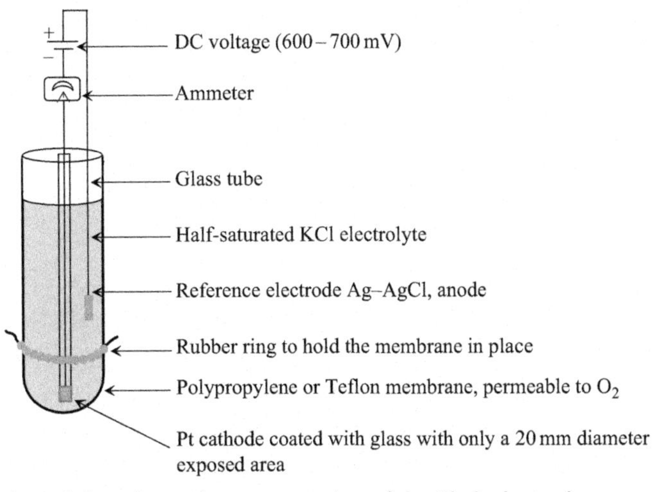

Figure 3.8 Side view of the schematic representation of the Clark electrode.

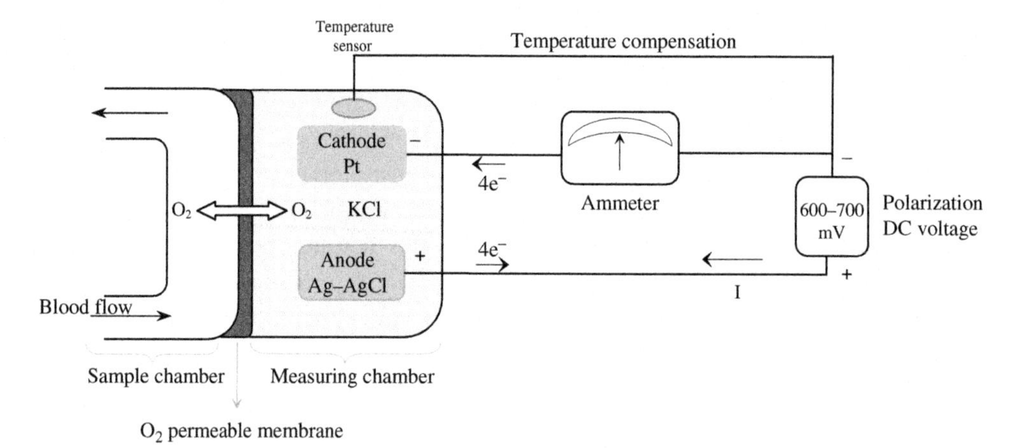

Figure 3.9 Schematic diagram of the Clark electrode operation.

The platinum cathode is biased negatively with respect to the Ag–AgCl anode with 600–700 mV DC. This voltage range corresponds to polarizing voltage values that allow the anode oxidation reaction to occur, maintaining the linear relationship between oxygen concentration and output current, without no other electrochemical reactions that would take place with higher voltages. Both cathode and anode are immersed in electrolytic solution (KCl) and separated from the blood sample by a permeable membrane that allows only O_2 molecules to go through. There is no electrical contact between the blood, where one wants to measure the pressure, and the metal electrodes; the permeable membrane, not the electrolyte, controls the O_2 diffusion between the sample and measuring chambers, according to O_2 differential pressure. The O_2 partial pressure is the pressure required to O_2 molecules to diffuse through the permeable membrane. In the measuring chamber, O_2 is reduced at the platinum cathode (Cobbold, 1974; Geddes & Baker, 1968; Webster, 2010):

$$O_2 + 2H_2O + 4e^- \rightarrow 4OH^- \tag{3.11}$$

And silver is oxidized at the Ag–AgCl anode:

$$4Ag \rightarrow 4Ag^+ + 4e^- \tag{3.12}$$

The number of electrons released, four for each molecule of oxygen, is proportional to the concentration of O_2 in the electrolyte and thus, the resulting current between anode and cathode is proportional to the concentration of dissolved O_2 in the blood. The ammeter reads an electric current value, which varies according to the DC voltage applied and the blood O_2 concentration. The current value is converted into mmHg, with temperature compensation, and the result is usually shown on a display.

The operation of the electrode for paO_2 measurement is dependent on the oxygen supply. The rate of O_2 reduction at the cathode (and thus the resulting current) depends on the concentration of oxygen in the sample chamber and depends on several other factors such as thickness and membrane permeability, temperature and viscosity of the sample. The oxi-reduction reactions are very sensitive to temperature changing and in order to maintain linearity of the relationship between the oxygen concentration and the measured current, the electrode temperature should be controlled within a range of $\pm 0.1°C$ (Cobbold, 1974; Geddes & Baker, 1968). This type of electrode is used in analyzers of dissolved gases in the blood in clinical laboratories and in ICUs. Blood sample must be recent, anaerobic and heparinized. The oxygen electrodes used in blood analyzers have characteristics similar to:

- O_2 permeable membrane 25 μm thick;
- Pt cathode 25 μm diameter;
- 99% of the response is achieved in 25 s;
- 20 pA/mmHgO_2 sensibility at 37°C;
- linearity 1%;
- insensibility to CO_2 molecules.

The paO_2 electrode can be constructed in miniature dimensions to be inserted into a catheter or syringe and perform blood paO_2 measurements *in vivo* (invasive and direct method of blood pressure measurement). Most *in vivo* detectors are comprised of very thin wires (anode and cathode) encased in sealed Teflon tubing filled with supporting electrolyte. The response time of the paO_2 electrode for catheter use depends on the diameter of the electrode and the thickness and diffusion coefficient of the membrane. It should have low sensitivity (<10%) to blood flow variation (from 0 to 100 cm/s) and high sensitivity to blood pressure ($\sim 10^3$ pA/mmHg, at 37°C) using a few units μm thick Teflon membrane.

Clark type microelectrodes can be constructed in a sharp needle format and also micromachined to do *in vivo* paO_2 measurements in living tissues, like brain, kidney. Microconstructed paO_2 electrodes (square shaped with side dimensions of about a few tens to a few hundreds of μm) have the cathode and anode formed as thin-film patterns on a glass substrate and a micro container for the internal electrolyte formed on a silicon substrate by anisotropic etching and a silicone rubber gas-permeable membrane. Their output current usually show reduced blood flow dependence than Clark macroelectrodes (the larger the cathode, the lower the current dependency on the blood flow) and the response time usually is <1 s (Bartlett, Saka, & Jones, 2008; Ndubuizu & LaManna, 2007; Suzuki et al., 2001).

Reusable paO_2 electrodes must be calibrated from time to time, with a known pattern, usually air or via standardized gas mixtures; most of laboratory blood analyzers use disposable electrodes.

The temperature influences the functioning of paO_2 electrodes. Considering blood temperature coefficient equal to 7%/°C and that the temperature coefficient of paO_2 electrode is typically 3%/°C, the paO_2 measurement will have a 10%/°C temperature coefficient. Thus, to obtain ± 1% accuracy in the paO_2 measurements, temperature regulation must be ± 0.1°C. Figure 3.8 shows a sensor temperature placed at the measuring chamber, which helps compensating any temperature variation (Cobbold, 1974; Geddes & Baker, 1968).

3.3.4.1 Optical fiber-based pO_2 microelectrodes

Microsensors made from optical fiber measure pO_2 directly in living tissues (tumors, vital organs, muscles, and wounds) and solutions with dissolved O_2 (e.g., *in vitro* dissolved oxygen monitoring in cell culture). When used directly in living tissues, the measurement of tissue oxygen tension ($ptiO_2$) provides a measure of oxygen availability at the cellular level; they are minimally invasive because the value of the electrode diameter is in the range 250–700 μm (as in OxyLab™, Oxford Optronix). Optical fiber-based paO_2 electrodes (or paO_2 optrodes) do not need to be recalibrated, do not suffer interference from ambient light (they are usually protected by an optical insulation), do not consume oxygen, which reduces problems of stability and drift, are sensitive even under hypoxic conditions and have integrated sensor for temperature variation compensation.

Optrodes are formed by a luminescent indicator and an optical system. Figure 3.10 shows the schematic diagram of a paO_2 optrode. At the tip of the sensor, there is a luminescent indicator, for instance, a platinum-based fluorophore (a fluorescent chemical compound that can re-emit light upon light excitation) impregnated in a membrane (porous sol–gel silica film, acrylic polymer, silicone rubber, polystyrene, etc.). Pulsed light from a blue LED (light emitting diode) and a reference red LED are sent over the optical fiber and reaches the luminescent

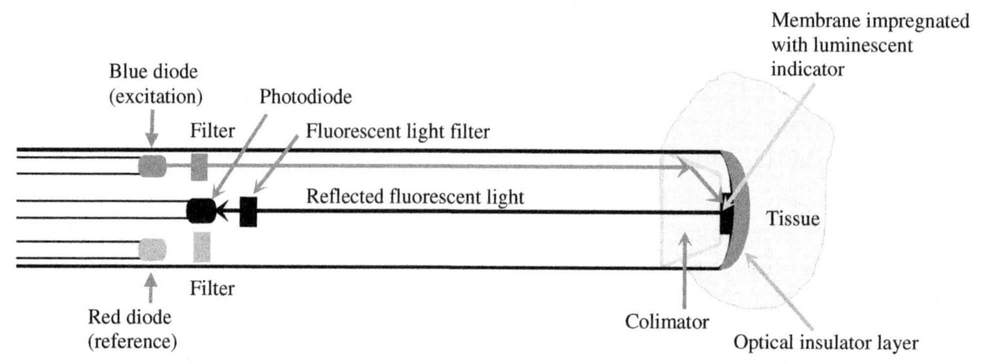

Figure 3.10 Simplified schematic diagram of the functioning of an optical fiber-based paO_2 electrode.

oxygen-sensitive indicator, which emits the luminescence to the measurement site (living tissue). Instead of an LED, a laser source can also be used. The fluorescent light that is not absorbed by the red cells is reflected, transmitted by the optical fiber and detected by a photodiode (or a photomultiplier), and then, processed in the instrument. The indicator is protected from the external environment with a black optical isolation layer (polystyrene carbonate), avoiding interference from external light sources. The lifetime of fluorescence is inversely proportional to the concentration of dissolved oxygen. Typical working range is 0–200 mmHg with response time <20 s and resolution 0.1 mmHg/0.1°C (McDonagh et al., 2001; Mesquita et al., 2011; Silva, 2007).

The functioning of optrodes for measuring blood pO_2 is based on the fluorescent quenching of oxygen-sensitive fluorescent dyes. The measurable intensity I of the excited light is described by the Stern–Volmer equation:

$$I = \frac{I_0}{(1 + k\mathrm{pO_2})} \tag{3.13}$$

where

I_0, intensity of the fluorescent light emitted in the absence of quenching

k, empirical constant.

The sensibility of the sensor is dependent on the pO_2 as shown in Eq. (3.14):

$$\frac{\mathrm{d}I}{\mathrm{dpO_2}} = \frac{-kI_0}{(1 + k\mathrm{pO_2})^2} \tag{3.14}$$

The optrode sensibility decays with pO^2 increasing values and its use is indicated for a pressure range from 0 to <150 mmHg (20 kPa). For values larger than 150 mmHg, the sensibility drops abruptly (Soller, 1994).

3.3.4.2 Measurement of electrolyte concentration

Blood plasma concentration of dissolved metabolites, such as glucose, lactate, glutamine, glutamate, urea, and cholesterol, are measured by biosensors, which are amperometric-based electrodes. The basic amperometric electrode is the oxygen electrode (Clark electrode), which consists of an oxygen-permeable membrane covering a platinum cathode. The metabolite electrode has an additional membrane (gel layer) with an immobilized enzyme, which is in contact to the O_2 permeable plastic membrane; this arrangement allows the set to become permeable to both, oxygen and the specific metabolite, and the electrode develops a current proportional to the analytic substance being measured. Figure 3.11 shows the schematic representation of the construction of a metabolite electrode.

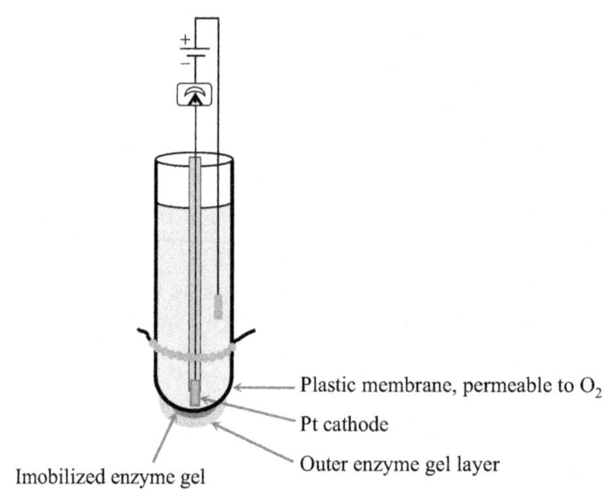

Figure 3.11 Schematic representation of the Clark-based metabolite electrode.

If the amperometric electrode is used to measure the concentration of glucose in blood plasma, the immobilized enzyme in the gel layer is glucose oxidase and the enzyme-catalyzed reactions are:

$$\text{glucose} + O_2 + H_2O \xleftrightarrow{\text{glucose oxidase}} \text{gluconic acid} + H_2O_2 \tag{3.15}$$

Thus, the concentration of glucose is proportional to the O_2 consumption, which is quantified by the resulting electrical current.

The enzymatic method is the principal method used for measuring cholesterol levels in plasma. If the amperometric electrode is used to measure the concentration of cholesterol in blood plasma, the immobilized enzymes used are cholesterol esterase and cholesterol oxidase, to first break the cholesterol ester into cholesterol and then, into cholest-4-ene-3-one, according to equations shown below:

$$\text{cholesterol esters} + H_2O \xleftrightarrow{\text{cholesterol sterase}} \text{cholesterol} + \text{fatty acids} \tag{3.16}$$

$$\text{cholesterol} + O_2 \xleftrightarrow{\text{cholesterol oxidase}} \text{cholesterol} + H_2O_2 \tag{3.17}$$

Again, the O_2 consumption can be used to quantify the analytic substance (cholesterol) concentration in blood plasma.

To measure the concentration of glucose and cholesterol and any other analyte that oxidize in the presence of a specific enzyme forming hydrogen peroxide, instead of measuring the amount of O_2 consumed in the reactions, one can measure the amount of hydrogen peroxide resulting from the analyte oxidation, instead of measuring the amount of O_2 consumed in the reactions (Chan, 2008; Cobbold, 1974; Robinet, Wang, Hazen, & Smith, 2010).

3.3.5 Electrodes for pCO_2 measurement

The potentiometric CO_2 electrode was developed by Stow in 1957 (Stow, Baer, & Randall, 1957) and modified by Severinghaus 1 year later (Severinghaus & Bradley, 1958), conferring a 100% improvement in sensitivity and diminishing the output drift. According to Eq. (3.2), CO_2 reacts with water in the blood plasma forming carbonic acid, which in turn dissociates forming bicarbonate and H^+ ion. Thus, it is possible to obtain the CO_2 concentration measuring the activity of the resulting H^+ ions from the carbonic gas dissociation. The potentiometric measurement of CO_2 concentration is made with an electrochemical cell, in which one half-cell is an H^+ ion sensitive electrode, a pH or glass electrode, and the other half-cell is the reference electrode (constant pH—calomel or Ag–AgCl), which is inert to H^+ ions. The output voltage, the difference between the Nernst potentials of the half-cells, is proportional to the dissolved CO_2 concentration in the blood plasma or pCO_2.

Figure 3.12 is the representation of the Stow−Severinghaus electrode for pCO_2 measurement.

This electrode uses a buffer solution of sodium bicarbonate and NaCl. The Teflon membrane selectively allows only CO_2 molecules to go through. The higher the CO_2 concentration in the blood sample, the higher the CO_2 diffusion through the semi-permeable membrane and the concentration of CO_2 in the buffer solution. The greater the concentration of CO_2 in the buffer chamber, the higher the concentration of H^+ ions, which in turn increases the voltage reading on the voltmeter (indicating a decrease in the pH of the sample).

The output voltage is proportional to the concentration of dissolved CO_2 in the blood plasma and depends on the hydrogen ion activity in the solution $[H^+_{blood}]$ (unknown) and the hydrogen ion activity in the electrolyte $[H^+_{ele}]$ (standard unit).

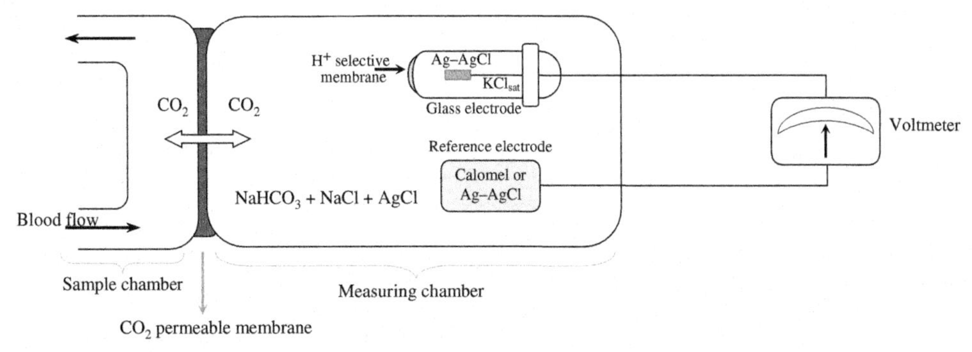

Figure 3.12 Schematic diagram of the Stow−Severinghaus electrode for pCO_2 measurement.

The relationship between PCO_2 and $[H^+_{blood}]$ is linear ($E = K - 0.059 \times pH$) in the pressure range from 1.3 to 12 kPa (10–90 mmHg). The typical response time of CO_2 electrodes, mounted in cuvette shape, used in laboratory blood analyzers achieves 98% of the final value within 45 s. The error is ± 1% and the resolution is 0.1 mmHg for the working range of 10–260 mmHg. The required volume of blood is 200 μl (Cobbold, 1974; Geddes & Baker, 1968).

3.4 REVIEW THE LEARNING

1. What are the main parameters obtained in gases? What parameters are measured with specific electrodes? What are the calculated parameters from the measured ones?
2. Why in the evaluation of pulmonary performance the arterial blood gasometry is used instead of venous?
3. How the amount of bicarbonate in the blood can be obtained?
4. Describe the functioning of the glass electrode.
5. Present the schematic diagram of the electrochemical cell used for pH measurement with glass electrode and reference electrode (hydrogen, calomel, or silver), explaining the function of the various components.
6. Explain the construction and functioning of the combined electrode used for pH measurement.
7. Explain what are the modifications made in the glass electrode, which allow its use to measure the concentration of other ions than H^+, dissolved in blood plasma to be measured.
8. Describe how the partial pressure of oxygen in a blood sample is measured using a Clark electrode.
9. Explain how amperometric-based electrodes measure the concentration of different metabolites in blood plasma.
10. Describe how the partial pressure of carbon dioxide in a blood sample is measured using a Stow–Severinghaus electrode.

REFERENCES

Bartlett, K., Saka, M., & Jones, M. (2008). Polarographic electrode measures of cerebral tissue oxygenation: Implications for functional brain imaging. *Sensors*, *8*, 7649–7670.

Chan, A. Y. K. (2008). *Biomedical device technology: Principles and design*. Springfield, Illinois: Charles C. Thomas.

Cobbold, R. S. C. (1974). *Transducers for biomedical measurements: Principles and applications.* John Wiley & Sons.

Cremer, M. (1906). Über die ursache der elektromotorischen eigenschaften der gewebe, zugleich ein beitrag zur lehre von polyphasischen elektrolytketten (About the cause of the electromotive properties of the tissue, a contribution to the teaching of polyphasic electrolyte chains). *Zeitschrift fur Biologie.*, *47*, 562.

Falck, D. (1997). Amperometrics oxygen electrodes. *Current Separations*, *16*(1), 19–22.

Graham, D. J., Jaselskis, B., & Moore, C. E. (2013). Development of the glass electrode and the pH response. *Journal of Chemical Education*, *90*(3), 345–351.

Geddes, L. A., & Baker, L. E. (1968). *Principles of applied biomedical instrumentation*. New York, NY: John Wiley & Sons.

Haber, F., & Klemensiewicz, Z. A. (1909). Uber elektrische phasengrenzkrafte (On the electrical forces at phase borders). *Zeitschrift für Physikalische Chemie*, *67*, 385.

Horovitz, K. (1923). Der Ionenaustausch am Dielektrikum I. Die Elektrodenfunktion der Gläser (The ion exchange on the dielectric I. The function of the glass electrodes). *Zeitschrift für Physik*, *15*(1-2), 369–398. <http://link.springer.com/journal/218>.

McDonagh, C., Kolleb, C., McEvoya, A. K., Dowlinga, D. L., Cafollaa, A. A., Cullena, S. J., et al. (2001). Phase fluorometric dissolved oxygen sensor. *Sensors and Actuators B*, *74*, 124–130.

Mesquita, R. C., Durduran, T., Yu, G., Buckley, E. M., Kim, M. N., Zhou, C., et al. (2011). Direct measurement of tissue blood flow and metabolism with diffuse optics. *Philosophical Transaction of the Royal Society A*, *369*, 4390–4406.

OxyLite™, Oxford Optronix. *In vivo* and *in vitro* oxygen monitoring. <http://www.oxford-optronix.com/product20/page501/Tissue-Vitality-Monitoring/Oxygen-Monitors/OxyLite-.html> Accessed 10.03.14.

Robinet, P., Wang, Z., Hazen, S. L., & Smith, J. D. (2010). A simple and sensitive enzymatic method for cholesterol quantification in macrophages and foam cells. *Journal of Lipid Research*, *51*, 3364–3369 <http://www.jlr.org/content/51/11/3364.full.pdf> Accessed 28.03.14.

Severinghaus, J. W., & Astrup, P. B. (1975). History of blood gas analysis II. pH and acid-base balance measurements. *Journal of Clinical Monitoring*, *1*(4), 259–277.

Severinghaus, J. W., & Astrup, P. B. (1986). History of blood gas analysis. IV. Leland Clark's oxygen electrode. *Journal of Clinical Monitoring*, *2*(2), 125–139.

Severinghaus, J. W., & Bradley, A. F. (1958). Electrodes for blood pO_2 and pCO_2 determination. *Journal of Applied Physiology*, *13*, 515–520.

Silva, K. R. B. (2007). *Optodos para a Determinação de SO2 e O2* (pp. 1–126). PhD thesis. University of Campinas. <http://biq.iqm.unicamp.br/arquivos/teses/vtls000434698.pdf> Accessed 10.03.14.

Soller, B. R. (1994). Design of intravascular fiber optic blood gas sensor. *IEEE Engineering in Medicine and Biology*, *13*(3), 327–335.

Stow, R. W., Baer, R. F., & Randall, B. (1957). Rapid measurement of the tension of carbon dioxide in blood. *Archives of Physical Medicine and Rehabilitation*, *38*, 646–650.

Webster, J. (Ed.), (2010). *Medical instrumentation: Application and design* (4th ed.). New York, NY: John Wiley & Sons.

Winker, L. W. (1888). Bestimmung des im Wassers Gelosten Sauerstoffes (Determination of dissolved oxygen in water). *Berichte der Deutschen Chemischen Gesellschaft*, *21*, 2843–2854.

CHAPTER 4

Temperature Transducers

Contents

4.1 INTRODUCTION

Two objects are in thermal equilibrium, that is, the same temperature, when the exchange of thermal energy is possible and no net flux occurs. The postulate of zero law of thermodynamics says that when two bodies are in thermal equilibrium with a third, they are in equilibrium with each other. The temperature of an object can be inferred by a thermometer, which is nothing more than a device that allows the comparison of the unknown temperature with known patterns, after thermal equilibrium has been reached, using calibration curves.

Temperature transducers are used in Biomedical Engineering in thermometers to measure, monitor, and control the temperature of patient's body and substances, such as electrolyte solution, plasma, blood, and air used in medical procedures; thermometers can be a stand alone device or part of a more complex equipment, such as infusion pump, extra-corporeal blood circulation pump, and anesthesia machine.

Principles of Measurement and Transduction of Biomedical Variables.
DOI: http://dx.doi.org/10.1016/B978-0-12-800774-7.00004-0

The body temperature is used as an indicator of physiological state of the patient and may highlight some pathologies, such as inflammation or infection. Another use of temperature transducers is in imaging by thermography, in which body regions with increased metabolism and thus higher temperature, indicative of the presence of a pathological process (e.g., breast cancer), can be identified. Some surgeries need the patient to be cooled, so there is a decrease in the metabolic process and blood circulation, and the temperature transducer is used to monitor the body temperature.

The patient's temperature can be obtained noninvasive or invasively. Invasive methods utilize catheters through which the sensor is inserted into regions of the body such as urethra and pulmonary artery, or hypodermic implants, in which a flexible and needle-shaped sensor is inserted beneath the skin or through internal organ tissues. Noninvasive methods measure the skin temperature, preferably in areas of great blood circulation and less influence of ambient temperature, such as mouth, armpit, rectum, and tympanum, with surface sensors. With respect to medical devices, the sensor is often used to indicate not only the temperature value but also to control the temperature in a closed loop system. Some examples of medical devices, which use the transducer for temperature control, are infant incubators used for life support, autoclaves used for sterilization, and Bier ovens used in thermotherapy, among others.

Temperature is a scalar quantity and the unit used to indicate its value varies according to the thermometric scale used. The three most common scales for measuring temperature are Celsius (°C), Fahrenheit (°F), and Kelvin (K). The temperature scales were defined according to three physical states of matter called fundamental fixed points, given in Table 4.1.

The basic unit of temperature in the International System of Units is Kelvin (K) 1/273.15 formally defined as the triple point of water temperature, that is, the temperature at which water can be in equilibrium in the solid state liquid and gas. 0 K is called absolute zero temperature corresponding to the point at which atoms and molecules have minimal thermal energy. Most current applications of day-to-day use is Celsius scale. On this scale, 0°C is the temperature at which water freezes and 100°C is the boiling point of water at atmospheric pressure at sea level. In both scales, the temperature difference is the same, that is, the temperature difference of 1 K is equal to the difference of temperature of 1°C.

Table 4.1 Thermometric scales and fundamental fixed points

Matter physical state	°C	°F	K
Absolute zero	− 273.15	− 459.67	0
Ice point of water (1 atm)	0	32	273
Boiling point of water (1 atm)	100	212	373

Absolute zero: The temperature at which the kinetic energy of atoms and molecules is minimal and adiabatic processes (no heat exchange with the environment) and isothermal (no temperature change) processes coincide.

There are several ways to infer the temperature of an object, each one with physical principles, applications, and different methods of use. Most temperature transducers use heat transmission by contact to come into balance with the energy of the medium, but there are also noncontact temperature transducers. Among them, in this text, the following types of sensors will be studied:

Contact transducers: Transduction by thermoexpansion, thermoresistive sensors (metal elements—RTDs (resistance temperature detector) and semiconductor elements—thermistors); thermoelectric sensors (thermocouples); capacitive transduction; transduction with diodes (PN junction); and thermochemical transduction (liquid crystal).

Contactless transducers: Optical pyrometers and infrared sensors.

4.2 CONTACT TRANSDUCERS

Contact temperature transducers perform the measurement of the temperature of an object by thermic conduction between the object and the thermosensitive element.

4.2.1 Thermoexpansion temperature transducers

The volumetric thermal expansion is one of the effects of temperature mostly used to measure its value. It is the basis of the operation of fluid expansion devices and bimetallic pair. Fluid expansion devices main classification includes the liquid mercury type thermometer and the organic liquid type. Versions employing gas instead of liquid are also available. Mercury is considered an environmental hazard, so there are regulations governing the shipment of devices that contain it. Fluid expansion sensors do not require electric power, do not pose explosion hazards, and are stable even after repeated cycling. On the other hand, they do not generate data that are easily recorded or transmitted, and they cannot make spot or point measurements.

4.2.1.1 Liquid mercury thermometer

The first thermometers of liquid column used water as thermosensitive element. Mercury has volumetric coefficients of expansion and contraction more sensitive and rapid than water (1 cm^3 mercury enlarges 1.8% its volume from 0 to 100°C), resulting in smaller and more efficient devices. The mercury thermometer has a bulb filled with liquid mercury, which expands through a narrowing to a capillary tube when submitted to a temperature increase (Figure 4.1A); the smaller the diameter of the capillary, the greater the sensitivity of the thermometer. When the bulb of the thermometer is put, for example, in the mouth, the volume of mercury expands proportionally to the temperature of the medium, and the new height of the metal column indicates, on a graduated scale, the temperature value. When the thermometer is removed from the mouth, the column height does not back to the original value, which facilitates reading the temperature value.

Both mercury and glass volumes change with temperature increase and the influence of glass expansion in thermometric measurements is minimized using glass with a low coefficient of expansion. To be able to show little temperature differences, fraction of a grade order, the capillary diameter must be <0.1 mm. Figure 4.1B represents a transversal section of the thermometer with construction details, showing that the thermometer has a frontal glass lens and a white background, which allow to read the height of the mercury column in thin capillary.

Mercury is an extremely toxic substance and its effects are cumulative, that is, they are not eliminated by the human body. Mercury poisoning can be fatal, and even small amounts can damage the nervous system. The mercury should never be touched with bare hands or its vapor be inhaled, situations able to occur in accidents where the thermometer breaks. In the last decades, the use of mercury thermometer has been replaced worldwide by electronic devices, as for instance, in the European Community, that was the largest world exporter of mercury in 2007, and banished its use in thermometers from 2011. Mercury is used in thermometers, also in mining, and in the production of PVC.

Alcohol and gases volumetric expansion are also used in temperature transducers. Alcohol has a coefficient of volumetric expansion higher than mercury, that is, expands more volumetrically per unit of temperature variation. Its working range is from −10°C to 150°C and is used in laboratories and residential thermometers.

Gas thermometers measure temperature through the ratio of the pressures exerted at the sensor by a constant gas volume, at reference and unknown temperatures. They may have a graduated scale in which each division corresponds to a

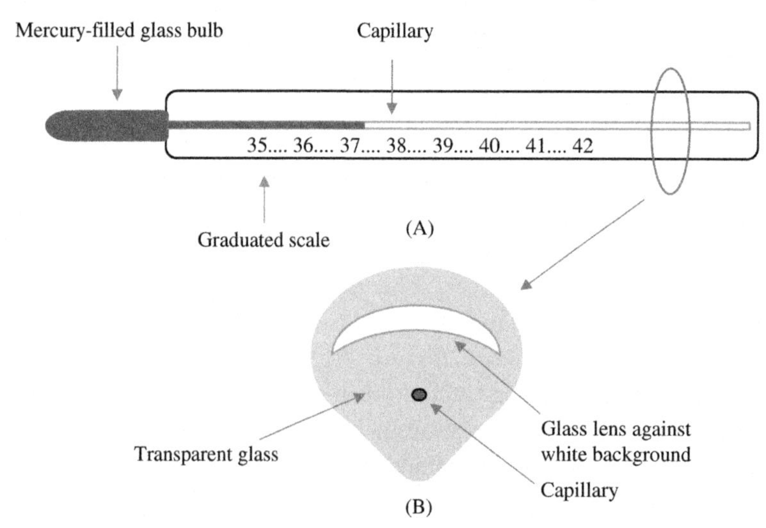

Figure 4.1 (A) Glass mercury thermometer with graduate scale and (B) construction detail showing the glass lens.

temperature value in a thermometric scale Celsius. This type of transducer is used for low temperature readings, with helium gas, whose condensation temperature at atmospheric pressure is next to $-269°C$. The reference point (P_1, T_1) is usually the triple point of water, at which its three states—ice, liquid water, and vapor, coexist in equilibrium ($P_1 = 610$ Pa and $T_1 = 273.16$ K). The unknown temperature T_2 is calculated by Eq. (4.1)

$$T_2 = T_1 \left(\frac{P_2}{P_1}\right)_{\text{volcte}} \tag{4.1}$$

where P_2 is the pressure of the constant volume gas (volcte) at the unknown temperature.

4.2.1.2 Bimetallic strip

Bimetallic strip thermometers are mechanical thermometers. They are widely used in industry, including medical equipment, in thermostats for measuring and controlling temperature. The thermal expansion coefficients of metals are different and if a pair of metallic strips (linear, circular, or helical configurations) of different materials (bimetallic) welded or heated, the strips dilate differentially and the resulting strip tends to bend toward the metal with the lowest expansion coefficient. Most bimetallic strips use a high thermal expansion alloy, such as steel or stainless steel, coupled with a low thermal expansion alloy such as Invar (64% Fe, 36% Ni) with one end fixed and the other free to bend. Bimetallic strips are used in thermostats for measuring and controlling temperature and also in mechanical switches.

Figure 4.2 shows two of the available constructions. In the first one, with a helical format, the bimetallic strips are coiled into a spiral and attached to a dial, which is

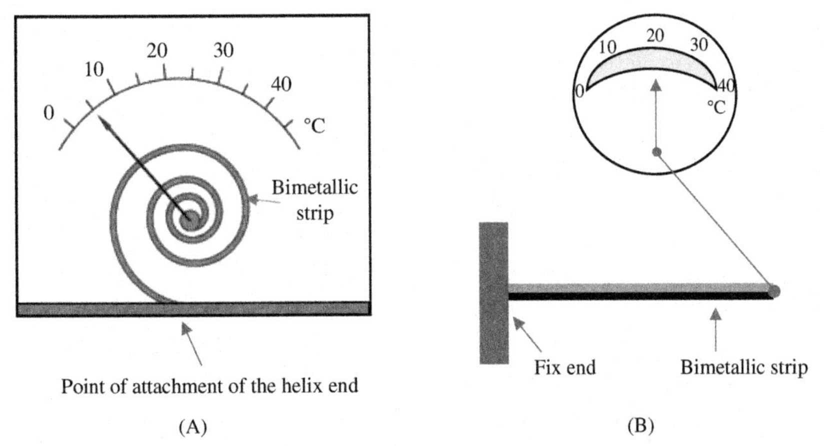

Figure 4.2 Available construction forms of bimetallic strip thermosensor: (A) helical and (B) cantilever.

calibrated for temperature indication. When the temperature changes the strips twist, moves the pointer, and indicates the temperature value. In the second, the bimetallic strips are bonded together in a cantilever and the temperature caused deflection can be used to activate a device temperature indicator or a switch.

The temperature changing is related to the strip linear expansion by the equation:

$$L_2 = L_1(1 + \gamma(T_2 - T_1)) \tag{4.2}$$

where γ is the coefficient of linear expansion of the assembly

T_1 is the initial reference temperature and L_1 is the initial length

T_2 is the final temperature and L_2 is the final length.

The bimetallic strip thermometer does not require a power source, is robust, easy to use and cheap, but not very accurate; it can be used from $-50°C$ up to $500°C$, with 1% of full-scale resolution and time of response 15–40 s. Its use is limited to applications where manual reading is acceptable, for example, a household thermometer. It is not suitable for very low temperatures because the expansion of metals tends to be too similar, so the device becomes a rather insensitive thermometer (Childs, Greenwood, & Long, 2000; McGee, 1988).

4.2.2 Thermoresistive and thermoelectric temperature transducers

The electrical resistance of several materials varies somewhat with temperature. This characteristic, often undesirable, is the basic principle of temperature measurement via thermoresistive elements. These elements exhibit a variation in their resistances with temperature very significant and easily measurable. They are made of metallic or semiconducting material. Temperature sensors made of conductive materials are traditionally known by its acronym in English RTD (resistance temperature detector) and the ones made of semiconductor, by thermistors.

The thermocouple, a thermoelectric temperature sensor, is a two wires device made of dissimilar metals or alloys with the ends tied forming junctions. The temperature difference between the two junctions causes the appearance of a potential difference, and this is the basic principle used in the measurement of temperature using thermocouples.

These concepts are explained below, showing how the transducers are used to measure temperature, their advantages and disadvantages and applications in biomedical engineering.

4.2.2.1 Thermoresistive temperature transducers

4.2.2.1.1 RTD—Resistance temperature detector

All metallic materials, even having good conductive characteristics, present an electrical resistance, which varies with temperature. All metals produce a positive variation in its resistance to an increase in temperature, which means that the resistance increases with temperature. This dependence of the electrical resistance with temperature is the fundamental principle used by an RTD. Despite this dependence, the relation between these two quantities (resistance and temperature) varies with the nature of the metal involved and does not necessarily occur linearly. The thermal behavior of most metallic resistive filaments may be expressed by a generic polynomial as follows:

$$R = R_0[1 + a_1(T - T_0) + a_2(T - T_0)^2 + \cdots + a_n(T - T_0)^n] \tag{4.3}$$

where

a_n is the coefficient of thermal resistivity

R_0 is the resistance at reference temperature T_0 (usually $T_0 = 0°C$).

Ideally, the polynomial equation has n terms, but a simplification is allowed depending on the application, type of metal or alloy used, required accuracy and temperature working range.

The higher the resistivity of a metal, the greater the variation of its resistance with increasing temperature. All metals can be used as thermal sensors, but some are more suitable for their characteristics of linearity, sensitivity, reproducibility, immunity to external influences and contamination, lifetime, robustness, etc. Figure 4.3 shows the curve of relative variation of resistance with temperature of the metals platinum, copper, and nickel, and the metallic alloy manganin, which is insensitive to temperature (0–400°C).

The metals traditionally used are platinum, nickel, and nickel alloys. Gold and silver are rarely used due to their low resistivity. Tungsten has a high resistivity but its use as RTD is reserved to very high temperature applications, because it is brittle, and so, difficult to use. Copper and copper alloys are also used as thermoresistive elements due to low cost, but its low resistivity makes RTD size greater than the high resistivity ones. Nickel and its alloys are also an economical choice but they are nonlinear and tend to drift with time.

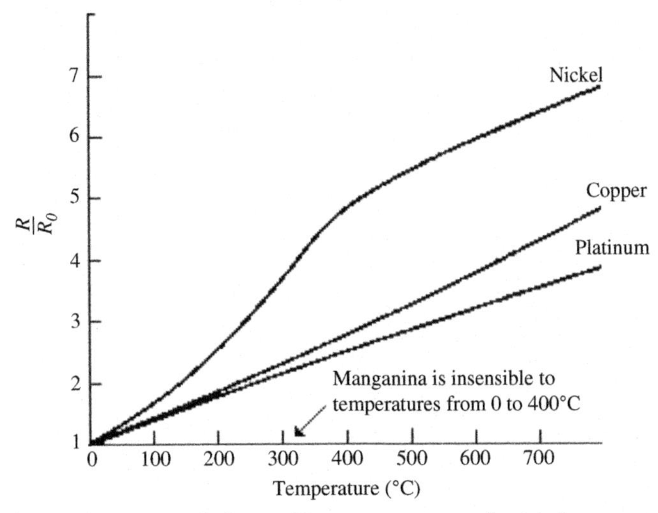

Figure 4.3 Relative resistance variation with temperature of nickel, copper, platinum, and manganin.

The polynomial equations of thermoresistive behaviors of platinum, copper, and nickel RTDs, in applications that require high accuracy, still can be simplified to just the first three terms of the equation, or even two, in the case of platinum. Platinum is the most used metal in the manufacture of temperature sensors, due to its high stability, immunity to contamination and wide working range (−277°C to 1,064°C).

The resistance of a metal is proportional to length and inversely proportional to the cross-sectional area of a wire used to fabricate an RTD of a required value. The resistivity property defines the length and cross-sectional area of the wire:

$$R = \rho \cdot L/A \tag{4.4}$$

where

ρ is the resistivity of the metal
L is the length of the wire
A is the cross-sectional area of the wire.

Platinum has a very high resistivity, which means it is necessary a small quantity of platinum to fabricate a thermoresistive sensor, making platinum cost competitive with other RTD materials. The platinum polynomial simplification with only the first two terms (a_0 and $a_1 \neq 0$) (Eq. (4.3)) has a maximum linearity error of 0.4% ± within the range of −70°C to 150°C and 0.2% ± within the range of 0–100°C, and in this last case, with an accuracy of approximately 0.001°C.

$$R = R_0[1 + a_1(T - T_0)] \tag{4.5}$$

4.2.2.1.1.1 RTD pattern platinum—PT100 In 1871, 50 years after Sir Humphrey Davy announcement of the metals resistivity dependence with temperature, Sir William Siemens used platinum in a resistance temperature sensor, but the classical resistance temperature detector construction using platinum was proposed by C.H. Meyers in 1932 (Price, 1959; The RTD, 2014). Figure 4.4 shows a representation of this first platinum RTD configuration: a helical coil of platinum wounded on

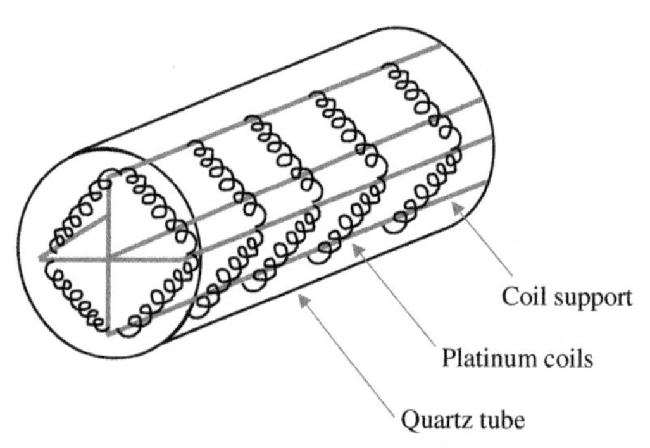

Figure 4.4 Representation of the platinum RTD constructed by Myers in 1932.

a crossed mica support mounted inside a glass tube. This construction minimized strain and maximized resistance on the wire.

Many improvements in the platinum RTD construction were made to minimize strain-induced and temperature effect on the material of the metal support. The most used platinum RTD, in medical, laboratorial, and industrial equipments, is the PT100. By definition, it has an electrical resistance of 100 Ω at 0°C with a sensibility of 0.385 Ω/°C. Figure 4.5 shows the PT100 calibration curve for a working range of −20°C to +120°C; the maximum linearity error in this range is <0.25%.

The equations obtained by the methods of first-order linear regression and second-order polynomial regression, describing the behavior of a platinum RTD for temperatures ranging from −20°C to +120°C, are, respectively:

$$R = 0.385T + 100 \tag{4.6}$$

$$R = -5.56 \cdot 10^{-5}T^2 + 0.391T + 100 \tag{4.7}$$

Figure 4.5 and Eqs. (4.6) and (4.7) show the great linearity of PT100 in the temperature range from −20°C to +120°C. The methods of second-order polynomial regression and first-order linear regression presented similar equations, due to the very small coefficient of thermal resistivity a_2 ($-5.56 \cdot 10^{-5}$ Ω/T^2) that contributed very little to the final result.

The platinum RTD has the best accuracy and stability among the common RTD materials. Platinum can be refined to high levels of purity and PT100 resistance values at any temperature are found in universal tables, so they do not vary according to sensor manufacturer. The following sections present details of construction and casing of

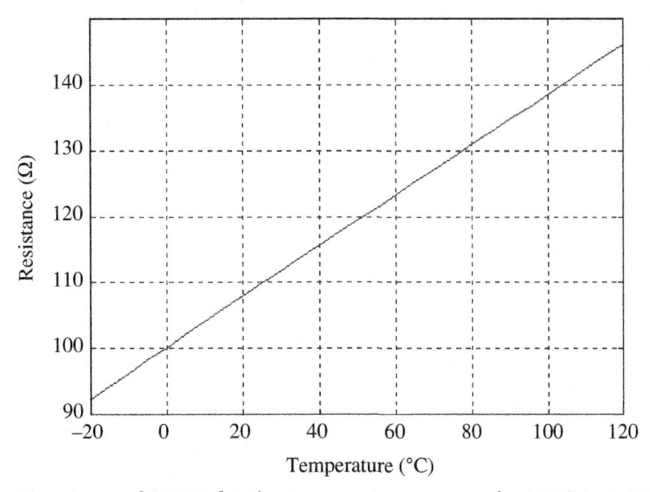

Figure 4.5 Calibration curve of PT100 for the temperature range of −20°C to +120°C.

platinum temperature sensing elements (Chan, 2008; Cobbold, 1974; Dally, Riley & McConnell, 1993; Doebelin, 1990; Geddes & Baker, 1968; OMEGA, 1983; RdF, 2014; The RDT, 2014).

4.2.2.1.1.2 Types of construction of RTD There are three types of construction of RTD, each one unique characteristics to suit different applications. The platinum sensing element can be obtained as wire wound, grid filament, and planar film.

Figure 4.6 shows some examples of wire wound platinum RTD (RdF, 2014). The platinum element can be unsupported, partially supported, or wrapped around an element support. The element support can be round or flat, but must be an electrical insulator, such as glass or ceramic, and should match the coefficient of thermal expansion of the sensing wire to minimize any mechanical strain that would result in an error in the temperature measurement due to strain-induced resistance change. In the unsupported design, the sensing element usually has a coil format, which allows the wire coil to expand and contract freely over temperature changes. The coil of platinum sensing wire is inserted into a packed insulating powder inside a mandrel to prevent it from shorting and to provide vibration resistance while using.

In the wire wound RTD, the sensing wire extremities are connected to larger wires, the lead wires. The material of these wires must be selected to be compatible with the platinum sensing wire, so the heating of the metals combination will not generate an emf (electromotive force), which would modify the temperature measurement. Whenever a strain-free method is used in the RTD construction, it contributes to produce a higher temperature coefficient and better stability temperature sensor.

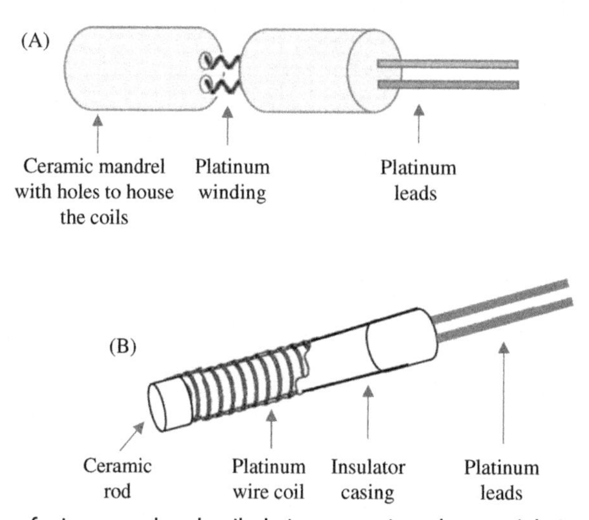

Figure 4.6 Examples of wire wound and coil platinum sensing element (platinum RTD) for temperature measurement.

Figure 4.7 shows examples of wire or filament grid and planar film platinum sensing element of RTD.

Filament grid RTD is obtained formatting a grid pattern with a thin platinum wire and fixing the grid with a support of an insulating material, ceramic for instance. The extremities of the grid are connected to lead wires and the resistance of the grid can be adjusted through little cuts to remove part of the material of the grid.

The planar film RTD is obtained depositing a thin layer of platinum on a ceramic substrate in a grid (or more complex) pattern, followed by very high temperature annealing and stabilization. As the filament grid, the film pattern usually has provisions for adjusting the final resistance by cutting the circuit in a trim area. Film grid extremities are connected to metal compatible lead wires. The grid pattern is coated by a thin glassy layer (or synthetic resin) and the lead connection is coated by a heavy glassy layer to mechanical reinforcement and moisture protection. The planar film type of sensing element allows getting greater resistances in smaller areas than with the other fabrication methods.

To measure the temperature in a solid, the thin planar film RTD can be fixed to its surface, which contributes to improve the response time of the assembly.

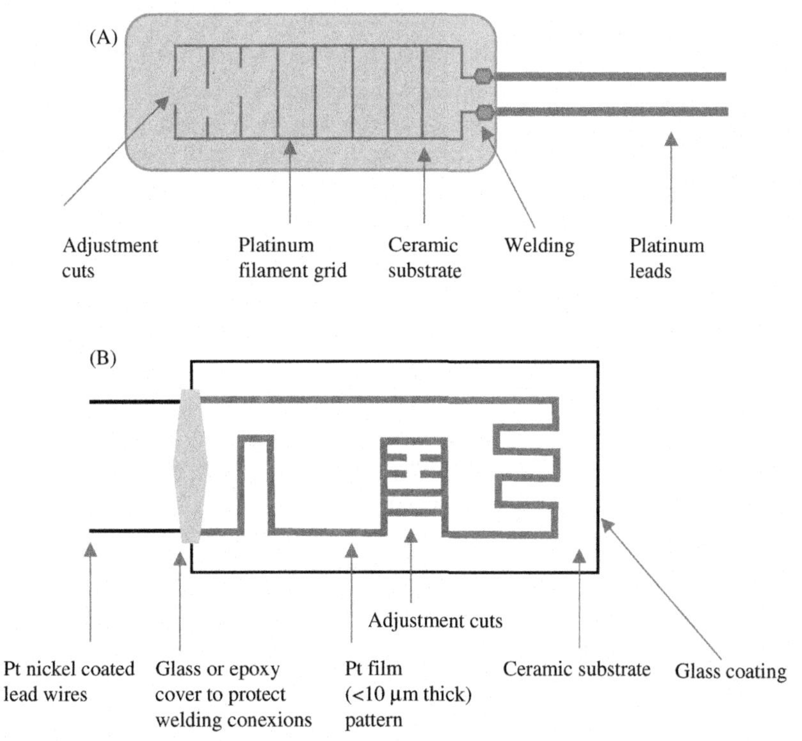

Figure 4.7 Examples of wire grid (A) and planar film (B) RTDs.

The response time results smaller, but makes the RTD susceptible to a "strain-gage effect," that is, if the solid deforms with any temperature changing, the film RTD will also deform, introducing a resistance modification related to physical dimensions modification.

4.2.2.1.1.3 RTD casing types To protect the RTD from damage caused by mechanical shock or from corrosion when the temperature measurement is made in environments with corrosive liquids, moist, or gases (e.g., sweat, blood, and exhaled air), the heat-sensitive resistive wire, filament, or film is covered by a protective case, usually made of ceramic, glass, synthetic resin, brass, or stainless steel.

The external case not only protects the transducer but also increases the final size and the response time of the temperature sensor. Typical RTD sizes for applications in biomedical engineering are around 1.5 mm diameter × 25 mm length. Although not too large, in direct and invasive measurements of temperature in which the sensor is placed inside the body through a catheter, for example, this size becomes quite significant. Physical dimensions become less important when dealing with the measurement in temperature control equipment such as Bier oven, infant incubators, and muffle furnace.

The casing can cause problems ranging from an increase in the time constant of the system to a decrease in the input impedance caused by the jacket in series association with the heat-sensitive filament. The time constant of the RTDs used in biomedical engineering applications is in the range 0.5–1 s (typical), while thermistors and thermocouples (type T) have time constant values typically round 0.1 s. The response time of the RTD is a limitation of usage of this sensor compared to thermistors and thermocouples. Still, the fact that it is a robust element and requires relatively easy measurement circuitry causes the RTD sensor to be of great importance, both in industry and medical applications.

RTDs are manufactured in the range of values from a few units Ω to tens of hundreds Ω. Higher values RTDs have the advantage of presenting smaller errors in relation to the resistance of the lead wires. The most used resistive temperature transducers are PT100 and then the PT1000, which is similar to the first, with the difference that its resistance in temperature 0°C is 1000 Ω instead of 100 Ω.

4.2.2.1.1.4 RTD measurement circuits The Wheatstone bridge is a widely used method for determining the resistance of the RTD. Figure 4.8 shows an example of the measurement circuit at 1/4 of the bridge. This bridge consists of a power supply (stable, constant intensity, DC or AC) and two parallel resistive voltage divider circuits with two resistors each. In this example, three branches are resistors with zero temperature coefficient (ideally), with constant and known values and the fourth branch is the RTD. In the deflexion mode of Wheatstone bridge operation, the constant resistors are chosen to balance the bridge (V_{out}—0 V) to a known temperature, for instance, 25°C. The output voltage V_{out} is equal to the voltage difference between the

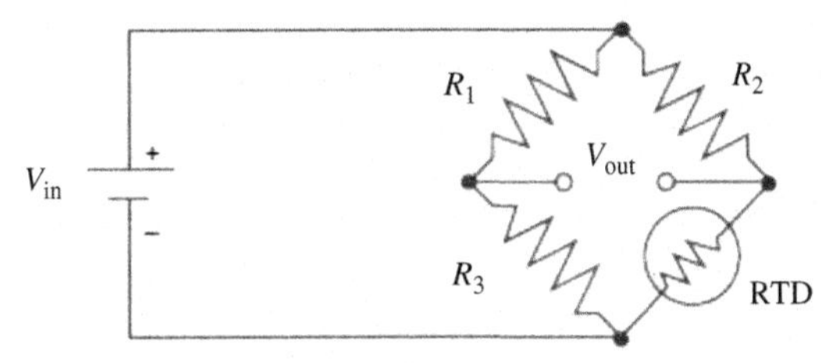

Figure 4.8 The Wheatstone bridge is a widely used RTD measurement circuit.

two dividers and depends on the RDT value, which varies with temperature. Any variation in the resistance of the RTD corresponds to a variation in the output voltage. The circuit bridge can also be used in the bridge null mode. In this case, two resistors are constant, one is variable and the circuit must be kept in the equilibrium condition (the current flowing through the sensor is zero). Initially the variable resistor is adjusted to balance the circuit to a known temperature (usually 25°C). When the temperature changes, the resistance of the thermistor also changes and the circuit loses its balance condition, which is restored adjusting the variable resistor, which value can be calibrated to indicate temperature range.

The output voltage is equal to

$$V_{out} = V_{in}\left(\frac{R_3}{R_1 + R_3} - \frac{\text{RTD}}{R_2 + \text{RTD}}\right) \tag{4.8}$$

and the RTD is calculated by

$$\text{RTD} = \frac{V_{in}R_3 - V_{out}(R_1 + R_3)}{V_{in}R_1 + V_{out}(R_1 + R_3)}R_2 \tag{4.9}$$

Equations (4.8) and (4.9) show that the output voltage value is directly proportional to the power supply, which either DC or AC, must be stable. If $R_1 = R_3$, Eq. (4.7) is simplified as

$$\text{RTD} = \frac{(V_{in} - 2V_{out})}{(V_{in} + 2V_{out})}R_2 \tag{4.10}$$

If the output voltage is zero, the bridge is said to be in balance, that is, the resistance values are such that each branch of the circuit has the same voltage division ratio. The ratio of resistors is

$$\frac{R_1}{R_3} = \frac{R_2}{\text{RTD}} \Rightarrow V_{out} = 0 \tag{4.11}$$

R_1, R_2, and R_3 should be high value resistors, typically 10 times the value of the RTD in the middle of the working range, so little current is drained from the power source. Typically a platinum RDT operating in the interval 0–100°C, using 10:1 resistance ratio, results in a nonlinearity close to 0.5°C. R_2 value is typically chosen so the output voltage is zero at the beginning or middle of the working range. If the 0°C temperature is part of the working range, it is customary to make the output voltage equal to zero at this point.

Usually, the measuring site is far away from the measuring circuit and the RTD is connected to the bridge circuit by a pair of wires, as is shown in Figure 4.9. This also prevents the entire measurement circuit to be exposed to large temperature variations.

The impedances R' of the connection wires ($\approx 5\ \Omega$) are significant (PT100 nominal impedance is 100 Ω), vary with the temperature changing, and are a probable error source, affecting the temperature reading. Considering the impedances R', Eq. (4.9) becomes

$$\mathrm{RTD}_{\mathrm{total}} = \mathrm{RTD} + 2R' = \frac{V_{\mathrm{in}}R_3 - V_{\mathrm{out}}(R_1 + R_3)}{V_{\mathrm{in}}R_1 + V_{\mathrm{out}}(R_1 + R_3)} R_2 \tag{4.12}$$

and

$$\mathrm{RTD} = \frac{V_{\mathrm{in}}R_3 - V_{\mathrm{out}}(R_1 + R_3)}{V_{\mathrm{in}}R_1 + V_{\mathrm{out}}(R_1 + R_3)} R_2 - 2R' \tag{4.13}$$

Equations (4.12) and (4.13) show that the measured resistance is $2R'$ greater than the actual value of the RTD, that is, the connection wires introduce an error of $2R'$. This problem is minimized by the use of three-wire bridge, as shown in the circuit of Figure 4.10.

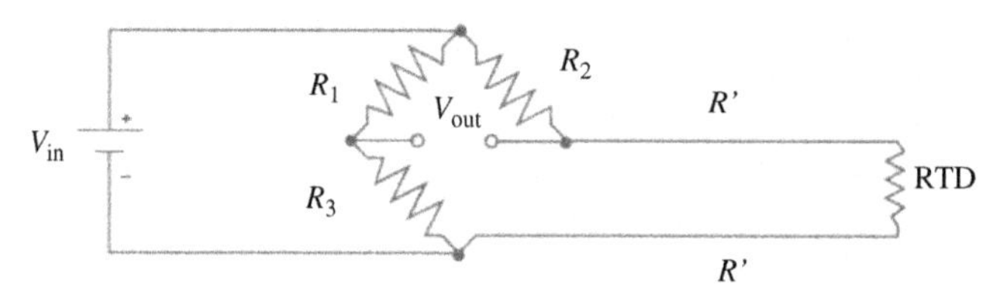

Figure 4.9 Measurement circuit with the temperature transducer connected to the Wheatstone bridge by a pair of wires of impedance R'.

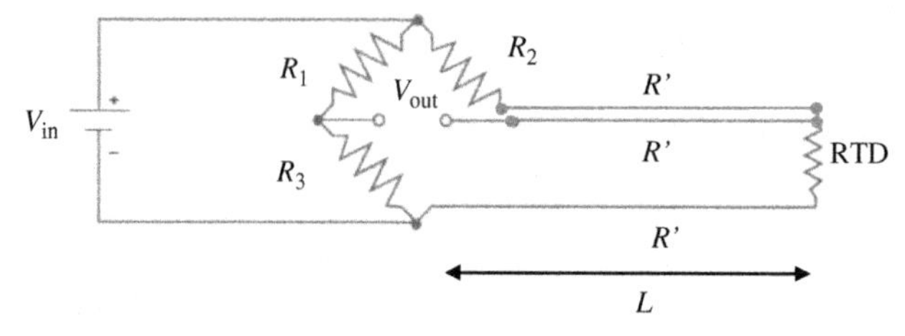

Figure 4.10 Measurement circuit with the temperature transducer connected to the Wheatstone bridge by three wires of impedance R'.

The error compensation of the three-wire bridge circuit works as follows: when the wires connecting the RTD are the same material, diameter and length, their resistances are almost equal. The resistance of the wire connecting one of the terminals of the RTD to the voltage measurement circuit can be neglected, because the input impedance of the latter should and is usually quite high, draining very little current in relation to the other elements of the bridge. The resistances of the other two wires are part of the bottom branch of the bridge, and one of them is added to the RTD resistance, while the other is added to the R_2 at the right top branch of the circuit. With this modification, Eq. (4.7) becomes

$$\mathrm{RTD_{total}} = \mathrm{RTD} + R' = \frac{V_{in}R_3 - V_{out}(R_1 + R_3)}{V_{in}R_1 + V_{out}(R_1 + R_3)}(R_2 + R') \tag{4.14}$$

and

$$\mathrm{RTD} = \frac{V_{in}R_3 - V_{out}(R_1 + R_3)}{V_{in}R_1 + V_{out}(R_1 + R_3)}(R_2 + R') - R' \tag{4.15}$$

Comparing Eqs. (4.7), (4.13), and (4.15), it is easily noted that the three-wire bridge circuit introduces smaller error than the two-wire circuit. Equation (4.13) shows that the smaller the output V_{out}, the smaller is the error in the RDT measurement, as when the bridge is close to balance. Three-wire bridge is better suited to resistive sensors that vary only a few percent its nominal resistance, like the strain gauges.

Another method of measuring the RTD resistance is the four-wire circuit, shown in Figure 4.11.

In the four-wire circuit configuration, two wires excite the transducer with constant current and the other two measure the voltage drop across the RDT. The constant current source assures that for whatever the values of R' and RTD, the current flowing through these elements does not vary. Moreover, by measuring the voltage across the RTD with a voltmeter (high impedance) the power drain is very small compared with the current flowing through the rest of the circuit. Thus,

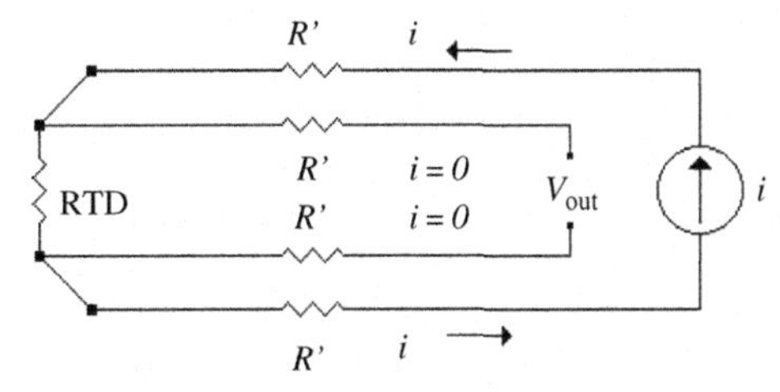

Figure 4.11 Four-wire circuit to measure the resistance of the RTD.

the resistance of the wires does not affect the temperature measurement. The value of the RTD is determined by Eq. (4.16):

$$\mathrm{RTD} = \frac{V}{i} \tag{4.16}$$

that is, the output voltage read by the voltmeter is proportional to the RDT value, which is easily calculated. The voltmeter is insensitive to the connection wires' length and can be placed remotely to the measuring site. The four-wire RTD circuit removes the effect of mismatched resistances on the lead wires, is the most accurate method to measure the RDT value, and introduces less error than the bridge solutions.

The Wheatstone bridges are widely used for its simplicity and good sensitivity to low signal, especially in circuits where the linearization, when necessary, is done in analog form. In circuits where the linearization is digital, based on tables or equations, the RTD is preferentially excited with current source.

The measurement of the RDT resistance using both, four-wire and bridge circuits, is susceptible to self-heating caused by the current flowing through the sensor. The relation $\mathrm{RDT} \cdot I^2$ gives the power dissipated over the RDT, which contributes to its heating and resistance increase. One way to circumvent this problem is the use of pulsed power. Thus, although the current may still cause self-heating, at the times when it is not flowing through the circuit, the RTD is allowed to cool down.

Another type of error that can occur in the RDT measurement is the voltage generated by the thermoelectric effect caused by the temperature difference between the various electrical contacts. This can be minimized by placing these contacts at the same temperature. The thermoelectric voltage is a DC value and another possible solution to this problem, and more feasible, is to use AC power and frequency filtering to eliminate the DC component of the output signal. Another advantage of AC power is the fact that the amplitude modulation causes the frequency spectrum of the output signal to be shifted to a region of higher frequency. Thus, high-pass filters can easily remove low frequency interference and 60 Hz noise and then, a simple demodulator circuit will restore the temperature information (RTD resistance value).

RTD is the most stable over time, most accurate, and linear (thermoresistive) temperature transducer. It is very resistant to contamination and to corrosion. It presents the disadvantages of high cost, relative large sizes, slow response time, and low sensibility to small temperature changes. It loses calibration if used beyond sensor's temperature ratings and is sensitive to vibration, which can strain the platinum element wire. Due to its linearity, stability, and robustness, RTD is largely used in biomedical applications that does not need very small temperature sensor.

4.2.2.1.2 Thermistor—Semiconductor temperature detector

Thermistors are temperature sensitive resistors, and are manufactured using semiconductor materials, such as metal oxide mixtures of nickel, cobalt, manganese, aluminum, titanium, iron, or copper and doped single crystals of silicon or germanium. When accuracy is less critical, they are a cheaper option of resistance temperature sensor than platinum thermometers. Usually they are less stable than RDTs, but they have larger temperature coefficients. The thermistor has a high sensibility but it is also an extremely nonlinear device.

Thermistors can be divided into three categories: NTC (negative temperature coefficient), whose resistances decrease with temperature increase and are manufactured by the sintering process of blends of metal oxides at high temperatures; PTC (positive temperature coefficient), made by sintering mixtures of barium, lead, and strontium, polycrystalline ceramic materials that are normally highly resistive, but made semiconductive by the addition of dopants, such as yttrium, manganese, tantalum, and silica; and PTC made from doped single crystal semiconductors (germanium and silicon), which have the largest temperature coefficients among thermistors. Single crystal PTC made of silicon is also named silistor, a thermally sensitive silicon resistor, or linear PTC (LPTC), due to its resistance-temperature characteristic. There is also a fourth type of thermistor, the polymer PTC, which consists of a slice of plastic embedded with carbon grains. When the plastic is cool, the carbon grains are all in contact with each other, forming a conductive path through the device. When the plastic heats up, it expands, forcing the carbon grains apart, and causing the resistance of the device to rise rapidly. Like the $BaTiO_3$ thermistor, this device has a highly nonlinear resistance/temperature response and is used for switching and thermal overcurrent protection in electronic circuits, not for proportional temperature measurement.

Thermistors of metallic oxide compounds were the first to be discovered. The negative temperature coefficient was observed by Faraday in 1833 when he measured the resistance variation with temperature of silver sulfide. However, it took until the 1940s before metallic oxides became available commercially. With semiconductor materials development after the Second World War, single crystal germanium and silicon thermistors were investigated.

NTC and PTC are widely found in industrial and medical applications, but NTC are the most used due to its resistance/temperature relationship and ease of use.

Thermistors are classified according to the method by which the electrodes are fixed in two classes, embedded contact and metallized surface contact and can be fabricated in many formats, such as bead, disk, rod, and chip.

Thermistors with bead format (Figure 4.12) are the most common within the class of embedded conductors. The bead is formed from a small amount of oxides mixture in paste form, to which a pair of parallel conductors (e.g., radially wired leads of copper) is applied. The bead undergoes a drying process and is sintered in an oven.

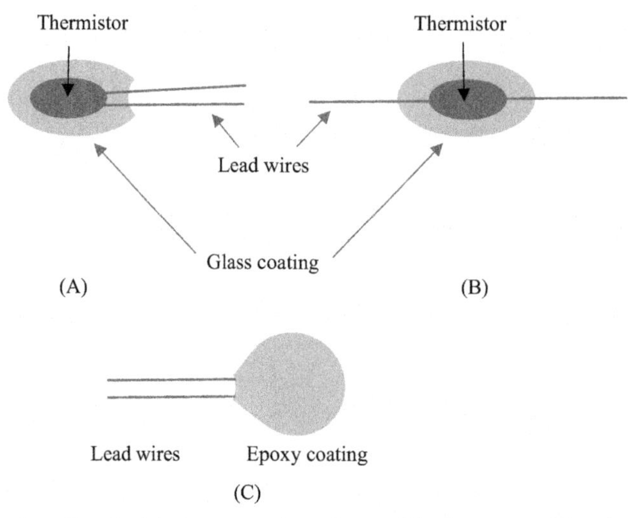

Figure 4.12 Examples of embedded contact thermistors: (A) glass coated bead with parallel leads; (B) glass coated bead with adjacent leads; and (C) epoxy coated bead.

While sintering, the metal oxides contract and form an excellent electrical connection with the wire leads (platinum alloys). The leads can then be arranged in two configurations, parallel (Figure 4.12A) or adjacent (Figure 4.12B). The beads are hermetically sealed and encapsulated with glass, ceramic, PVC, or epoxy. This external coating improves the thermistor stability, avoiding water absorption by inner metal oxides.

Disk thermistors are a representative example of contact with metallized surface class. The disc-like PTC thermistors are manufactured by compressing a combination of oxides powder under high pressure. The discs are sintered and their flat surfaces are electrolyzed. After electrolysis, the discs are submitted to heating and drying process. The resistance nominal values are obtained adjusting the disk diameter before establishing contact with the lead wires. Metallized contacts are applied to the surface of the device by painting, dipping, sputtering, or flame spraying. Every step of the manufacturing process is important to the final characteristics of stability and working temperatures range. Figure 4.13 shows examples of thermistors of the metallized surface contact type. Disk and chip thermistors are generally larger than the bead types and so they exhibit response times that are comparatively slower.

Thermistors are also manufactured in waffers, rods, washers, and other formatting to produce sensors of various sizes and models for the most varied applications, among them, medical thermometers. A thermistor is chosen based on its nominal resistance at the operating temperature range, on the size, and on the time constant, which are typically in the range 5–10 s. Thermistors are usually designated by their resistance at 25°C, with common resistances ranging from 470 Ω to 100 kΩ.

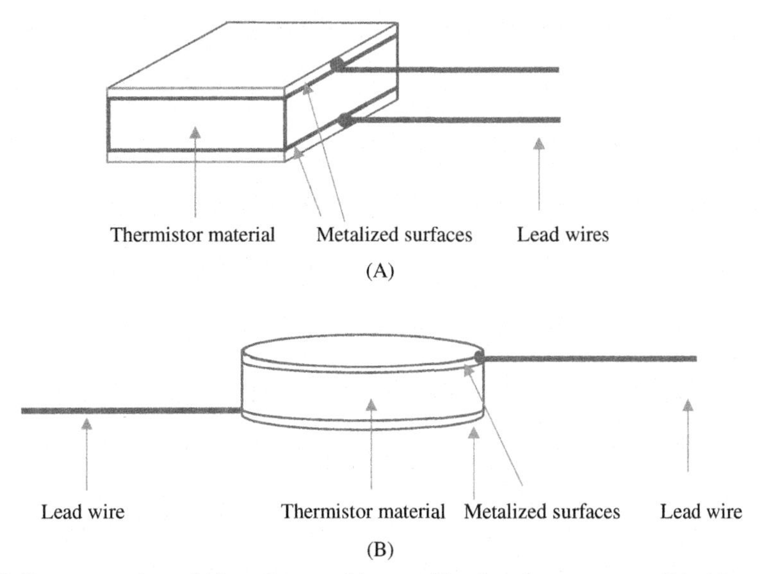

Figure 4.13 Representation of thermistors with metallized surface contact: (A) chip and (B) disc formats.

NTC thermistors have temperature coefficients within the range −3 to −5%/°C, about 10 times greater than the RDTs (Pt_{100} 0.39 Ω/°C). Depending on the encapsulation used, glass, for example, stability may be ±2% of the nominal resistance per year, corresponding to a temperature stability of about 0.05°C per year. Changes in their electrical characteristics can be obtained varying the oxides used, their relative proportions and sintering conditions. Thus a wide range of resistance and sensitivity can be obtained (a few kiloohms to tens of megaohms). Thermistor sizes can be very small (diameter from 125 μm to 1.5 mm); they also have excellent stability and large temperature coefficient, which make them suitable to be used in numerous biomedical engineering applications: respiration rate monitoring, temperature measurements in chemical reactions (enzymology), gas analyzers, flow meters, infusion pump, and other.

4.2.2.1.2.1 Resistance versus temperature Figure 4.14A shows a characteristic curve of resistance versus temperature for an NTC with nominal resistance at 25°C equal to 320 Ω. Figure 4.14B shows the resistance temperature characteristic for a PTC on a semilogarithmic coordinate graph due to PTC high sensibility and resistance values. The NTC resistance always decreases nonlinearly with increasing temperature while resistance of most PTC thermistors exhibits their common behavior only after "switching" at a certain critical temperature, when their resistance rises suddenly.

Ceramic PTC devices are made of a mixture of oxide powder that is compacted and formatted under high pressure and then sintered to form a doped polycrystalline ceramic, which usually contains barium titanate ($BaTiO_3$, a ferroelectric material) and

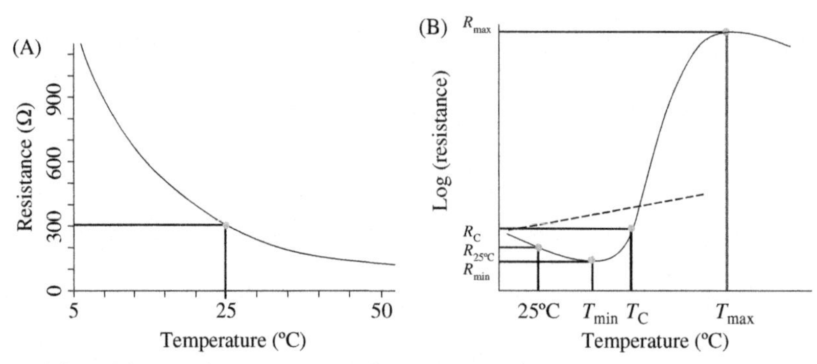

Figure 4.14 (A) NTC (nominal resistance 320 Ω at 25°C) and (B) PTC nonlinear characteristic curves (dashed line: silistor; solid line: switching PTC).

other compounds. The dielectric constant of this ferroelectric material varies with temperature. Below the Curie point temperature, the high dielectric constant prevents the formation of potential barriers between the crystal grains, leading to a low resistance. In this region, the device has a small negative temperature coefficient. At the Curie point temperature, the dielectric constant drops sufficiently to allow the formation of potential barriers at the grain boundaries, and the resistance begins to increase sharply. Figure 4.12B highlights important points of the behavior of PTC: maximum and minimum resistance and temperature values, as well at 25°C and Curie point. R_{min} is value of the PTC resistance at the beginning of the temperature range (T_{min}) with a positive temperature coefficient. The temperature value at which the resistance is twice R_{min} is the Curie switching point; an exact value to temperature switching point is difficult to assign and manufacturers assume different ratios, like 10 times. At even higher temperatures than T_{max}, the material reverts to NTC behavior; this usually occurs at an extremely high temperature beyond the normal operating range for which the device has been designed or specified. The equations used for modeling this behavior were derived by W. Heywang and G.H. Jonker in the 1960s (Childs et al., 2000; Cobbold, 1974; Dally et al., 1993; Doebelin, 1990; Geddes & Baker, 1968; OMEGA, 1983).

The NTC characteristic can be empirically modeled by an equation that describes a single crystal semiconductor behavior. The electron density n of an intrinsic semiconductor (that do not contain impurities) increases with temperature according to Eq. (4.17):

$$n \propto T^{3/2} e^{(-Eg/2kT)} \tag{4.17}$$

where

n is the electron density of an intrinsic semiconductor

Eg is the energy gap between conduction and valence bands

k is the Boltzmann constant

T is the absolute temperature (K).

Furthermore, the mobility of carriers (electrons and holes) in intrinsic semiconductors varies with $T^{-3/2}$ and the resistivity, as a function of temperature, is given by

$$\rho \propto e^{(\beta/T)} \tag{4.18}$$

where $\beta = \text{Eg}/2k$ (K), is a constant, temperature characteristic of each material (typical values are in the range 3,000–5,000).

Finally, the equation that describes the temperature dependence of the thermistor resistance is

$$R_T = R_0 e^{[\beta((1/T)-(1/T_0))]} \tag{4.19}$$

where

R_T is the thermistor resistance at temperature T and

R_0 is the thermistor resistance at temperature T_0 K (298 K = 25°C).

Differentiating Eq. (4.19) with respect to R_T and dividing the result by R_T, leads to an expression for α, the temperature coefficient of resistance or sensibility of a thermistor:

$$\alpha = \frac{dR_T}{R_T dT} = -\frac{\beta}{T^2} \tag{4.20}$$

Typically for an NTC at 300 K, $\alpha = -0.044\ (\text{K})^{-1}$ or $\alpha = -4.4\%/\text{K}$. The temperature dependence of the thermistor resistance can be approximated to a more digitally feasible equation through the Steinhart–Hart equation:

$$\frac{1}{T} = A + B \ln R_T + C(\ln R_T)^3 \tag{4.21}$$

where A, B, and C are curve fitting coefficients, determined from calibration curves of voltage versus current, for different environmental conditions and constant power dissipation, to each type of material from which the thermistor is made.

4.2.2.1.2.2 Self-heating When a current flows through a thermistor, it will generate heat, which will raise the temperature of the thermistor above that of its environment. Both PTC and NTC dissipate power due to the heat produced by the passage of electric current in the circuit where they are placed. If the thermistor is being used to measure the temperature of the environment, this electrical heating may introduce a significant error if a correction is not made. If nothing is done, the cumulative effect of the self-heating causes the NTC resistance to decrease more and more and the current through it to increase even more, which eventually leads to the destruction of the sensor by excessive power dissipation (Thermal avalanche). An increase in the PTC temperature causes an increase in its resistance, and with it, a reduction in the production of heat and power dissipated in the thermistor, stabilizing its operation (regenerative cycle). Instead of correcting it is better to prevent self-heating by limiting the current flow and minimizing the power dissipation in the sensor.

A typical NTC with nominal resistance $R_T = 500\ \Omega$ is able to dissipate 1 mW at each 1°C of temperature increase. This corresponds to a self-heating factor $F = 1°C/mW$. If the temperature measurement should have an accuracy equal to 0.5°C, the dissipated power must be <0.5 mW. Equation (4.20) shows the relationship between the current flowing through a resistive element and the dissipated power:

$$i = \sqrt{p/R_T} \tag{4.22}$$

Substituting the values above in Eq. (4.20), the current through the thermistor should be limited to

$$i = \sqrt{0.0005/5000} = 316\ \mu A$$

In practice, current values even smaller than those calculated by Eq. (4.20) should be used due to high sensibility of the thermistor. The self-heating factor or the maximum current to avoid overheating is usually indicated in the thermistor data sheet.

For most thermistor applications, the self-heating effect is undesirable and the sensor should work as close to zero power as possible. The zero-power resistance of a thermistor at a specified temperature is the DC resistance measured when the power dissipation is negligible (i.e., a further decrease in power will result in not more than 0.1% change in resistance).

4.2.2.1.2.3 Linearization The resistance versus temperature characteristic of a thermistor NTC is negative and nonlinear (Figure 4.14A and Eq. (4.19)). If thermistor is used only in a small range of temperature, resistance characteristic can be considered linear, but in a long range, the nonlinearity can be a problem. The nonlinear characteristic can be overcome, if necessary, by using two or more matched thermistors packaged in a single device, so the nonlinearities of each device offset each other.

There are analog techniques that use external matching resistors to linearize the thermistor characteristic curve to a limited range of temperatures. The first technique uses a shunt resistor and a constant voltage supply as is shown in Figure 4.15A. The parallel combination results in a new characteristic curve with an inflexion at the half of the temperature range, as can be seen in Figure 4.15B. Note that S-shaped curve is almost linear over its region around the mid-temperature.

The expression to the parallel arrangement resistance R is indicated by Eq. (4.23):

$$R = \frac{R_P R_{Th} e^{\beta/T}}{R_P + R_{Th} e^{\beta/T}} \tag{4.23}$$

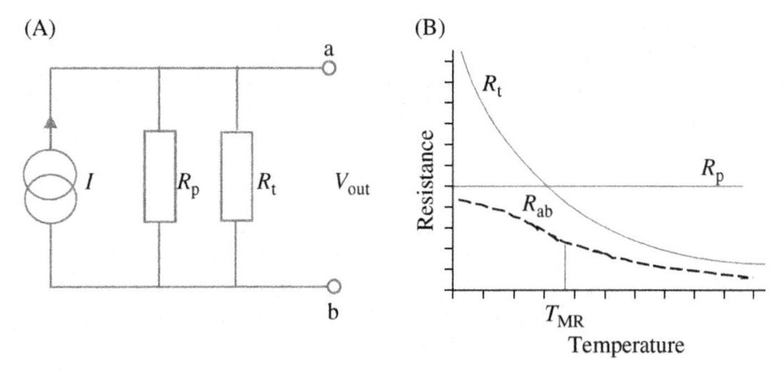

Figure 4.15 Shunt linearization of resistance versus temperature characteristic of NTC thermistors.

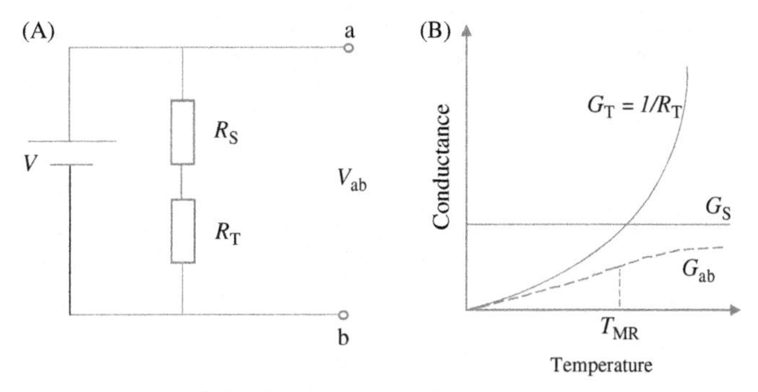

Figure 4.16 Series linearization of the thermistor conductance versus temperature characteristic.

where

R_P is the shunt resistor for parallel linearization

R_{Th} is the thermistor resistance

β is the thermic constant of the thermistor.

The shunt resistor is determined by deriving Eq. (4.23) twice and then equaling the result to zero, to find the inflexion point of the equivalent resistance curve in Figure 4.15B, which results in Eq. (4.24):

$$R_P = R_{TMR}\left(\frac{\beta - 2T_{MR}}{\beta + 2T_{MR}}\right) \tag{4.24}$$

where

R_{TMR} is the thermistor resistance at the mid-range of temperature

T_{MR} is the mid-range temperature.

The second analog linearization method uses a constant current supply and a series resistor (Figure 4.16A). Its objective is to produce an inflection point in the resulting conductance curve at the mid-range of temperature (Figure 4.16B), which produces an almost linear resistance temperature response around this point.

In a similar way to what was done to shunt linearization, it can be shown that the value of the series resistance R_S, necessary to make the thermistor conductance versus temperature characteristic approximately linear, is given by

$$\frac{1}{R_S} = G_S = G_{Ti}\left(\frac{\beta - 2Ti}{\beta + 2Ti}\right) \tag{4.25}$$

where

G_S is the series conductance to linearize the thermistor characteristic

G_{MR} is the thermistor conductance at the mid-range of temperature.

The effective temperature coefficients for the linearization circuits in parallel and in series can be obtained by differentiating the expressions of R_P and R_S resulting in Eqs. (4.26) and (4.27), respectively:

$$\alpha_{eff} = \frac{(\beta T_m^2)}{[(R_{Tm} R_P) + 1]} \tag{4.26}$$

$$\alpha_{eff} = \frac{(\beta T_i^2)}{[(G_{Ti} G_S) + 1]} \tag{4.27}$$

Comparing these coefficients to Eq. (4.20) and looking at Figures 4.15B and 4.16B, it is easily noticed that linearization improves the transfer function linearity of the thermistor, but both solutions, parallel and series, reduce its sensibility.

Thermistor curves can be linearized by incorporating the thermistor and a compensating thin film resistor in a hybrid assembly on a single casing. Digital linearization can be performed in the digital domain using look-up tables containing the manufacturer's device characteristics to linearize the thermistor output. Most of modern medical equipment have microcontrolled systems with digital data acquisition and processing, which can compensate any lack of signal nonlinearity by digital circuitry and software, making the linearization with analog circuits unnecessary. There are digital integrated circuits, like AD7711, a signal conditioning analog-to-digital converter from analog devices, which allow voltage or current thermistor excitation, linearization, and also digitalization of the thermistor output (AD7711, 2014).

4.2.2.1.2.4 Measuring circuits As in the case of RTD, the Wheatstone bridge is a widely used method for measuring the resistance of the thermistor. In the deflection method, the appropriate choice of constant resistors in three branches of the circuit allows balancing the bridge at a given reference temperature at which the thermistor resistance is known. If the temperature changes, the thermistor resistance also changes, the circuit becomes unbalanced and the current through the sensor is used to determine the temperature value. Figure 4.17A shows a bridge circuit with the thermistor mounted in one branch. Depending on the voltmeter sensibility, temperature readings

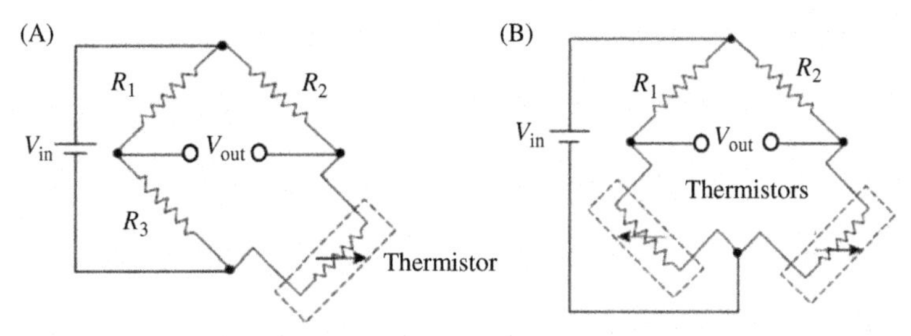

Figure 4.17 Wheatstone bridges used to measure thermistor resistance changing (A) ¼ bridge and (B) differential bridge circuit.

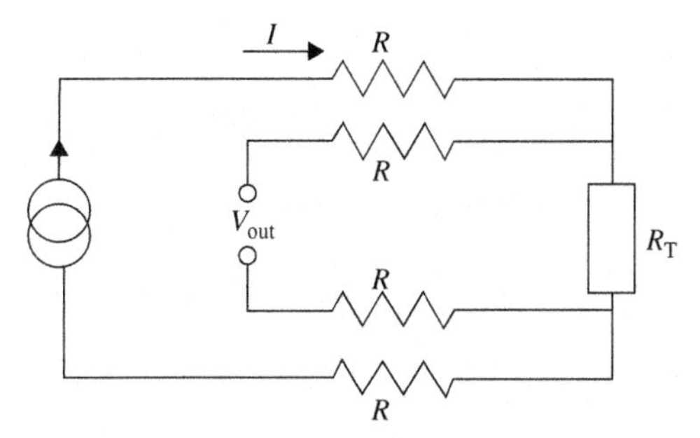

Figure 4.18 Four wires circuit to high accuracy measurement of thermistor resistance. The four wires have equal resistances *R*.

of 1°C can be made. Figure 4.17B shows a differential bridge with two thermistors mounted in two branches of the circuit, which allows very accurate temperature measurement, with readings as little as 10^{-3}°C. The temperature difference of the two sensors unbalances the bridge circuit. The use of two and three wires bridge circuits is unnecessary due to high resistance values of thermistors (tens to hundreds 10^3 Ω compared to 100 Ω of PT100), so the resistances of the connection lead wires can be neglected.

The four wires circuit (Figure 4.18) with constant current source is used in cases of high accuracy measurement, as in calibrations made in laboratory, where the temperature needs to be measured and controlled with close margin of tolerance. In this method of measurement, the constant current flows through the thermistor, but does not flow through the wires used to measure the voltage drop across the sensor. The voltmeter and conditioning circuit have high input impedance and the resistances of the connecting wires (*R*) are negligible.

4.2.2.1.2.5 General characteristics, advantages, and disadvantages of thermistors Table 4.2 resumes some characteristics of NTC and PTC.

One disadvantage of thermistors compared to other resistive temperature sensors (RTD and thermocouple) is their instability and drift due to changes in the characteristics of the semiconductor materials, when used for long periods or at high

Table 4.2 Typical ranges of values of the characteristics of NTC and PTC thermistors

NTC	$PTC_{ceramic}$	$PTC_{semiconductor}$
Temperature range 200–700 K	Temperature range −60°C to +150°C	Germanium—< 100 K Silicon—up to 250 K
α: −3 to −5%/°C	α: 10–60%/°C	α: 0.5–1%/°C (according to crystal doping)
β: 3,000–5,000	β: 3,000–5,000	β: 3,000–5,000
Stability of ±0.05% to 0.2% per year in resistance nominal value and ±0.01 to 0.05% per year in nominal temperature	Unknown long-term stability	Excellent long-term stability ≤0.01°C per year
Manufactured in dimensions smaller than 0.5 mm	Manufactured in dimensions smaller than 0.5 mm	Manufactured in dimensions smaller than 0.5 mm
Values of nominal resistance from some units Ω up to MΩ	Values of nominal resistance from a few tens Ω to a few kΩ	Values of nominal resistance from a few hundred Ω to a few kΩ
Response time from 200 ms to 10 s (according to casing and size)	Response time up to a few tens s for surface mount elements	Response time up to a few tens s for surface mount elements
Commonly encapsulated in glass, Epoxy, PVC, polyimide, or stainless	Most are intended to operate without insulating coating (surface mounting); glass casing when required	Most are intended to operate without insulating coating (surface mounting); glass casing when required

temperatures. The use of thermistors is generally limited to a few hundreds degree Celsius, which usually is not a problem in most of medical applications.

As well as other temperature sensors, thermistors must have characteristics of interchangeability according to accuracy standards, so one sensor could be replaced, in case of damaging, without having to recalibrate the whole circuit of which it is part. The reproducibility or interchangeability of a thermistor is related to manufacturing techniques. β and R_0 are determined by the proportions and quality control of the components used, sintering process, etc. Resistance of thermistors can be affected by oxides composition, quality control of components, thermal treatment, thickness and diameter (disc type), distance between wire leads (bead type), impurity doping (silicon single crystal type), substrate material (thin film type), heterogeneity in diffusion of the contact material in the case of thermistors with metallized surface (chip type), etc. The resistance tolerance of thermistors is reduced producing them in "matched units pair," which consists of an arrangement of two thermistors (drop type, chip or thin film) connected in series or in parallel that results in better tolerance for a given temperature range. Accurate temperature sensing within wide temperature range can be obtained by mounting both high and low resistance thermistors in the same casing.

Thermistors, mainly NTC type, of different formats, sizes, and casings are used in medical electronic thermometers for monitoring the patient temperature with skin probes, for central temperature measurement (e.g., esophageal and rectal) with internal probes, and for direct temperature measurement (e.g., inside blood vessels and heart chambers) with invasive probes with mini and microsensors inserted in catheters. Thermistors are also used for liquid immersion temperature measurements (blood, saline, drug solutions, etc.).

The main advantage of the use of thermistors as temperature transducers is their high sensibility to small temperature changes. Thermistors are less expensive than RTD, copper or nickel extension wires can be used and they become more stable with use. Some disadvantages may also be mentioned, such as their limited working temperature range, the initial accuracy drift, the lack of standards for replacement, and the possibility of loss of calibration, if they are used beyond temperature ratings.

4.2.2.2 Thermoelectric temperature transducers

4.2.2.2.1 Thermocouple

A thermocouple is a temperature sensor that consists of two wires of different metallic materials put in thermal contact (Figure 4.19). The thermal contact, called a junction, is made by fusing or welding two different materials. If these materials are in thermal equilibrium with each other, there will be a tendency of electrons to diffuse across the junction. The electric potential of the receptor material may become more negative in the junction while the electron emitter material may become more positive. Diffusion continues until an equilibrium condition is reached by the action of the electric field on the electrons (similar to the mechanism that generates a potential barrier at the semiconductor PN junction). Since the forces of diffusion are temperature dependent, the electric potential developed at the junction provides a measurement of this temperature.

If two different and homogeneous materials form a closed circuit and the two junctions are kept at the same temperature (Figure 4.20A), the electric field at each

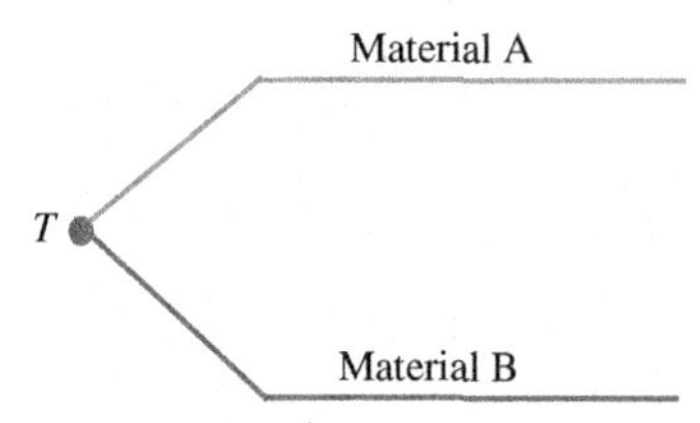

Figure 4.19 Simple junction thermocouple.

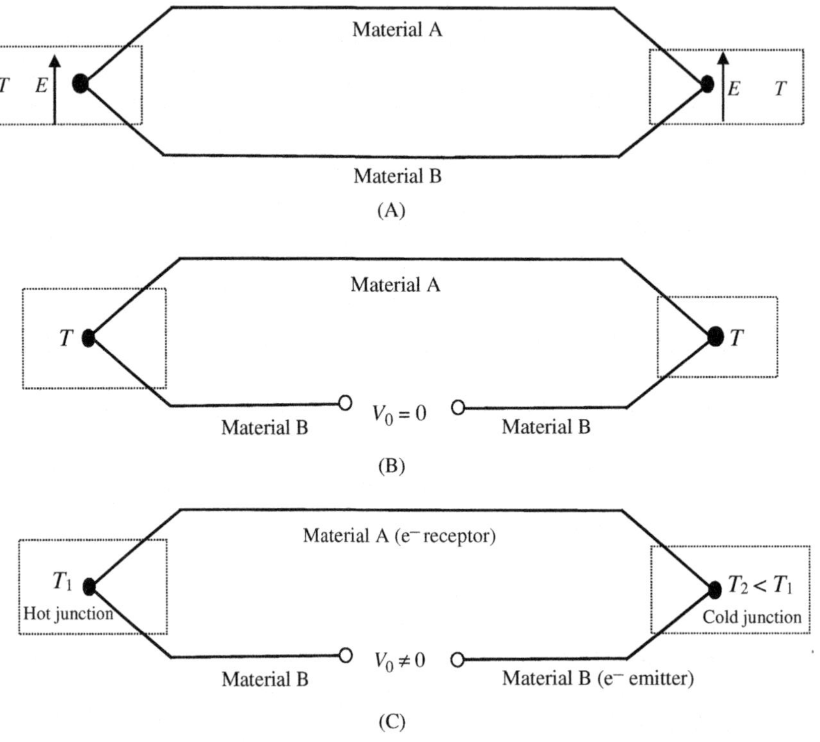

Figure 4.20 (A) simple junction thermocouple; (B) thermocouple circuit with the two junctions at the same temperature; and (C) thermocouple circuit with the two junctions at different temperatures.

junction has the same intensity and polarity and there will be no electrons flowing through the circuit. Opening the circuit anywhere along the loop (Figure 4.20) the potential difference measured will be null. Submitting the junctions at different temperatures, the electric fields at each junction will be different and the difference is measured with a voltmeter as an open circuit voltage V_0 anywhere along the loop (Figure 4.20C). As temperature goes up, the output of the thermocouple rises, though not necessarily linearly. V_0 is function of the temperature difference and the materials of the wires and the thermocouple does not require voltage or current excitation. Thermocouple converts thermal energy into electrical energy (Chan, 2008; Cobbold, 1974; Dally et al., 1993; Doebelin, 1990; Geddes & Baker, 1968; Khandpur, 2005; McGee, 1988; OMEGA, 1983; Webster, 2010).

The open circuit voltage produced by the electrons diffusion in the junction of the dissimilar materials is called "Seebeck voltage" or "Seebeck emf," in honor of Thomas Johann Seebeck, who discovered this thermoelectric phenomenon in 1821 ("Seebeck effect").

The thermoelectric voltage V_0 is a nonlinear function of temperature that can be approximately represented by

$$V_0 = c_1(T_1 - T_2) + c_2(T_1^2 - T_2^2) \tag{4.28}$$

where c_1 and c_2 are dielectric constants dependent of materials 1 and 2

T_2 is the temperature of the hot junction

T_1 is the temperature of the cold junction.

In addition to the Seebeck effect, two other basic thermoelectric effects occur in the thermocouple circuit: Peltier effect and Thomsom effect, which are represented in Figure 4.21.

The Peltier effect was discovered in 1834 by Jean Charles Athanase Peltier, who found out that an electrical current would produce heating or cooling at the junction of two dissimilar metals, and this was caused by the heat transfer that occurs due to current flow in the thermocouple circuit. This amount of heat is given by

$$q_P = \prod_{AB} \cdot i \tag{4.29}$$

where

q_P is the amount of heat transfer in watts

Π_{AB} is the Peltier coefficient from A to B in the junction AB.

Equation (4.29) is a vector equation and changes its polarity with the current flow direction.

In 1854, William Thomson (later Lord Kelvin) described a third thermoelectric effect, Thomson effect, the thermoelectric effect that less affects the thermocouple circuit. This effect involves the generation (cooling) or absorption (heating) of heat (q_T) whenever there is a temperature gradient due to the current i flowing in a material. The amount of heat transferred is given by

$$q_T = R_0 \cdot (T_1 - T_2) \tag{4.30}$$

where R_0 is the Thomson coefficient (related by thermodynamics to Seebeck coefficients).

Both effects, Peltier and Thomson, produce voltage in the output of the thermocouple circuit and affect the accuracy of the temperature measurement; therefore they

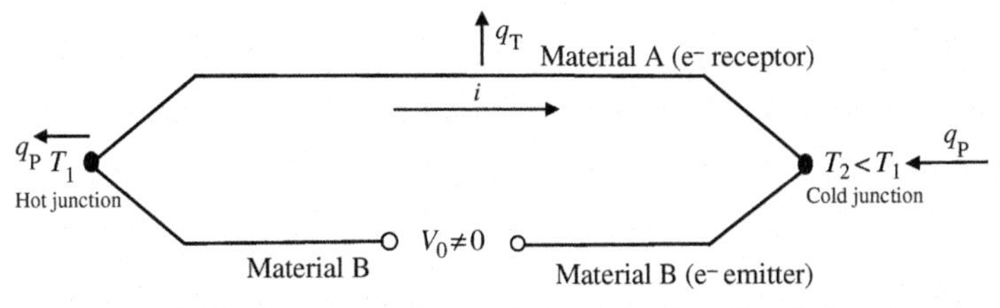

Figure 4.21 Heat transfer in the thermocouple circuit due to Peltier effect (q_P) and Thomson effect (q_T).

should be minimized, limiting the current flowing through the junction during the measurement of V_0.

The thermocouple circuit of Figure 4.21 is used to measure the unknown temperature T_1 of junction J_1, while the junction J_2 is maintained at a known reference temperature T_2. Thus it is possible to determine the temperature T_1 by measuring voltage V_0 with Eq. (4.28). Most often this equation is not enough to accurately represent the characteristic curve voltage versus temperature of a thermocouple and look-up tables or high-order polynomial equations are used. Polynomial equation is in this form:

$$T_1 - T_2 = a_0 + a_1 V_0 + a_2 V_0^2 + \cdots + a_n V_0^n \tag{4.31}$$

where

$a_0, a_1, \ldots, a_n$ are calibration coefficients taken from the NIST (National Institute of Standards and Technology) database of thermocouple values for a specific common type of thermocouple (e.g., J type or K type)
T_1 is the thermocouple temperature (in °C)
T_2 is the cold junction temperature (usually 0°C)
V_0 is the thermocouple voltage (in millivolts).

4.2.2.2.1.1 Empirical laws of thermocouples operation The operation and practical use of thermocouples are based on six fundamental principles that are explained below.

- a thermocouple circuit must contain at least two different materials and at least two junctions;
- output voltage of a thermocouple circuit only depends on the junction temperatures difference $(T_2 - T_1)$ and is independent of temperature along the material, provided that no current flows through the circuit;
- if a third material C is inserted along the material A or B, the output voltage V_0 is not affected, since the two new junction temperatures are the same;
- the introduction of a material C on the junction J_1 and J_2 does not affect the output voltage V_0 if the new junctions J_{CA} and J_{CB} are at the same temperature;
- a thermocouple circuit with junctions J_1 and J_2 at T_1 and T_2, respectively, has $V_{0(2-1)} = f(T_2 - T_1)$ and with junctions J_1 and J_2 at T_2 and T_3, respectively, has $V_{0(3-2)} = f(T_3 - T_2)$. If the same junctions are exposed to T_1 and T_3, the output voltage is $V_{0(3-1)} = V_{0(3-2)} + V_{0(2-1)}$;
- if a thermocouple circuit manufactured with materials A and C generates an output V_{0AC} when exposed to temperatures T_1 and T_2, and a similar circuit made of materials C and B generates an output V_{0CB}, then a thermocouple made of materials A and B generates an output $V_{0AB} = V_{0AC} + V_{0CB}$.

These principles show that the output voltage V_0 of the thermocouple circuit is not influenced by the temperature distribution over the materials, except at the points where connections are made to form the junctions. They also show that V_0 is independent of the lengths of the connecting wires and that they may be exposed to the environment.

4.2.2.2.1.2 Thermocouple materials Many metals and metallic alloys are suitable to be used in thermocouples as thermoelectric effect occurs when two materials are put in contact forming a thermal junction. However, thermocouple materials are chosen according to some important characteristics: maximum sensibility over the entire operating range, long-term stability including high temperatures, cost, and compatibility with the available instrumentation. Most often thermocouple materials are metallic alloys with two or more components to achieve the desired characteristics to a range of temperatures. Platinum, for example, can be combined with other metals resulting in positive and negative sensibilities (μV/°C) as is given in Table 4.3 (ASTM Standards, 1974; Mosaic Ind., 2014; Thermocouple Reference tables, 1983).

Some types of metal combinations were developed to create thermocouples that would fit specific applications. There are noble metal and base metal thermocouples and according to their formulations, they are assigned some capital letters. Table 4.4 gives pattern noble metal and base metal thermocouples, their composition, range of measurement temperatures and sensibilities at 20°C with reference junction at 0°C (ASTM Standards, 1974; Mosaic Ind., 2014; Thermocouple Reference Tables, 1983).

The noble metal thermocouples, types B, R, and S, are all platinum-based thermocouples, which are the least sensible, but are the most stable among thermocouples. The base metal thermocouples, known as types E, J, K, T, and N, have higher sensibilities than the noble metal. They comprise the most commonly used category of thermocouple and the conductor materials in base metal thermocouples are made of common and inexpensive metals such as nickel, copper, and iron. The same combination of metals is available in different compositions to fit specific needs of voltage versus temperature curve. Constantan is a generic name for a whole series of copper–nickel alloys and the constantan used in the type E (chromel–constantan) thermocouple is different from the type J (iron–constantan) thermocouple and is not the same as the constantan used in the type T (copper–constantan) couple.

Table 4.3 Sensibility of thermocouples made from platinum combined with other metals

Platinum with	Sensibility (μV/°C) (or Seebeck coefficient)	Platinum with	Sensibility (μV/°C) (or Seebeck coefficient)
Silicon	440	Gold, silver, copper	6.5
Germanium	300	Mercury	0.6
Iron	18.5	Nickel	− 15
Tungsten	7.5	Constantan	− 35

Table 4.4 Characteristics of pattern noble metal and metal based thermocouples

Type	Positive material	Negative material	Sensibility at 20°C (μV/°C)	Range of temperature (°C)
E	Chromel (nickel 10% chromium)	Constantan (nickel 45% copper)	58.7	−270 to 1,000
G	Tungsten	Tungsten 26% Rhenium	19.7 (600°C)	0 to 2,320
C	Tungsten 5% rhenium	Tungsten 26% rhenium	19.7 (600°C)	0 to 2,320
D	Tungsten 3% rhenium	Tungsten 26% rhenium	19.7 (600°C)	0 to 2,320
J	Iron	Constantan (nickel 45% copper)	50.4	−210 to 760
K	Chromel (nickel 10% chromium)	Alumel (nickel 5% aluminum and silicon)	39.4	−270 to 1,372
$N_{(AWG\ 14)}$	Nicrosil (84.3% Ni, 14% Cr, 1.4% Si, 0.1% Mg)	Nisil (95.5% Ni, 4.4% Si, 0.1% Mg)	39	−270 to 400
$N_{(AWG\ 28)}$	Nicrosil (84.3% Ni, 14% Cr, 1.4% Si, 0.1% Mg)	Nisil (95.5% Ni, 4.4% Si, 0.1% Mg)	26.2	0 to 1,300
B	Platinum 6% Rhodium	Platinum 30% Rhodium	1.2	0 to 1,820
R	Platinum 13% Rhodium	Platinum	5.8	−50 to 1,768
S	Platinum 10% Rhodium	Platinum	5.9	−50 to 1,768
T	Copper	Constantan	38.7	−270 to 400

The chemical composition affects thermocouple sensibility and also the diameter of the lead wires can influence the sensibility value. Type N couple has its sensibility indicated in Table 4.4 for wires with 1 mm (AWG 14) and 1.6 mm (AWG 28) diameters. Tungsten–rhenium thermocouple types C, D, and G comprise a third category of thermocouples, refractory metal thermocouples, which were developed to be used at high temperatures, in reduced atmosphere or vacuum environments, and should never be used in the presence of oxygen at temperatures above 260°C due to high reaction rates. They are expensive, difficult to manufacture, brittle, and must be handled carefully.

All types of thermocouple show a positive proportionality between the output emf and the rising temperature (except type B, which output voltage exhibits a double-value region to temperatures raising from 0 to 42°C) and have a very large range of working temperature, considering the normal range of measurements for biomedical applications. The right choice of a thermocouple should consider stability, linearity, and accuracy in the temperature of interest range, size, inertness of the casing material, response time, and cost. Thermocouples usually are smaller than thermistors and RTDs and their smaller thermal mass implies in faster response times than these larger temperature transducers.

The long-term stability is an important characteristic if the thermocouple should monitor temperature for long periods. Thermal instability causes a cumulative drift in the output voltage of the thermocouple during its exposition to high temperatures for long periods. This error is due to changings in the composition of material in the junction caused by internal and external oxidation. Thermal instability appears, in some cases, after a hundred to a thousand hours of use. Thermocouple type N was developed to eliminate internal oxidation and minimize external oxidation. It presents high thermal stability and stays stable even after more than 1500 h being submitted to temperatures higher than 700°C.

The thermocouple casing is frequently made from a metal or ceramic shield that protects it from the environments. Metal-sheathed thermocouples are also available with many types of outer coatings, such as polytetrafluoroethylene, which permits its use in corrosive solutions. At high temperatures, metal shield and sheath can vaporize and the metallic vapor is able to diffuse into the thermocouple material, which can change, for example, platinum wire calibration; therefore, platinum wires should never be used inside a metallic sheath, but nonmetallic materials, such as high-purity alumina, are allowed. A sheath made of platinum could be used, but this solution is prohibitively expensive.

4.2.2.2.1.3 Measurement circuits The temperature measurement with thermocouples uses a standard scale were 0°C (32 F) corresponds to the standard cold junction temperature and 0 mV output. Thermocouple output V_0 is proportional to the difference $(T_1 - T_2)$ and T_2 is the temperature of the cold junction or reference temperature. It is essential to the thermocouple operation that the temperature (T_2) at the cold junction (J_2) stays constant or precisely controlled. Some methods used to maintain the cold junction temperature controlled are explained below:

1. to keep J_2 immersed in a balance water/ice mixture ($T_2 \approx 0.1$°C);
2. to use the Peltier refrigeration method to keep J_2 at 0°C;
3. to apply the electric-bridge method to compensate the cold junction temperature;
4. to keep the cold junction at a constant temperature above room temperature;
5. to use the double oven method to emulate a 0°C reference.

In the first method, the cold junction is kept in a bath inside a thermic closed reservoir with the ice and water mixture, to avoid losses and temperature gradients. The water must be periodically removed and ice should be added to keep the temperature constant. This mixture of water and ice keeps the junction temperature to 0.1°C, but is not a practical solution. In practice, to determine the temperature of the reference or cold junction, it can be kept it in contact with an isothermal block, of aluminum, for example, at a known temperature (replacing the bath water and ice).

The second method uses a Peltier cooler. The thermocouple is stored in a tank containing deionized distilled water and kept at 0°C. The external walls of the tank are cooled by thermoelectric cooling elements. When the water starts to freeze, its volume increases and expands bellows connected to a microswitch that deactivates the cooling elements. The "water freezing and ice defrosting" cycle in the tank maintains the temperature of the water precisely at 0°C.

The schematic diagram shown in Figure 4.22 represents the electric-bridge method application. The temperature T_2 of the environment, where the cold junction is placed (usually room temperature), is monitored by a temperature transducer (RTD). The RTD is used in a temperature compensation circuit to create a voltage, with the same intensity but opposite polarity, that cancels any thermocouple output voltage caused by changings in the cold junction temperature T_2.

In the fourth method, the cold junction temperature is controlled and maintained above the room temperature and the voltage values of the table voltage temperature of the thermocouple must be shifted to correct the cold junction temperature different from 0°C.

In the double oven method, four new junctions are added to the circuit (Figure 4.23) and each one is heated to a controlled temperature, one at 65°C and the other at 130°C, in a way that the emf created at the new junctions is canceled, resulting in the net effect of a voltage equivalent to the thermoelectric effect of a simple cold junction at 0°C.

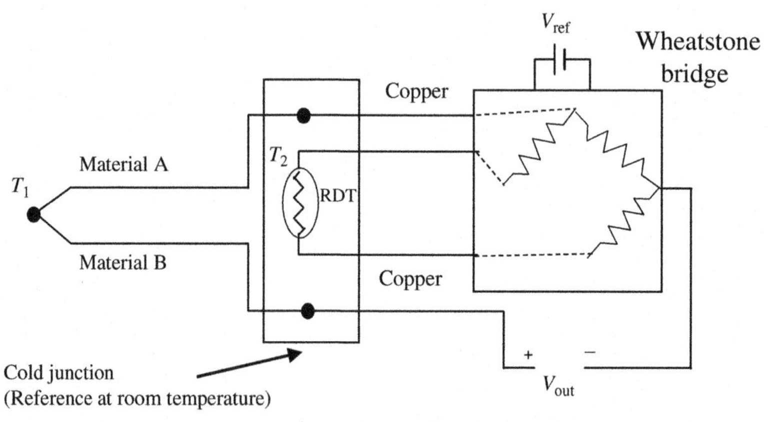

Figure 4.22 Electric-bridge method to establish a cold junction constant temperature.

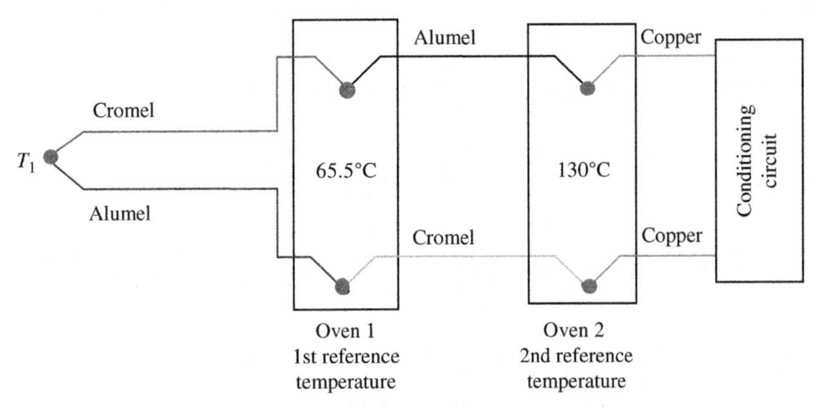

Figure 4.23 Double oven method to establish a cold junction with constant temperature T_2 to measure T_1.

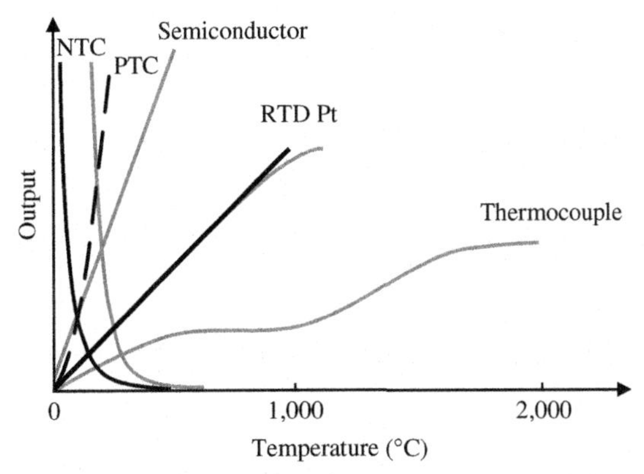

Figure 4.24 Comparison of the relative output of thermoresistive and thermoelectric temperature sensors.

Figure 4.24 presents the transfer functions of thermoresistive and thermoelectric temperature sensors emphasizing the low voltage output of thermocouples compared to other temperature sensors. To increase the sensibility of temperature measurement with thermocouples, a thermopile (series association of thermocouples) can be used. Figure 4.25A shows a representation of a thermopile.

If all J_2 junctions are at the reference temperature T_2 and all J_1 junctions are at T_1, the Seebeck output voltage of the series arrangement of thermocouples is

$$V_{\text{out}} = n\alpha_{\text{AB}} \cdot (T_1 - T_2) \tag{4.32}$$

where n is the number of thermocouples in the pile.

The thermopile V_{out} is the sum of the emf of each thermocouple; it increases the sensibility of the temperature measurement and allows to detect little temperature

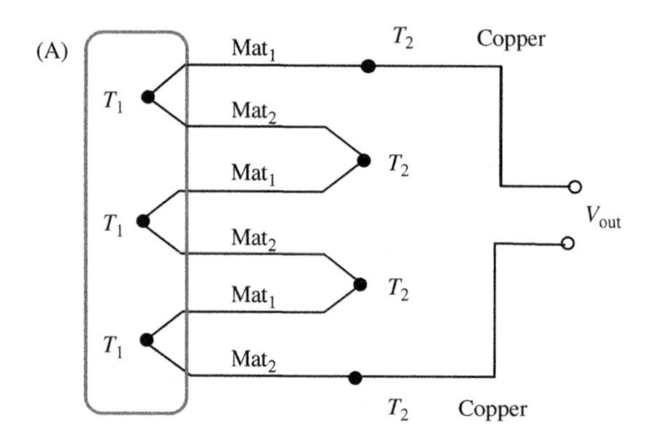

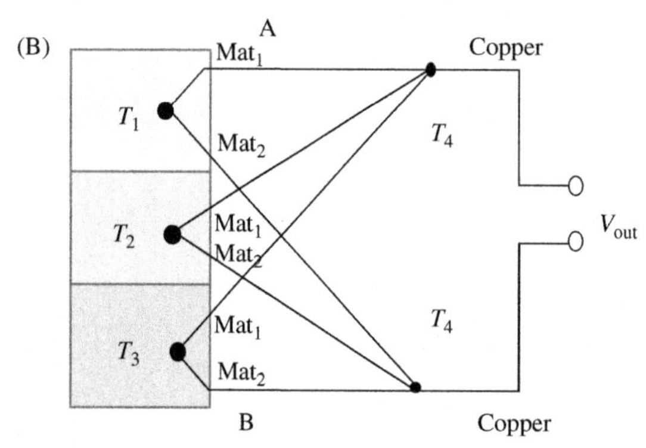

Figure 4.25 (A) Series association of thermocouples in a thermopile. (B) Parallel association of thermocouples.

differences. A typical chromel/constantan thermopile with 20 thermocouples has sensibility of ≈ 1 mV/F.

A parallel association of thermocouples, as shown in Figure 4.25B, generates an output voltage that is the average of the emf of all thermocouples:

$$V_{\text{out}} = \alpha_{\text{AB}} \cdot \left(\frac{T_1 + T_2 + T_3 + \cdots + T_n}{n} \right) - T_{\text{ref}} \qquad (4.33)$$

where T_{ref} is the temperature of the reference (cold) juctions of all thermocouples.

The output voltage of a parallel association of thermocouples gives information about the average temperature.

Thermocouples require linearization or linearity calibration, which is done in firmware and software. Firmware calibration requires a stable and known reference temperature or cold junction temperature; above in this chapter, some options to obtain a cold junction reference were presented. Software linearity calibration reduces linearity errors through the use of look-up tables and high-order polynomial equations to calculate the temperature value correspondent to the measured Seebeck voltage.

As advantages of thermocouples, one can say that they are simple, low cost, rugged and do not have problems with lead wire resistances and they respond quickly to temperature changes. Thermocouples are least stable, least repeatable, and have the lowest accuracy compared to RTD and thermistors. Lead wires must be of the same thermocouple material and the reference junction temperature must be monitored and controlled.

Due to its long-term stability, response time of the order of microseconds and little size, thermocouples are extensively used in biomedical applications. Thermocouples can be manufactured in micrometric dimensions (350 μm thickness and 400 μm diameter), through the vacuum deposition of two metals on an appropriate substrate, allowing their insertion in hypodermic needles and catheters to be placed inside blood vessels and heart chambers to do direct and invasive temperature measurements.

4.2.3 Semiconductor-based temperature transducer

A quite simple method for temperature measurement utilizes the current versus voltage characteristic of a semiconductor PN junction. The direct-biased PN junction of a diode and the base–emitter junction of a NPN transistor have a transfer function similar to that shown in Figure 4.26. Keeping the current constant, as the temperature increases, the voltage drop across the junction decreases. Keeping the voltage constant, as the temperature increases, the current across the junction also increases. The temperature sensor can

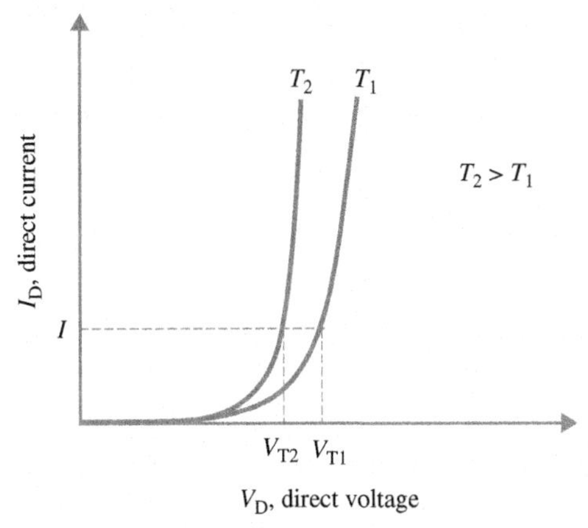

Figure 4.26 Current versus voltage of a typical PN semiconductor junction and the temperature effect.

be obtained applying constant voltage in the PN junction and measuring the resultant current or applying constant current and measuring the output voltage variation with temperature (Cobbold, 1974; Doebelin; 1990; Geddes & Baker, 1968).

Equation (4.34) describes the relation between current I_D and voltage drop V_D in a direct-biased PN junction at temperature T:

$$I_D = I_S(e^{(V_D/V_T)} - 1) \tag{4.34}$$

where

$I_S = cAT^{(3/2)}e^{(E_g/2kT)}$ is the reverse saturation current
c is a constant that depends on the fabrication technology of the PN junction
A is the transversal area of the junction
E_g is the energy gap to the element at 0 K (absolute temperature)
k is $8.62 \cdot 10^{-5}$ eV/K
$V_T = (kT/q)$ is the thermal voltage
q is the electron charge ($1.60217657 \times 10^{-19}$ C).

Equation (4.35) gives the voltage drop V_D across a direct-biased PN junction:

$$V_D = V_T \ln\left(\frac{I_D}{I_S} + 1\right) \tag{4.35}$$

Equation (4.35) can be simplified as

$$V_D \approx V_T \ln\left(\frac{I_D}{I_S}\right) \tag{4.36}$$

In Eqs. (4.34) and (4.36), temperature variations affect thermal voltage (V_T) and reverse saturation voltage (I_S). A temperature increase shifts the curve in Figure 4.26 to the left and a decrease shifts it to the right. Plotting V_D versus T to a constant current I_D, the resultant curve is similar to that shown in Figure 4.27. It is easily noticed that the voltage across the junction changes linearly with temperature variation to temperatures above ≈ 40 K. To a silicon semiconductor PN junction, fed by 1 mA constant current, the voltage drop decreases 2 mV/°C. If the current is 10 μA, the voltage variation with temperature is −2.8 mV/°C.

Figure 4.28 shows a typical configuration of bipolar transistor working as temperature sensor. The base of the transistor is shorted to the collector. A constant current flowing in the remaining PN junction, the base–emitter junction, produces a direct voltage drop V_D proportional to temperature. Compared to the diode configuration, the transistor configuration as temperature sensor presents the advantage of the transistor current gain (β).

Semiconductor-based temperature sensors are used in integrated circuit temperature transducers.

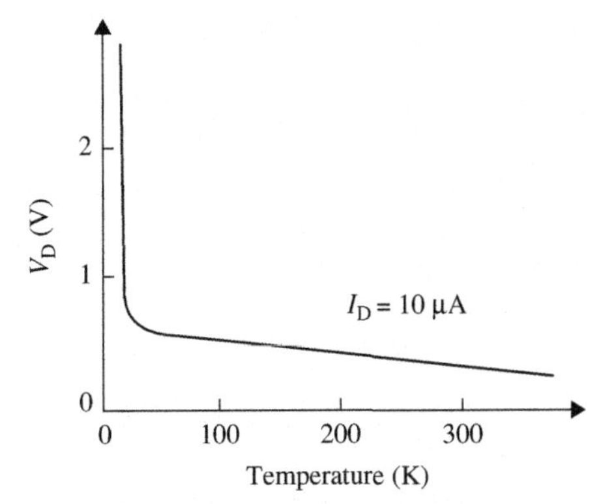

Figure 4.27 Direct drop voltage versus temperature when a constant current flows through the semiconductor PN junction.

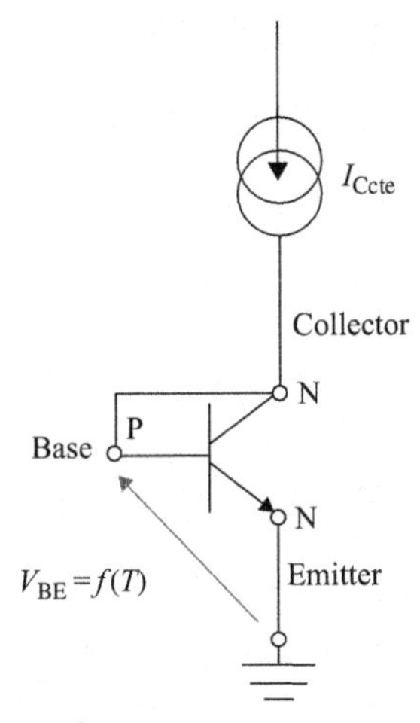

Figure 4.28 Bipolar transistor configured as a temperature sensor.

4.2.4 Integrated circuit temperature transducers

Integrated circuit temperature transducers are available in both voltage and current output configurations, with typical sensibility values of 10 mV/K (LM335, 2014) and 1 μA/K (AD590, 2014), respectively. Both configurations supply an output that is linearly proportional to absolute temperature. Some integrated circuit sensors even represent temperature in a digital output format that connects directly to a microprocessor or microcontroller input to digital processing, like LM75 (LM75/76, 2014), which have I^2C interface compatible output.

The AD590 (AD590, 2014) is an integrated circuit temperature transducer which utilizes the difference of two base–emitter voltage drops of transistors configured as temperature sensors. It produces an output current proportional to absolute temperature. For supply voltages between 4 and 30 V, the device acts as a high impedance, constant current regulator with 1 μA/K sensibility. It has a wide temperature range, −55°C to +150°C, and shows a typical nonlinearity error of ±0.3°C over full working range.

The LM335 (LM335, 2014) operates by sensing the difference of the base−emitter voltage of two transistors running at different current levels and acts like a Zener diode whose reverse breakdown voltage V_Z is proportional to absolute temperature, $V_Z = 10$ mV/K (or $2.73 + 0.01T$, T in °C) and its accuracy is around ±3°C. This temperature sensor acts like a Zener diode and it needs a bias current between 400 μA and 5 mA, according to LM335 data sheet. It is important to note that self-heating can be a significant problem, and a high bias current should be used carefully. LM335 is linear with respect to absolute temperature and introduces little error (typical nonlinearity error ±0.3°C) over full working range (−55°C to 150°C).

Highly sensitive and fast temperature sensors arrays with very little sensitive areas, for medical applications, can be made from thin films of semiconductor material, like amorphous germanium (a-Ge), over glass, alumina or polymer substrates, with high temperature coefficient of resistance (2%/K at room temperature) (Urban et al., 1989).

Semiconductor-based temperature transducers offer a linear output with temperature, but these integrated circuit sensors share all the disadvantages of thermistors. They are semiconductor devices and thus have a small temperature range compared to thermocouples and RTDs; self-heating problem must be prevented and they require an external power source, but they can be quite inexpensive. These small devices provide a convenient way to produce an easy-to-read output that is proportional to temperature or easily integrated to other electronic devices; they are used, for example, to monitor the temperature of the thermocouple junction reference. Some integrated circuit temperature sensors have a high degree of integration and include in the same chip A/D converters, multiplexers, voltage reference, digital I/O, logic fault detector and registers for processing and storing data and instructions.

4.2.5 Capacitive temperature transducer

Some types of ceramic capacitors have their capacitance values dependant on temperature. The way the capacitance varies with temperature is the temperature coefficient, which can be defined in the capacitor manufacturing process. These capacitors are used as temperature sensors usually as part of oscillating circuits (LC), whose resonance frequencies (Eqs. (4.37) and (4.38)) become temperature dependent (Cobbold, 1974; CS-501 GR, 2014).

$$f_0 = \frac{\omega_0}{2\pi} \tag{4.37}$$

$$\omega_0 = \frac{1}{\sqrt{LC}} \tag{4.38}$$

where

ω_0 is the angular frequency

L is the inductance

C is the temperature dependant capacitance.

The behavior of the oscillation frequency is approximately linear if the temperature variation occurs within a small range, for example, $\pm 5°C$. The oscillation frequency that varies with the temperature is compared to the output of a reference oscillator of constant frequency. The difference between these two frequencies is due to the variation of temperature at which the capacitor is subjected, and can be fed to a microcontrolled circuit to digital processing and display of the temperature. Figure 4.29A shows a typical capacitance versus temperature curve. Derivating $C(T)$ relative to T results in the sensibility of the capacitive temperature sensor can be as good as a few pF/K (to a few nF nominal capacitance). Figure 4.29C shows a schematic diagram of a capacitive temperature transducer (Lake Shore Cryotronics, Inc.; Cobbold, 1974). Figure 4.29B shows the current versus frequency curve of an LC circuit with a ressonace frequency at f_0; this ressonance frequency changes with temperature if the capacitor is temperature sensitive.

Capacitive temperature transducers are used mainly in industrial applications and are well suited to temperature monitoring and control in high magnetic fields environments, since their capacitance do not show magnetic field dependence. Although a long-term stability is expected, care must be taken to account for aging and hysteresis due to repeated heating and cooling cycles.

4.2.6 Liquid crystal temperature transducer

The liquid crystal thermometer allows measuring the temperature of a solid object surface, and the human body, without providing a corresponding electrical signal, making use of special material (heat-sensitive, thermochromic liquid crystal) contained in plastic strips, which are placed against the object or skin surface and that change their color while absorbing heat.

The aligned molecular structure of some organic liquids can be altered by electric or magnectic fields. In addition to electric and magnetic field sensitive organic liquids, there are also temperature sensitive organic liquids. These liquids known as liquid crystals look like liquid in terms of mechanical properties, but have optical properties of single crystals.

The temperature sensitive liquid crystal is an organic material that exists between the solid and the isotropic liquid phase, according to its temperature. The material is in the amorphous solid phase below a determined temperature, and above an upper

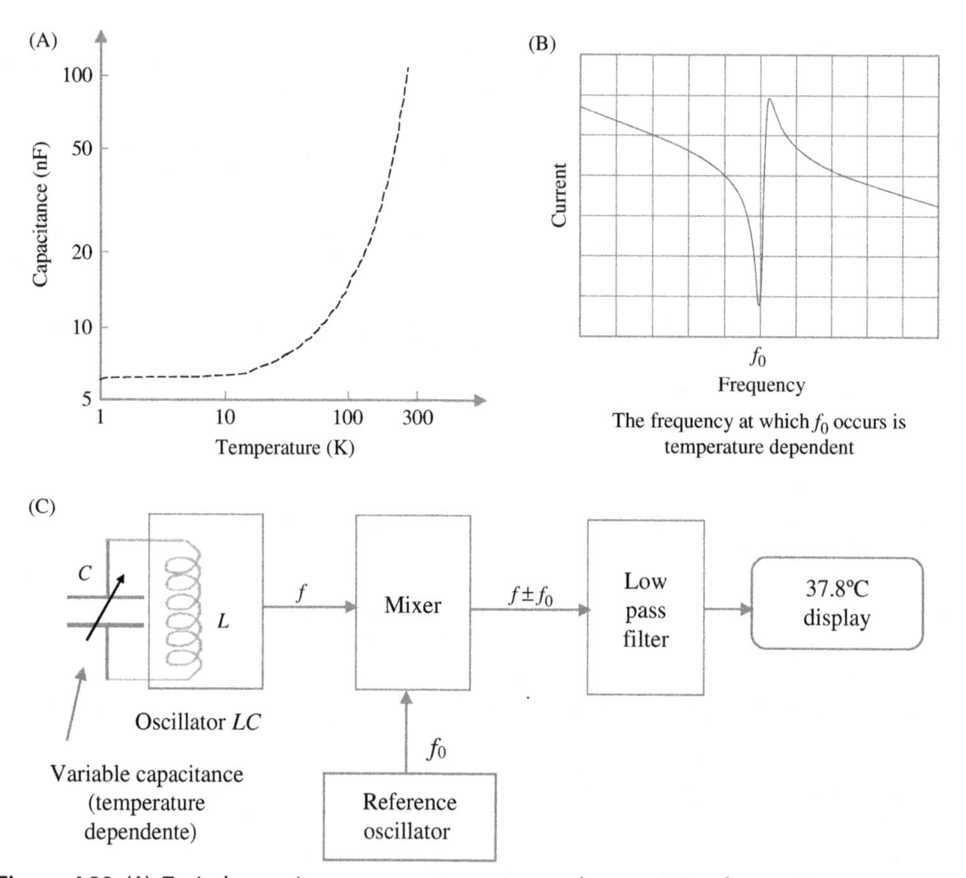

Figure 4.29 (A) Typical capacitance versus temperature characteristic of capacitive temperature sensor. (B) Typical current versus frequency curve of an oscillator LC circuit showing the resonance frequency, which changes with temperature. (C) Schematic diagram of a capacitive temperature transducer.

limit, it enters in the liquid state. In between these temperature limits, it shows different molecular organizations that resemble crystalline states. The transition between the crystal and liquid phases (melting point) occurs at a well-determined temperature and depends on the material composition and by combining different ratios of the mixture components that make up the crystal it is possible to control the temperature of phase transition.

Liquid crystal compounds are called "cholesteric" because they have a molecular structure similar to cholesterol. Cholesteric compounds have a helical structure with a characteristic pitch and the length of this helix pitch is in the range of the wavelength of visible light. The pitch changes (reversably) with an external stimulus such as

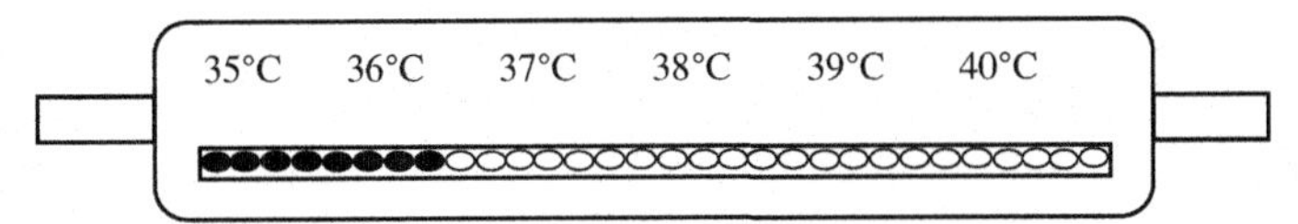

Figure 4.30 Flexible strip liquid crystal thermometer measuring 36.4°C (resolution 0.2°C). The liquid crystal compartments with composition sensitive to the temperatures below 36.4°C change from solid to transparent liquid state allowing viewing the black background.

temperature. The cholestric helical structure of liquid crystals has optical properties: each pitch of the helical structure is sensible to a wavelength in such a way that combining the proportion of the compounds of the liquid crystal is possible to control at which temperature the phase shift between solid and liquid happens. Confining these compounds inside an optical transparent plastic compartment of parallel walls, which maintains the right optical orientation of the liquid crystal, the optical effect is enhanced. Combining compounds, separated a few microns in compartments along the plastic strip, of slightly different compositions, is possible to obtain a transducer sensible to 0.1°C different temperatures. The temperature is identified visually in the strip (Figure 4.30) because the compartments have different liquid crystal compositions sensible to determined temperatures, in a crescent value order. When the strip is placed against the forehead, each of the strip compartments sensible to temperatures below the body surface temperature changes from the solid to liquid phase, that is, from the opaque to the transparent state and are viewed against a nonreflecting (black) background. The external stimulus, temperature, does not affect the chemical structure of the liquid crystal and it can respond repeatedly to molecular pitch changings, that is, it can be reused many times as a reliable temperature transducer, although disposable liquid crystal thermometers have been also developed for home and medical use (Cobbold, 1974; Turner, 2009; Webster, 2010). Gregory, Horrow, and Rosenberg (1990) investigated the performance of forehead crystal liquid compared to other temperature technology thermometers, during open heart surgeries, and concluded that it has the ability to reflect core temperature during noninvasive temperature monitoring.

4.3 NONCONTACT TEMPERATURE TRANSDUCERS (RADIATION THERMOMETERS)

The most common way to measure the temperature of an object is through the heat conduction between the object and the heat-sensitive element, and therefore requires contact between the transducer and the object. This can be a problem if the object is moving, like an incandescent piece in the industrial production line, or the contact of the object with the heat-sensitive element is not allowed due to its fragility, as for example, the surgical field during cardiac revascularization.

Every object with temperature above 0 K emits electromagnetic radiation with an intensity that depends on its temperature, that is, electromagnetic energy radiates from all matter, regardless of its temperature. Different materials radiate with different levels of efficiency. This efficiency is quantified as emissivity, a decimal number or percentage ranging between 0% and 1% or 0% and 100%. Most organic materials, including skin, are very efficient, frequently exhibiting emissivities of 0.95 and this amount of radiation emitted by the skin is used to quantify the human body temperature. Polished metals tend to be inefficient radiators at room temperature, with low emissivity or efficiency (20% or less).

The highest possible emissivity, unity, is accounted to the ideal emitter of electromagnetic radiation, called black body; black because it is not reflective at any wavelength and it is not transparent, but opaque. The radiation intensity varies with temperature and with the wavelength. Figure 4.31 shows the spectral power of a black body at different temperatures in the wavelength range from 0.1 to 2 μm. Within this electromagnetic radiation range lies the visible light (0.4–0.724 μm) and part of the infrared spectrum (0.724–100 μm).

When the temperature of a black body increases, the overall radiated energy increases and the peak of the radiation curve moves to shorter wavelengths. The spectral power of a black body as a function of temperature and wavelength is described by Max Planck's Law:

$$E_\lambda = \frac{C_1}{\pi\lambda^5(e^{C_2/\lambda T} - 1)} \tag{4.39}$$

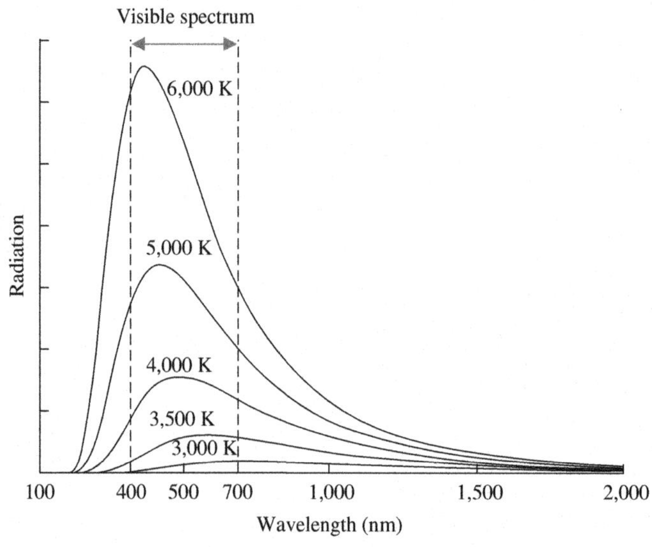

Figure 4.31 Spectral power of a black body at different temperatures and wavelengths.

where

C_1 is a constant $= 3.75 \times 10^{-16}\ \mathrm{Wm}^2$

C_2 is a constant $= 1.44 \times 10^{-2}\ \mathrm{mK}$.

According to Plank's radiation formula the radiant energy is maximum at a certain wavelength for each radiation temperature and that the product of the peak wavelength and the temperature is found to be a constant (Wien's displacement law):

$$\lambda_{\max} \times T = 2898(\mu\mathrm{m\ K}) \tag{4.40}$$

where 2898 is an approximation of $(2.8977685 \pm 51) \times 10^{-3}\ \mathrm{mK}$ (Mohr & Taylor, 2005).

From Eq. (4.39) and Figure 4.31, we see that the wavelength at which the irradiation peak occurs varies for each temperature and the higher the object temperature, the lower is the wavelength of the electromagnetic radiation emitted by the object. The area under a given curve corresponds to the total radiated power or the total radiant energy W_T at that temperature. Integrating Planck's equation for λ from zero to infinity, and assuming ε constant, results in the Stefan–Boltzmann equation:

$$W_\mathrm{T} = \int_0^\infty W_\lambda \mathrm{d}\lambda = \varepsilon \tau T^4 \tag{4.41}$$

where τ is Stefan–Boltzmann constant $= 5.7 \times 10^{-12}\ \mathrm{W\ cm}^{-2}\ \mathrm{K}^{-4}$.

To a black body, the emissivity is 1 and Eq. (4.41) becomes

$$W_\mathrm{T} = \int_0^\infty W_\lambda \mathrm{d}\lambda = \tau T^4 \tag{4.42}$$

The relationship between the ideal behavior of the black body and a real object is its emissivity or emittance, which is frequently considered being constant to each type of material, although its value depends, on the same material, according to its shape, surface oxidation state, etc. It is possible to determine the temperature of an object from the measurement of the intensity of spectral radiation W_λ or the total radiant energy W_T, if the emissivity of its surface is known.

Pyrometers are temperature sensors that use the information of electromagnetic radiation emitted by an object and do not require physical contact between the sensor and the object. There are many types of pyrometers, optical pyrometers, radiation pyrometers, total radiation pyrometers, automatic infrared thermometers, ear thermometers, fiber optic thermometers, two-color pyrometers, infra-snakes, and many more. According to the wavelength range to which pyrometers are sensible, they are classified as optical pyrometers and radiation pyrometers. Optical pyrometers are sensible to the visible electromagnetic spectrum; this method compares the radiation of a heated object surface with a known standard. Radiation pyrometers are sensible to longer wavelengths, in the infrared electromagnetic spectrum (mostly in short infrared); this method uses detectors that measure the flux density of the radiation emitted from the heated object surface (Cobbold, 1974; Dally et al., 1993; Doebelin, 1990; Geddes & Baker, 1968; Gruner, 2003; Webster, 2010).

4.3.1 Optical pyrometers

Optical pyrometers operate within the visible spectrum to measure temperatures typically in the range from 700°C to 4,000°C by comparing the photometric brightness of the heated object against the brightness of a standard source, such as an incandescent tungsten filament. A monochromatic filter for the red wavelength radiation (630 nm) is used to support the operation; the comparison of the brightnesses is dependent on the sensitivity of the human eye (on manual versions) to distinguish the brightness difference between two surfaces of the same color. The brightness comparison is made adjusting the current through the filament of the standard brightness source until its brightness becomes equal to that of the measured object. It is possible to obtain measurements with accuracy better than 1%. There are also commercial automatized versions of optical pyrometers.

Because this type of pyrometer operates in the visible spectrum, it is necessary that the object radiates at wavelength from 400 to 720 nm, which correspond to temperatures higher than 700°C, making it impossible to measure the lower temperatures of the working range of the most applications of thermometers in Biomedical Engineering. This does not occur with infrared radiation pyrometers, as discussed later.

4.3.2 Radiation pyrometers (infrared sensors)

The radiation pyrometers detect the emission of energy from the surface of an object in a range of wavelengths longer than the optical pyrometers reviews. They are used for measuring temperatures lower than 700°C. A thermal detector collects the radiation in the infrared region emitted by the object and focuses it in a secondary temperature sensor. The absorption of radiation causes the sensor temperature to increase and then it converts the temperature value sensed into an electric signal, which is conditioned, processed, and displayed. Figure 4.32 shows a schematic diagram of an infrared pyrometer.

The various types of radiation pyrometers are differentiated according to the type of radiation detector they use. Radiation sensors are classified as thermal detectors and photon detectors. Although both types of radiation detectors are photon detectors, here we call thermal detector the one that receives photons and turns the photon energy into heat; photon detector will be the detector that receives photons and uses this energy to create charge carriers. Photon detectors are subdivided in photoconductive, photovoltaic, and photoemissive detectors according to the electrical effect (current or voltage) produced (Kruse, 1995; Rogalski, 2010; Smith, Jones, & Chasmar, 1968).

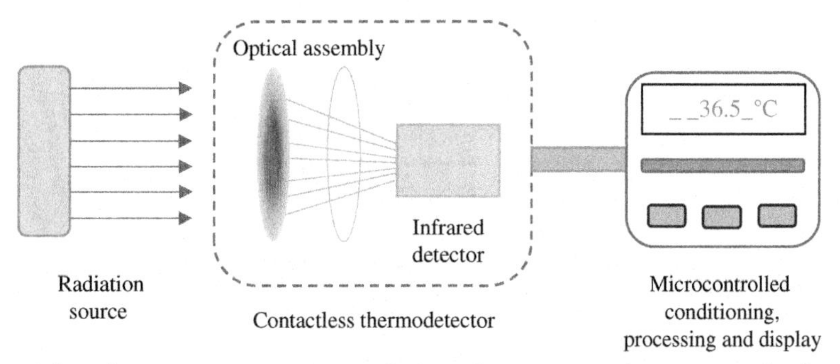

Figure 4.32 Infrared sensors are noncontact devices that measure the amount of infrared energy radiation emitted by the surface of an object. Thermodetectors collect the radiation and focus it on a secondary temperature sensor which converts the temperature value into an electric signal.

4.3.2.1 Thermal detectors

They are blackened elements designed to absorb the maximum amount of incident radiation at all wavelengths. The absorbed radiation causes an increase in the detector temperature until equilibrium is reached; then, the measurement of the equilibrium detector temperature, caused by the amount of radiation absorbed, gives the temperature of the radiating surface. There are heat losses and temperature interference from the neighboring environment; they are compensated through periodically sampling the ambient temperature.

Thermal detectors measure the temperature mostly using thermistors (bolometers) or thermocouples (thermopile) and the response time is relatively large (1–15 ms for bolometers and 1–2 s for thermopiles). Pyroelectric detectors are also used and their response times are faster than bolometers and thermopiles. Figures 4.33A and 4.34 show examples of thermal detectors with thermistor and thermocouple, respectively.

The thermal detector shown in Figure 4.33A is constructed with Sb–Bi thermocouples in cascade forming a thermopile. Each Sb–Bi thermocouple has a sensibility of 6.4 mV/°C. In this configuration, the darkened element (specimen) has a large surface area exposed to absorb a large amount of radiation. The temperature of the specimen is measured in relation to the temperature of a reference body through the cascade of thermocouples. Figure 4.33B shows the block diagram of an infrared thermometer that uses a thermopile as thermodetector and the temperature of the environment as reference.

In the radiation bolometer, the darkened element is a thermistor that is heated by the radiation at which it is exposed. An electronic circuit with a bolometer type thermal detector is shown in Figure 4.34. There is a second thermistor that is protected from incident radiation and whose function is to make the temperature compensation caused by self-heating.

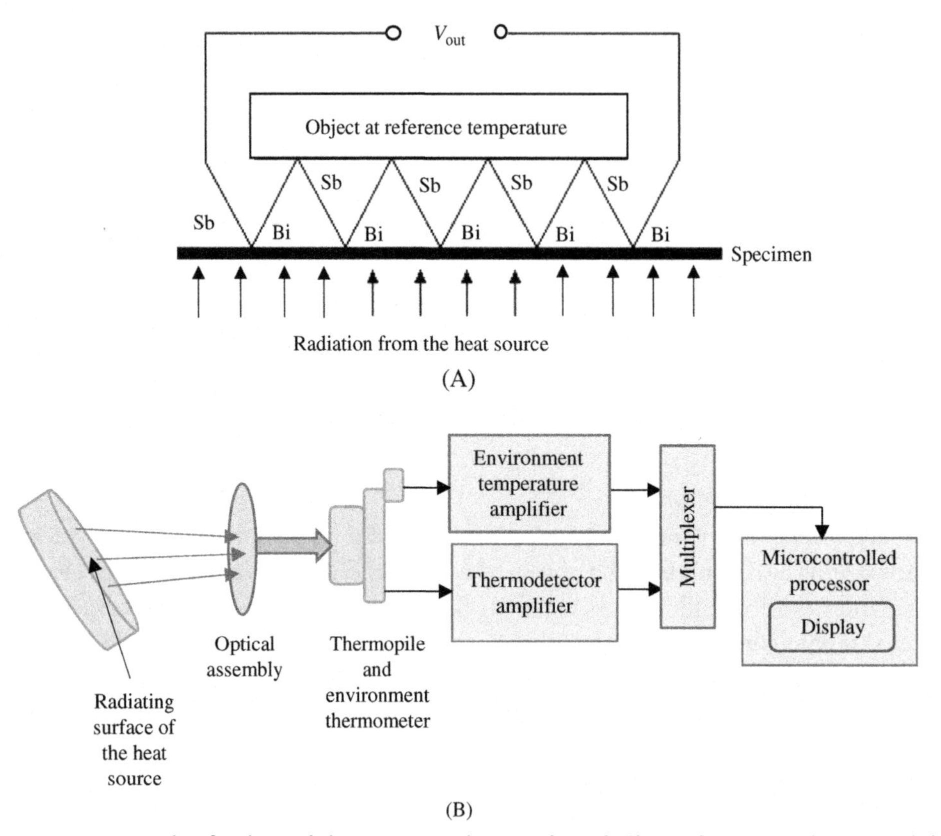

Figure 4.33 Example of a thermal detector type thermopile with Sb–Bi thermocouples (A) and the block diagram with the main components of an infrared thermometer.

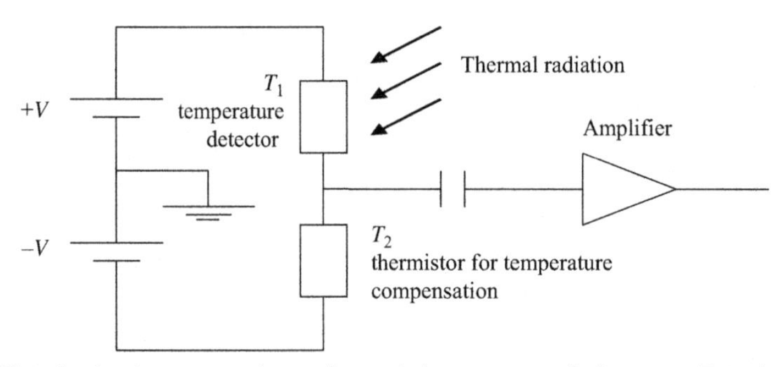

Figure 4.34 Electric circuit representing a thermal detector type bolometer. T_1 is the temperature sensor and T_2 is a thermistor used for compensation.

Thermal detectors respond uniformly to all wavelengths and have fairly simple physical principles of operation. The absorption of thermal radiation alters the temperature of the material of the detector, which can be manifested as a change in thermistor resistance, the development of an emf as thermocouple, or a change in the dipole moment of a ferroelectric crystal as the pyroelectric detector. Except for the last, thermal detectors have slow response times when compared with photon detectors.

4.3.2.2 Photon detectors

The incident radiation releases electrons in the structure of the detector yielding a measurable electrical effect. The basic feature of the operation of photon detectors is the intensity variation of the electric effect according to the amount of radiation (photons) absorbed. The individual incident photons directly interact with the electrons of the crystal lattice of the detector, creating charge carriers that cause different effects, such as changes in conductivity, as in the case of photoconductive cells or, in the potential difference across the junction of materials, such as the photovoltaic cells.

Some photodetectors can operate at room temperature, but the majority need to be cooled to reduce noise and increase the directivity of the measurement. The sensibility of both types of photodetector varies with the wavelength of the thermal radiation to be measured and its spectrum must be taken into account when selecting the thermometer to be used. Their typical time response is around 1 ms. Figure 4.35 shows a schematic diagram of a photon detector.

4.3.2.2.1 Photoconductive detector

Photons are absorbed in the semiconductor material of photoconductive detectors generating free carriers, thereby increasing the conductivity of the material. Photoresistors are the simplest example of photoconductive detectors. An electric current can be generated applying an external electric field to the detector circuit. The semiconductor material used may be intrinsic or extrinsic (larger number of charge

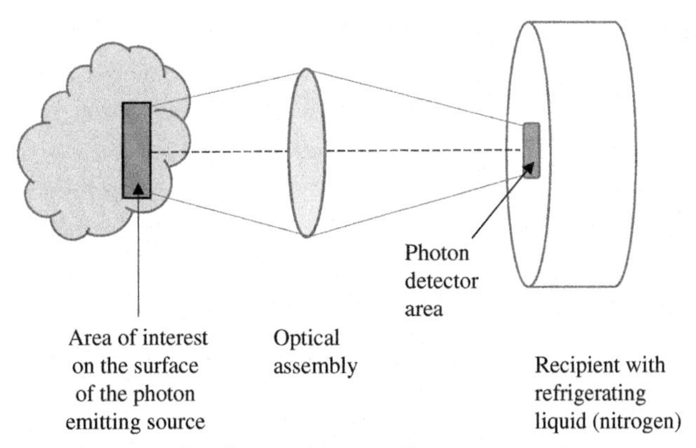

Figure 4.35 Schematic diagram of a photon detector showing its main components.

carriers) depending on the range of the wavelength of the radiation to be measured. Photon energy (E_p) depends on its wavelength:

$$E_p = 1.24/\lambda \text{ eV } (\lambda \text{ in } \mu\text{m}) \quad (4.43)$$

Intrinsic photodetectors respond well up to 10 μm (big wavelength, small energy gap). In extrinsic photodetectors, the impurity atoms occupy intermediate levels of energy, close to the donor (conduction band) or receiver (valence band) levels.

4.3.2.2.2 Photovoltaic detector

The photovoltaic detector consists of a semiconductor PN junction at which is generated a potential difference when the junction is exposed to radiation. The thermal radiation causes the release of free electron-hole pairs that are allocated near the junction, increasing the depletion region. This charge separation produces a potential difference, which is related to the temperature of the radiating body. Free charge carriers are attracted to opposite sides of the junction, causing flow of electrical current. Photodiodes and phototransistors are examples of photovoltaic detectors.

The photoconductive cells require a bias voltage to detect the change in conductivity caused by the incident radiation (proportional to temperature). In photovoltaic cells, incident radiation causes the flow of electric current (or electric potential difference) without using an external source. The current generated by the photodetection can be amplified by a current amplifier.

The energy radiated by an object depends on the emissivity (ε) of its surface. It is maximal for a black body ($\varepsilon = 1$), and close to zero for a polished surface. Radiation pyrometers are calibrated against a black body, and a correction factor must be applied when the measurement is performed in an object with different emissivity. To function properly, an infrared detector must take into account the emissivity of the surface being measured. Although the emissivity can be found in reference tables for different materials, its value is a factor of uncertainty as it varies with the state (oxidation and roughness) of the radiating surface, with its temperature, etc. A practical way to measure temperature with infrared, when the emissivity level is not known, is to "force" the emissivity to a known level, by covering the surface with a highly emissive mask (emissivity of 95%) such as a tape or paint. Another factor of uncertainty in the measurement of objects with emissivity lower than 1 is the influence of the surrounding objects. Some of the sensor input may consist of energy that is not emitted by the equipment or material whose surface is being targeted, but instead is being reflected by that surface from other equipment or materials. Emissivity pertains to energy radiating from a surface, whereas "reflection" pertains to energy reflected from another source.

Another aspect of the performance of infrared thermometers is related to the material of the lens used to focus the radiation on the detector. Materials such as glass do not transmit radiation at wavelengths >2.8 μm; quartz transmits only up to 4 μm; fluoride calcium transmits up to 10 μm; and thallium bromide iodide up to 30 μm (Klocek, 1991). When measuring lower temperatures, as the typical working ranges of Biomedical Engineering applications, these characteristics should be kept in mind to help choosing the proper pyrometer.

The infrared approach is also attractive when one does not wish to make contact with the surface whose temperature is being measured. Thus, the temperature of fragile or wet surfaces, such as painted surfaces coming out of a drying oven or biological tissue during an open chest surgery, can be monitored in this way.

Compared to thermal detectors, infrared detectors are faster, smaller, and have better accuracy and stability over time (although it is affected by background radiation, smoke, etc.). Main disadvantages of infrared detectors are wavelength-dependent sensibility, more complex electronic support and higher cost than thermal detectors.

4.3.2.2.3 Photoemissive detector

When the incoming radiation over the surface of a material (metal), kept in vacuum, has photons with sufficient energy, the excited electrons can overcome the potential barrier of the material surface and escape to the vacuum as free electrons. This process in which photogenerated electrons are liberated from the metal surface as free electrons is called photoelectron emission and is the principle of functioning of photoemissive detectors. Phototubes and photomultipliers are examples of this type of thermal radiation detector. Photomultipliers are the most sensitive photodetectors and have response time better than 10 ns, but in many applications, they can be replaced by photodiodes.

4.3.2.3 Medical application of radiation detectors

The main medical applications of the use of temperature measurement by radiation emission are the noninvasive determination of internal temperatures and thermography. The measurement of body temperature via the tympanic membrane is an example of noninvasive measurement of internal temperature. In addition to being noninvasive, the fact that there is no physical contact constitutes a protection against possible eardrum perforations and infections. The infrared thermometer captures the heat radiated from the body, in the form of infrared energy, through the tympanic membrane, and a detection optical system focuses the energy on a detector. The detector converts the energy into an electrical signal, which in turn is amplified, linearized, digitally converted, and displayed (usually a liquid crystal display) after 2–3 s.

When the whole object is at same temperature, the measurement may be made at any point of its surface without loss of information. In the presence of a temperature gradient on the surface of the object, for example, the gradient caused by metabolic differences in a biological tissue or organ, the temperature measurement must be made over the entire surface. According to the size of the area to be analyzed and the speed required to obtain the measurement, the radiation detector used may be a single sensor, which scans the area, or multiple sensors arranged in an array, which measure the radiation from different points at the same time. The array performs far more rapidly, but may lose resolution (finite number of transducers) and accuracy (different physical behavior for each transducer).

The emissivity of a biological tissue is difficult to determine and can vary greatly along its surface. Thus, the temperature measurement by scanning the tissue surface has little quantitative significance. Its result has qualitative value when the scanning results in a map of radiation quantification, usually represented in pseudo-color or gray scale. The infrared radiation mammography is an example of application of thermography, at which a map of infrared radiation wavelengths is obtained, allowing to identify areas of increased metabolism (warmer areas) that may indicate the presence of some pathological process.

Medical applications of images obtained by thermal scanning have increased significantly, especially in the area of diagnosis in orthopedics, diabetes, skin diseases (since it is possible to make a thermal image of the surface of the human body), vascular diseases, research on chronic pain, sportive medicine, etc.

4.4 REVIEW THE LEARNING

1. Describe the physical principles involved in the transduction of temperature with RDT. What are some of the characteristics of RDT that make it suitable for use in biomedical applications?
2. Describe the physical principles involved in the transduction of temperature with thermistors. What are the main characteristics of the thermistors that make them suitable to be used in biomedical applications are?
3. Describe the physical principles involved in the transduction of temperature with thermocouples. What is Peltier effect? What is Thompson effect?
4. Which are the main characteristics of thermocouples that make them suitable for use in biomedical applications? What are some of the empirical properties of the thermocouples that facilitate its use in temperature measurement?
5. Explain the functioning of the semiconductor-based (PN junction) thermosensor?
6. Self-heating is one of the problems commonly encountered in the use of temperature sensors. How self-heating affects the operation of thermistors and RDTs and how can it be avoided?
7. The Wheatstone bridge is an electrical circuit suitable for measuring sensors to work with low temperature sensitivity. Why? Show an example and explain its operation.
8. Explain the functioning of the liquid crystal temperature transducer.

9. Describe three types of thermometer function without contact between the sensor element and the body. Compare their functioning and give examples of medical applications of these thermometers.
10. Compare the functioning and performance of the following temperature sensors: thermistor, RTD, and thermocouple. Suggestion: Organize a table with accuracy, linearity, working range, size, shape excitation, measurement circuit, etc.

REFERENCES

AD590, Analog Device. AD590: 2-Terminal Temperature Transducer Data Sheet. <http://www.analog.com/en/mems-sensors/digital-temperature-sensors/ad590/products/product.html> Accessed 16.04.14.

AD7711, Analog Device. Technical Note Temperature Measurement using a Thermistor and the AD7711 Sigma Delta ADC by Albert O'Grady. <http://www-corp.analog.com> Accessed 16.04.14.

ASTM Standards (1974). *Manual on the use of thermocouples in temperature measurement.* ASTM Special Publication 470A, Omega Press.

Chan, A. Y. K. (2008). *Biomedical device technology: Principles and design.* Springfield, Illinois: Charles C. Thomas Publisher Ltd.

Childs, P. R. N., Greenwood, J. R., & Long, C. A. (2000). Review of temperature measurement. *Review of scientific instruments, 71*(8), 2959–2978. Available from: <http://hdl.handle.net/10044/1/7036> Accessed 01.04.14.

Cobbold, R. S. C. (1974). *Transducers for biomedical measurements: Principles and applications.* New York: John Wiley & Sons.

CS-501GR, Lake Shore Cryotronics, Inc. Capacitance Temperature Sensors. <http://www.lakeshore.com/products/Cryogenic-Temperature-Sensors/Capacitance/Pages/Overview.aspx> Accessed 20.04.14.

Dally, J. W., Riley, W. F., & McConnell, K. G. (1993). *Instrumentation for engineering measurements* (2nd ed.). New York, Chichester: John Wiley & Sons.

Doebelin, E. O. (1990). *Measurements systems—Application and design* (4th ed.). New York: McGraw Hill.

Gregory, C. A., Horrow, J. C., & Rosenberg, H. (1990). Does forehead liquid crystal temperature accurately reflect "core" temperature? *Canadian Journal of Anaesthesiology, 37*(6), 659–662. Available from: <http://www.infinitimedical.dk/upload/Studie/Sharn/LC%20and%20Core%20Temp.pdf> Accessed 22.04.14.

Gruner K.-D. (2003) Principles of non-contact temperature measurement. Raytek Corporation. <http://support.fluke.com/raytek-sales/Download/Asset/IR_THEORY_55514_ENG_REVB_LR.PDF> Accessed 25.04.14.

Geddes, L. A., & Baker, L. E. (1968). *Principles of applied biomedical instrumentation.* New York, NY: John Wiley & Sons.

Khandpur, R. S. (2005). *Biomedical instrumentation: Technology and applications.* New York, NY: McGraw Hill.

Klocek, P. (Ed.), (1991). *Handbook of infrared optical materials.* New York: Marcel Dekker Inc.

Kruse, P. A. (1995). A comparison of the limits to the performance of thermal and photon detector imaging arrays. *Infrared Physics & Technology, 36*, 869–882.

LM335, Texas Instruments. LM335/335A Precision Temperature Sensors Data Sheet. <http://www.ti.com.cn/cn/lit/ds/symlink/lm135.pdf> Accessed 20.04.14.

LM75/76, Texas Instruments. Digital Temperature Sensor and Thermal Watchdog with Two-Wire Interface. <http://www.ti.com/product/lm75a> Accessed 20.04.14.

McGee, T. D. (Ed.), (1988). *Principles and methods of temperature measurement.* New York: John Wiley & Sons [ISBN 0 471-62767-4].

Mohr, P. J., & Taylor, B. N. (2005). CODATA values of the fundamental constants 2002. *Reviews of Modern Physics*, 77(1), 1–107.

Mosaic Industries, Inc. Efficient Thermocouple Calibration and Measurement. <http://www.mosaic-industries.com/embedded-systems/microcontroller-projects/temperature-measurement/thermocouple/calibration-table> Accessed 16.04.14.

OMEGA, OMEGA® Engineering Inc (1983). *Omega temperature measurement handbook*. Stamford, CT: Omega Press.

RdF, RdF Industrial Platinum RTDs. Platinum RTD Probe Construction. <http://www.rdfcorp.com/anotes/pa-r/pa-r_02.shtml> Accessed 06.04.14.

Price, R. (1959). The platinum resistance thermometer—A review of its construction and applications. *Platinum Metals Review*, *3*(3), 78−87.

Rogalski, A. (2010). *Infrared detectors* (2nd ed., ISBN 978-1-4200-7671-4). Boca Raton, FL: CRC Press, Taylor & Francis Group.

Smith, R. A., Jones, F. E., & Chasmar, R. P. (1968). *The detection and measurement of infrared radiation*. Oxford: Clarendon Press.

Thermocouple Reference Tables, NBS Monograph 125, National Bureau of Standards, Washington, DC, 1979. Also, Temperature-Millivolt Reference Tables-Section T, Omega Temperature Measurement Handbook. Omega Press, 1983.

The RTD. Omega Engineering Inc. <http://www.omega.com/temperature/z/pdf/z033-035.pdf> Accessed 10.04.14.

Turner, J. (Ed.), (2009). *Sensors technology series, automotive sensors*. New York, NY: Momentum Press [ISBN-13: 978-1-60650-009-5].

Urban, G., Jachimowicz, A., Kohl, F., Kuttner, H., Olcaytug, F., Kamper, H., et al. (1989). High-resolution thin-film temperature sensor arrays for medical applications. *Sensors and Actuators A: Physical*, *22*(1−3), 650−654.

Webster, J. (Ed.), (2010). *Medical instrumentation: Application and design* (4th ed.). Hoboken, NJ: John Wiley & Sons.

CHAPTER 5

Displacement, Velocity, and Acceleration Transducers

Contents

5.1 INTRODUCTION

Displacement transducers are used in both direct and indirect measurements of biomedical variables. The direct displacement measurement is used in biomedical applications, for example, to measure cardiac muscle contractility (in isolated muscle preparations), to detect changing in the diameter of blood vessels and in the volume of heart chambers, and in the study of the properties of bones submitted to mechanical stress. The displacement measurement, as part of indirect determination of other variables, is common in biomedical application: pressure and force transducers usually measure the displacement of a rod, a piston, or diaphragm, for example, to determine the secondary values of pressure and force. Most of displacement

Principles of Measurement and Transduction of Biomedical Variables.
DOI: http://dx.doi.org/10.1016/B978-0-12-800774-7.00005-2

transducers are classified as resistive, capacitive, inductive, and ultrasonic, according to their principle of operation. The functioning of a few of these displacement transducers is explained later.

5.2 DISPLACEMENT TRANSDUCERS

5.2.1 Resistive transducers

There are two major groups of resistive transducers: potentiometers and strain gages. They are dissipative devices, classified as zero-order systems, as they do not accumulate energy. Their output is immediately available and the response time is null.

5.2.1.1 Potentiometric transducer

A potentiometer-like transducer of displacement is an electromechanical device of variable resistance and usually is part of an electric circuit with a constant voltage source (DC or AC). It determines the position of an object, which is connected to its movable segment, or cursor, and gives an output voltage that is linearly proportional to the object displacement regarding to an absolute position or origin (Figure 5.1A). There are translation and rotational potentiometers, according to their construction (Figure 5.1A and B). In the translation potentiometer, a sliding contact displaces linearly while in the rotational potentiometer a moving shaft displaces angularly rotating the sliding contact. Rotational potentiometer can have a single turn or multi turns. Translation and rotational potentiometers are passive devices and when inserted in an electric circuit, respond to linear and angular displacement, respectively, with a linearly proportional output voltage (Figure 5.1C). There are also logarithmic potentiometers, whose output resistance is logarithmically related to the sliding contact displacement (Chan, 2008; Cobbold, 1974; Dally, Riley, & McConnell, 1993; Geddes & Baker, 1968; Khandpur, 2005; Webster, 2010).

The potentiometers are discrete or continuous variable resistors. Discrete type are made of metal wires helically coiled (or wire wound) around a rod; while the cursor slides due to displacement, it doesn't touch continuously the wire, giving the output a discrete characteristic. Continuous type is made from metal film, almost always carbon, ceramic (Cermet), or conductive plastic. The potentiometer resistance varies in a sinusoidal, linear, or logarithmic way.

Generic potentiometer-like transducers are able to detect displacements as little as a few millimeters and as large as hundreds of millimeters, if the translational type is used; the range is 10° to $\approx 270^\circ$ for the single-turn rotational or 50 turns, for the multi-turn rotational. Their accuracy is usually better than $\pm 1\%$ to both, continuous and discrete types and the maximum linearity error is better

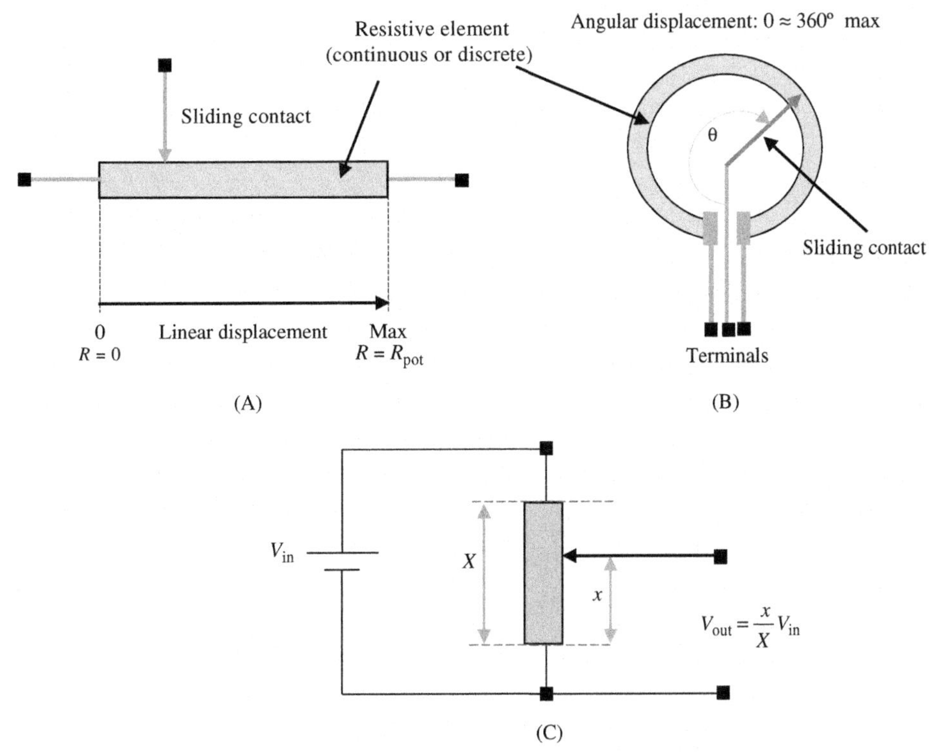

Figure 5.1 Resistive transducers type potentiometers (A) linear translation; (B) angular translation (single turn rotational). They usually respond to a linear or angular displacement with a linearly proportional output voltage (C).

than $\pm 0.1\%$ to translational discrete and $\pm 0.02\%$ if the rotational single-turn discrete is used.

5.2.1.1.1 Nonlinearity error

For biomedical applications, the linearity error should be maintained below $\pm 1\%$ to avoid nonlinearity distortion in the value being read. The device that reads the variable resistance value must have input impedance several times larger than the transducer output impedance, otherwise, it can load the transducer causing distortion. Input impedance of measuring circuits is usually large and the nonlinearity is a problem mainly if the nominal value of the transducer resistance is high. Figure 5.2A shows the effect of the input impedance of the measuring device in the transfer function of the potentiometric transducer. The input impedance of the multimeter, R_{in}, must be several times larger than the transducer output impedance R_{out}, and that usually happens when good reading devices are used. If $R_{out}/R_{in} \approx 0$, the influence of R_{in} is practically null. However, if the impedance

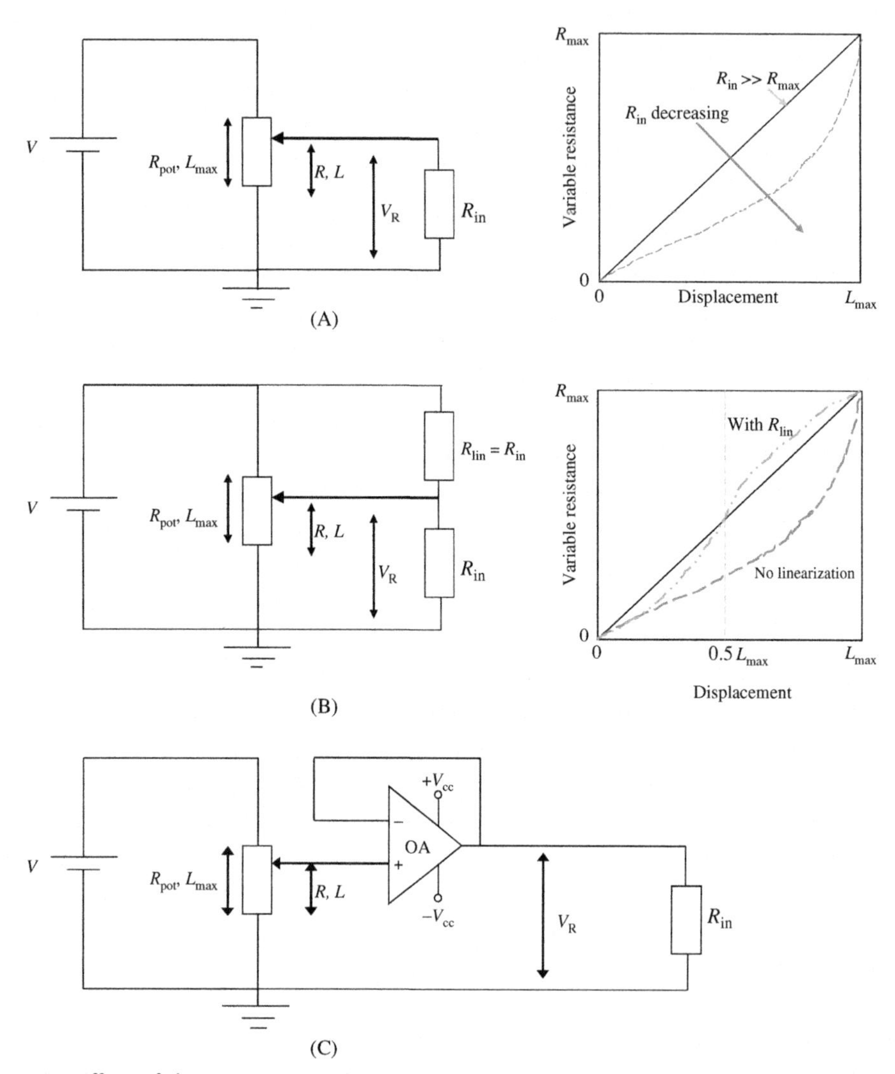

Figure 5.2 Effect of the resistance (R_{in}) "seen" by the output terminals of the resistive transducer of displacement on the linearity of its response (A) and the passive solution for minimize the nonlinearity error (B). (C) Active linearization solution with operational amplifier (OA).

values are of the same order, the effect will be an increase in nonlinearity of the output for different displacements. The introduction of a resistance R_{lin} of the same value as R_{in}, as shown in the circuit of Figure 5.2B, reduces the influence of R_{in}, linearizing the response of the transducer. Another solution to achieve error minimization is the active linearization with the use of operational amplifier (OA), as is shown in Figure 5.2C. The OA buffer circuit has unit voltage gain, a large input impedance seen by the potentiometer and a low output impedance seen by the reading device.

5.2.1.1.2 Variable resolution

The continuous potentiometric transducer of displacement has infinite resolution while the discrete potentiometric transducer has variable resolution. This variable resolution depends on the diameter of the metallic wire coils, the distance between coils, and the size of the cursor tip (Figure 5.3A). The output resistance shows steps of variable values as the cursor slides over the wire coils (Figure 5.3B). The better resolution that can be achieved is 20 μm with a 500 turns/cm potentiometer (Webster, 2010).

The ideal value of the input impedance of a potentiometric transducer is zero; the mass of the cursor and the ease with which he slides over the contact (continuous or

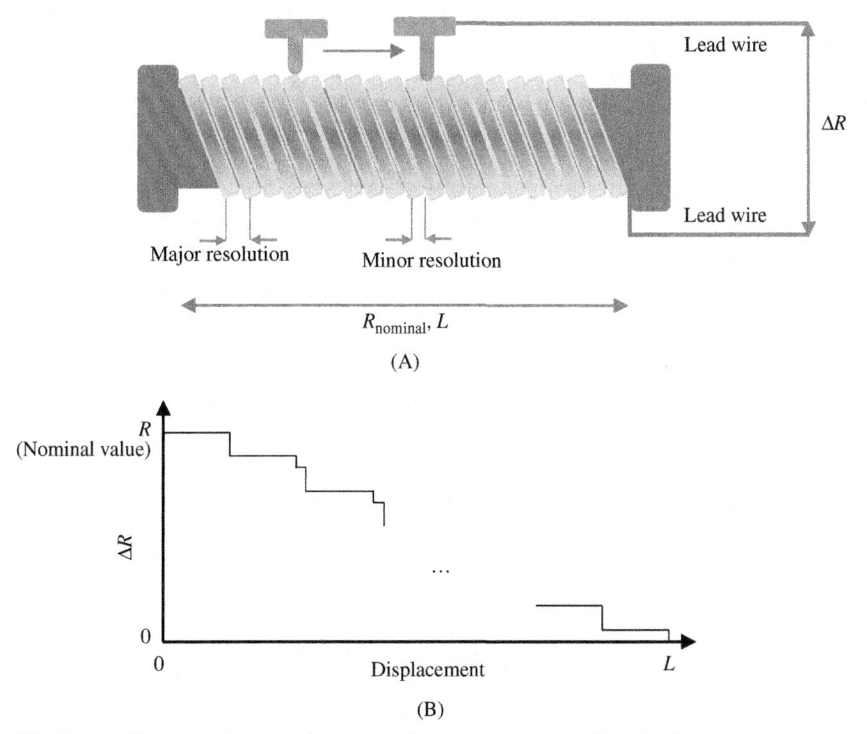

Figure 5.3 Non-uniform resolution of wound wire potentiometer-like displacement transducer. The contact touches one or two wire coils while slides over the helically wounded wire (A). When it touches two coils, they are short-circuited resulting in a different resistance value than if only one coil is touched (B).

coiled wire) is an important factor to be considered in its operation. For transducers of rotational type, the initial torque, the torque during movement and moment of inertia of the cursor should be small (ideally zero). For transducers of translation type, the initial strength and strength in movement of the cursor should also be small (or zero). However, in practice, this does not occur and initial torques have typical values of 5–50 g cm and initial force around 200 g, respectively. Specially designed devices can show good characteristics as initial torque <0.5 g cm and initial force <50 g.

Potentiometric displacement transducers are used in surface scanning devices like the one shown in Figure 5.4. Micro and nanoindentation can be performed locating the indenter probe with a XYZ resistive positioner. A similar device, developed with variable multi-turn potentiometers, is used to locate microprobes in the deep cerebral tissue during neurosurgical procedures.

Resistive displacement transducers of potentiometric type are used in the measurement of body segment orientations and inertial motion sensors of wearable assist devices. The miniaturization of electronics has allowed the creation of biofeedback assistive devices that can be worn on a belt and even embedded into clothing without affecting the wearer's ability to perform normal daily activities. To detect and predict balance instabilities in individuals with acquired brain injury, algorithms track and interpret human movement using miniaturized motion sensors, which provide real-time 3D orientation data.

Displacement transducers can be used in the construction of artificial limbs or robotic prostheses and in the determination of the position of precision instrumentation used in neurological and orthopedic surgeries. A XYZ micropositioner with resolution of 0.0004″ and linearity error equal to $\pm 0.3\%$ along a 2″ full-scale displacement can be constructed with a multi-turn potentiometer. This type of micropositioner helps locating microelectrodes during Parkinson's disease surgery.

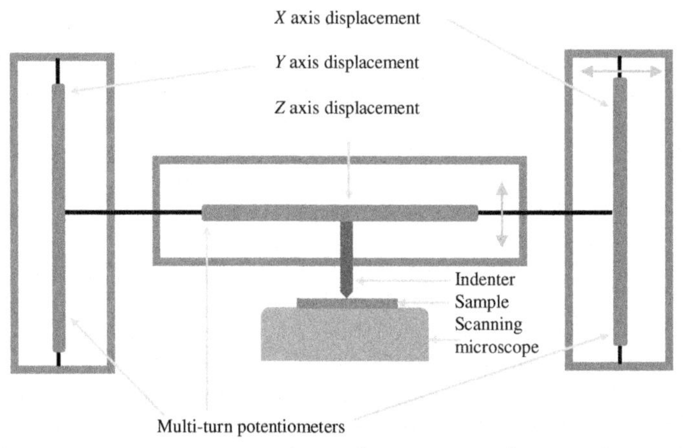

Figure 5.4 XYZ potentiometric positioner for surface micro and nanoindentation. A multi-turn potentiometer defines the displacement along each of the axes (*XYZ*).

5.2.1.2 Strain gage

The displacement transducers of the extensometer type are widely used in biomedical applications. They are commonly called strain gauges or strain gages and can be classified as elastic, metal, and semiconductors. The elastic strain gages are used to measure large displacements. An example application is their use in breathing monitor: placing an elastic band with a strain gage around the abdomen of a newborn, whose diameter varies with the phase of the ventilation cycle, the breathing can be monitored by the resistance variation of the elastic strain gage. Strain gages of metal and semiconductor are well suited to measure small displacements, smaller than 20 μm and even of the order of nanometer. This displacement range is typically found in studies of the bone surface mechanic and in investigations of the deformation of other softer human tissues such as muscles and tendons. Metallic and semiconductor strain gages are devices that require a large actuation force and the displacement value is often used as an indirect measurement used in force, pressure, and acceleration transducers (Barlian, Park, Mallon, Rastegar, & Pruitt, 2009; Cobbold, 1974; Geddes & Baker, 1968; Giorgino, Tormene, Lorussi, De Rossi, & Quaglini, 2009; OMEGA, 2014a,b; Webster, 2010).

Consider a stationary solid with plane surface area A and length L submitted to an external tensile force F as in Figure 5.5A. The mechanical responses to the applied force are stress, a traction resulting from the internal resistance of the object, and strain, the resulting deformation per unit length due to stress. If a compressive force is

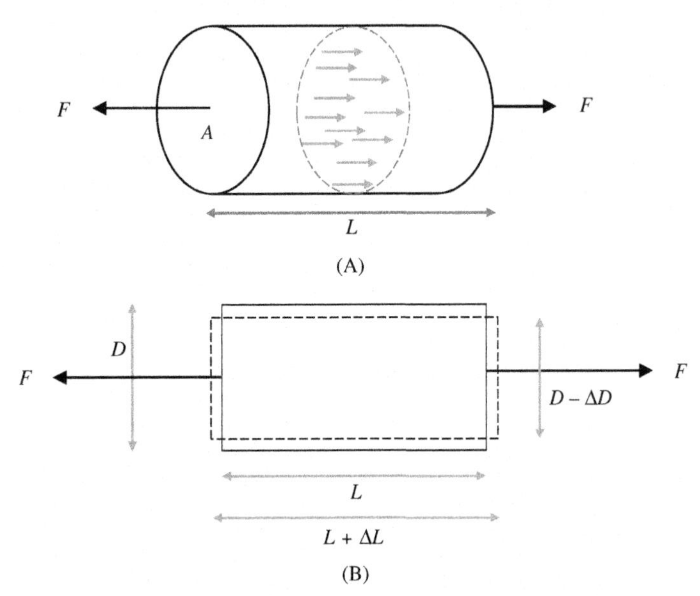

Figure 5.5 Stationary solid with plane surface area *A* and length *L* submitted to an external force *F* (A). Lateral view showing the deformation resulting from stress and longitudinal and transversal strain (B).

applied, instead of tensile, the resulting stress would be a compressive tension. For small displacements, for which the elastic limit of the extensometer material is not exceeded, the strain is directly proportional to stress.

$$\text{Stress}(\sigma) = \frac{\text{force}}{\text{unit area}} = \frac{F_\text{n}}{A} \tag{5.1}$$

$$\text{Strain}(\varepsilon) = \frac{\text{length changing}}{\text{initial length}} = \frac{\Delta L}{L} = \frac{\sigma}{E} \tag{5.2}$$

where

σ is the normal stress ((Pa) N/m^2, psi)
F_n is the normal component force (N, lb$_f$)
A is the area (m^2, in^2)
ΔL is the change of length (m, in)
L is the initial length (m, in)
ε is the unit less measure of engineering strain
E is the Young's modulus or modulus of elasticity (Pa, psi).

Equation (5.1) is valid if the internal resistive forces are uniformly distributed all over the area. The solid also suffers transversal deformation, in addition to longitudinal deformation, and so, strain can be of longitudinal and transversal types (Figure 5.5B):

$$\varepsilon_\text{L} = \frac{\Delta L}{L} \tag{5.3}$$

$$\varepsilon_\text{T} = \frac{\Delta D}{D} \tag{5.4}$$

Poisson's ratio ν is defined as the ratio between longitudinal (or lateral) and transversal (or axial) stress:

$$\nu = -\frac{\varepsilon_\text{L}}{\varepsilon_\text{T}} \tag{5.5}$$

The negative sign is introduced for convenience so that ν comes out positive. For structural materials ν $0.0 \leq \nu < 0.5$. For most metals ν lies in the range $0.25-0.35$; for ceramics, $\nu \approx 0.10$ and for rubber, $\nu \approx 0.5$. A material for which $\nu = 0.5$ is called incompressible.

Typical values of strain $\Delta L/L$ are very little. The strain can be compressive or tensile and is usually measured by strain gages, which are designed to convert mechanical displacement in electronic signal proportional to the change experienced by the sensor, usually electrical resistance when properly inserted into an electronic circuit.

The functioning of the elastic, metallic, and semiconductor strain gages is based on the variation of electrical resistance of a conductive fluid volume (elastic strain gage), a wire, tape, or thin metal film (metallic strain gage), or semiconductor material (semiconductor strain gage), inserted, bonded, or deposited on an insulating, flexible, and thin surface which is subjected to mechanical stress. The equation below is presented considering the material of the strain gage as having cylindrical shape, such as a wire, with much smaller diameter than its length. The electrical resistance of a wire is defined by Eq. (5.6):

$$R = \left(\frac{\rho L}{A}\right) \tag{5.6}$$

where

ρ is the resistivity of the strain gage material
L is the length of the wire
A is the area of the wire section.

For a wire with diameter D and length L, $A = \pi D^2/4$ and Eq. (5.6) can be written as

$$R = R(\rho, L, D) = \frac{4 \cdot L \cdot \rho}{\pi \cdot D^2} \tag{5.7}$$

Equation (5.7) shows that the resistance of the wire is function of its length, diameter, and resistivity. A incremental variation of the resistance is calculated by partial derivatives and can be simplified by Eq. (5.9):

$$\frac{\Delta R}{R} = \frac{\Delta L}{L} - 2\frac{\Delta D}{D} + \frac{\Delta \rho}{\rho} \tag{5.8}$$

Replacing Eqs. (5.3)–(5.5) in Eq. (5.7), we get Eq. (5.9):

$$\frac{\Delta R}{R} = (1 + 2\upsilon)\frac{\Delta L}{L} + \frac{\Delta \rho}{\rho} \tag{5.9}$$

The left-hand side of Eq. (5.10) is the incremental variation of the wire resistance due to the stress. In the right-hand side, the first component reflects the dimensional effect of the stress and the second component, the piezoresistive effect. Dividing both sides of Eq. (5.7) by $\Delta L/L$:

$$G = \frac{\Delta R/R}{\Delta L/L} = 1 + 2\upsilon + \frac{\Delta \rho/\rho}{\Delta L/L} \tag{5.10}$$

where G is the sensitivity of the strain gage, also called gage factor or sensitivity of deformation.

Metallic strain gages have no effective piezoresistive effect and their sensitivity depends only on Poisson's ratio. The semiconductor strain gages, on the contrary, have significant piezoresistive effect. The average Poisson's ratio of metals is 0.3 and the sensitivity of most metallic strain gages is ≈ 1.6. The sensitivity of semiconductor strain gages depends on the material used and its level of impurity.

5.2.1.2.1 Elastic strain gages

The elastic displacement transducers are made from elastic and flexible tubes (silicon or rubber) filled with conductive fluid, such as mercury, copper sulfate, and electrolyte paste (e.g., same as used for EEG). The ends of the tube are sealed by electrodes of copper, silver, or platinum (Figure 5.6) and are used to measure the change in resistance of the conductive fluid due to the displacement of the tube. They usually have larger dimensions than the strain gages of metal or semiconductor and are used for measuring large linear and volumetric variations.

The strain gage shown in Figure 5.6 can be coupled to an elastic band that is wrapped around the leg or the arm of the patient in order to conduct member plethysmography tests that evaluate the variation of the blood volume in isolated limb segment. If the conductive fluid inside the elastic tube is liquid mercury, which is essentially incompressible, a tensile force applied between the extremities of the tube stretches it (as in the blood income in the limb during cardiac systole) and reduces the tube diameter, with the volume remaining constant. Equation (5.6) can be written as

$$R = \left(\frac{\rho L^2}{V}\right) \tag{5.11}$$

where

V is the volume of mercury inside the elastic tube

L is the length of the tube

A is the cross-sectional area of the tube filled with mercury.

The variation in mercury resistance to a length stretching can be approximated by

$$\frac{\Delta R}{\Delta L} = \frac{2\rho L}{V} = \frac{2R}{L} \tag{5.12}$$

Equation (5.12) shows that the fractional change in resistance is twice the fractional change in length. If the mercury strain gage is stretched by 1%, its resistance increases by 2%. This is valid for all liquid strain gages, since all liquids are incompressible.

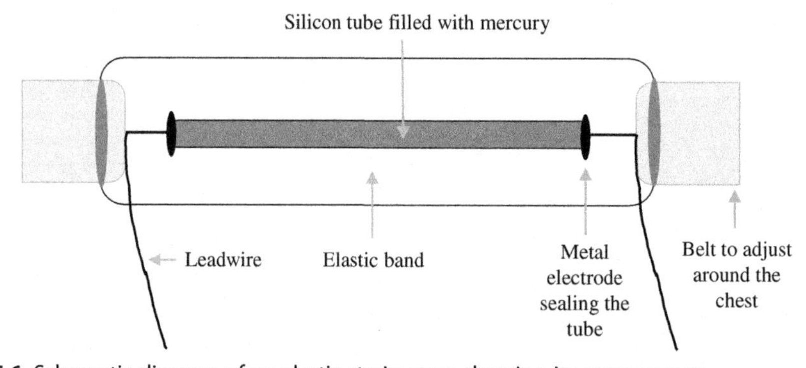

Figure 5.6 Schematic diagram of an elastic strain gage showing its components.

Elastic displacement transducers are used with less frequency in biomedical engineering than metal and semiconductor strain gages. Mercury strain gages were used in hospitals for blood pressure monitoring (arterial pulse plethysmography). A rubber tube filled with mercury was stretched around a leg or arm and the pressure fluctuations were recorded on strip-chart recorders. Such devices were replaced by solid state strain gage or other modern technology instruments. Elastic displacement transducers are also used to monitor, typically in neonates, the displacement of the chest during breathing, which is useful to avoid death by respiratory arrest of the sleep apnea test that typically affects premature neonates. The elastic strap with the extensometer is adjusted around the chest of the baby and allows monitoring breathing through the displacement of the chest wall: the elastic tube filled with mercury stretches during inspiration and returns to the initial end-expiratory position, with variation of electrical resistance of the conductive fluid.

Typical characteristics of elastic strain gages are internal diameter equal to 0.5 mm; external diameter 2 mm; length from 3 to 25 cm, and resistance values from 0.02 to 2 Ω/cm. The nonlinearity error varies with the distension percentage with regard to the original length: for deformations up to 10%, the error is in the range $\pm 1\%$ of full scale; above 30% of the resting value, the error is $\pm 4\%$. They respond well to frequencies <10 Hz; frequency components above 30 Hz are considerably distorted (Cobbold, 1974; Geddes & Baker, 1968; Webster, 2010).

5.2.1.2.2 Metallic strain gages

The metallic strain gage is basically a resistor whose electrical resistance varies proportionally to the variation of its length (Eq. (5.7)). Metallic strain gages must to be coupled to the specimen under test and according to the way they are coupled, they are classified as bonded and unbonded. Bonded strain gages are constructed with resistance wires as plane grids (Figure 5.6A) and wound grids (Figure 5.6B), or depositing thin metallic films on a substrate to form foil grids (Figure 5.6C). Plane, wound, and thin film grid strain gages must be carefully bonded to the surface of the material under stress, called the test specimen (All About Circuits 1, 2014; Cobbold, 1974; Dally et al., 1993; Geddes & Baker, 1968; OMEGA, 2014a,b; Webster, 2010).

5.2.1.2.2.1 Bonded strain gages Plane grid strain gages were developed in the end of the 1930s. The resistance wire is formatted like a plane grid; then the grid is bonded to a flexible substrate and receives a thin layer of insulating material (Figure 5.7A). The substrate can be a thin layer of paper or epoxy and the insulating covering can be a thin layer of paper, felt, or varnish.

Wound grid strain gages are constructed by winding the strain-sensitive metal wire around a support made of paper, for instance, and then recovering the set with an insulating material (Figure 5.7B).

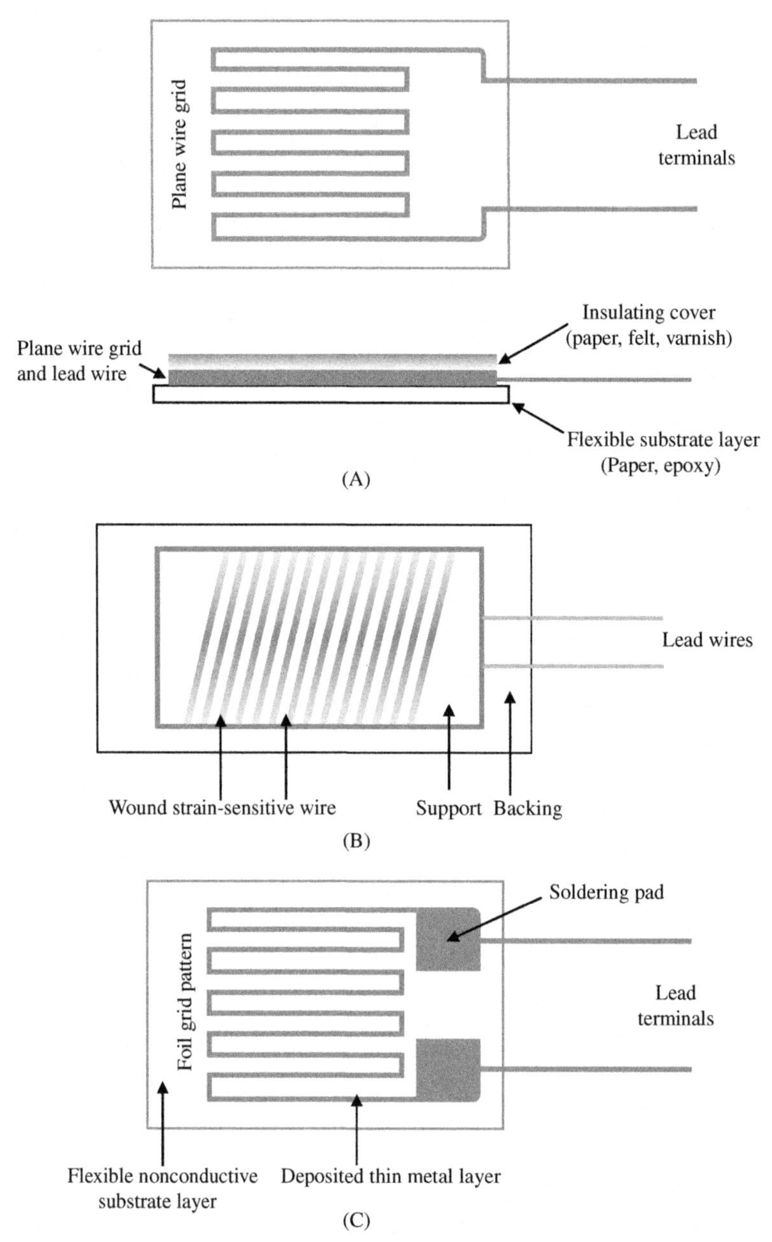

Figure 5.7 Metallic strain gages. (A) Plane wire grid, top view and lateral view. (B) Wound wire grid. (C) Foil grid. An insulating material recovers the bodies of the gages.

Foil grids can be fabricated with printed circuit technique (etching), allowing complex and varied metallic grid formats that can be bonded to a proper substrate material, called the carrier, for instance, a thin layer of ceramic; alternatively thin strips of metallic film are deposited on a nonconducting substrate without the need of using any cement or glue (Figure 5.7C). They are the most used strain gages since 1950, when they were developed. They are constructed with lengths varying from 20 μm to 10 mm and grid thickness ~25 μm, to get nominal resistance values from a few tens of Ω to a few units of kΩ (unstressed).

The strain gage size must be small enough to be deformation sensitive in the maximum tension point of the specimen. Ideally, its rigidity should not interfere with reinforcement or damping, and its resistance should vary linearly with the tension being measured. Measurements obtained with strain gage must be repeatable, reproducible, stable, and insensitive to environment conditions, mainly temperature. Moreover, the strain gage also should present low transversal sensitivity and hysteresis, small response time, low cost, and the ability to do static and dynamic measurements.

Real bonded resistive strain gages can be used to do static and dynamic measurements with very low hysteresis; they are relatively low cost and temperature insensitive; their accuracy is better than ±0.10% and are constructed with nominal resistances ranging from 100 Ω to 1 kΩ in sizes small as a few millimeters and ΔL_{max} as large as a few μm. The strain gage sensitivity varies according to the metal or metallic alloy composition used in its grid. Table 5.1 shows some examples of commercial grid materials and their sensibility values (Cobbold, 1974; Geddes & Baker, 1968; Johnson, 1997). Isoelastic strain gage is indicated to dynamic measurements, even the impact type, but is very sensitive to temperature changing.

When the direction of the main deformation of the specimen under test is known, a uniaxial extensometer (Figure 5.8A) can be used and it must be adequately bonded to specimen surface, that is, along the direction of the main deformation, cause the strain gage insensitive to lateral forces. If deformation occurs in two main directions, and these directions are known, a two-direction rosette can be used, like the one shown in Figure 5.8B, in this case, sensitive to deformation in orthogonal directions; both strain gages are constructed on the same substrate. If the main deformation directions are unknown, multiple direction rosettes can be used. Figure 5.8C shows three strain gages constructed in the same substrate, each one sensitive to a different direction.

Table 5.1 Metal strain gage grid composition and sensitivity

Grid material	Composition	Sensitivity G
Nicromel	80% Ni; 20% Cr	+2.0
Constantancopel	45% Ni; 55% Cr	+2.0
Isoelastic	36% Ni; 8% Cr; 0.5% Mo; 55.5% Fe	+3.5
Manganine	4% Ni; 12% Mn; 84% Cu	+0.47
Iridium–platinum	5% Ir; 95% Pt	+5.10
Monel	67% Ni; 33% Cu	+1.9
Nickel	100% Ni	−12.0

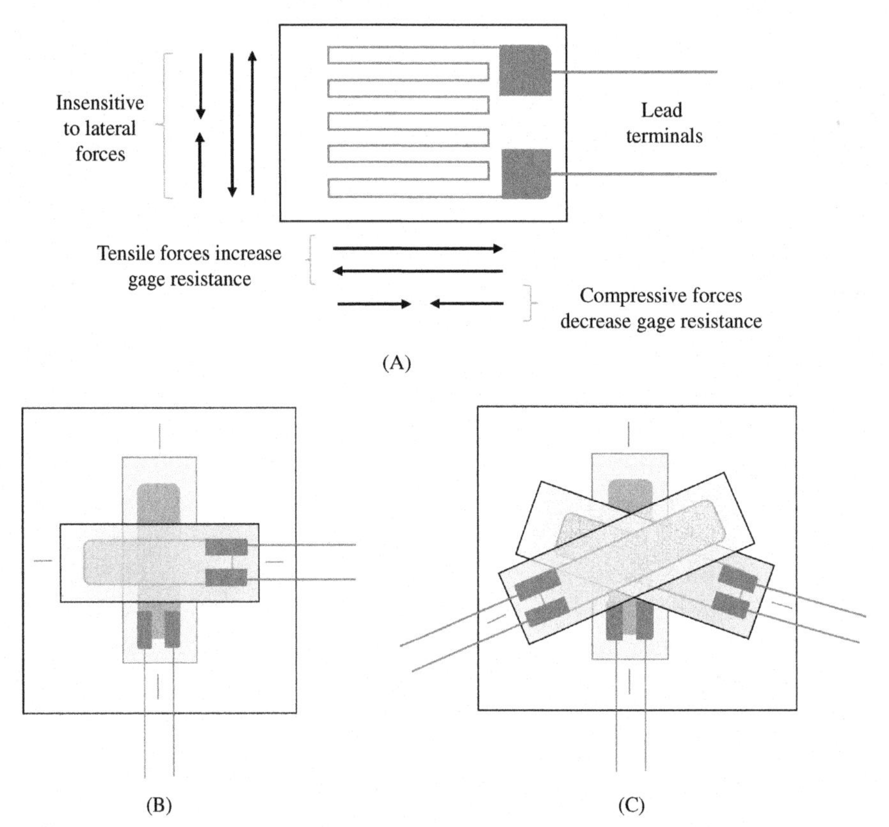

Figure 5.8 (A) Uniaxial, (B) biaxial, and (C) triaxial bonded extensometers.

The metallic material of the grid of the bonded strain gage and the wires used in unbonded strain gages should have high sensitivity (G) and resistivity (ρ), low sensitivity to temperature variation, low thermal emf (electromotive force) when connected to another material and to be corrosion resistant.

5.2.1.2.2.2 Unbonded strain gages Bonded strain gages must to be adequately glued, usually to the surface of a larger structure under test, to obtain accurate and stable strain measurements. In many applications, it is not practical the displacement sensor to be glued to the specimen under test, as for instance, during direct blood pressure measurement.

Metal strain gages can also be obtained with a structure similar to that shown in Figure 5.9A, where flexible wires are assembled between a fixed frame and a movable armature, without being glued to the surface of the specimen. In this example, four sets of thin strain-sensitive wires are wrapped around two electrically insulated supports forming four resistors of the same value (unstressed); in each set, one support is

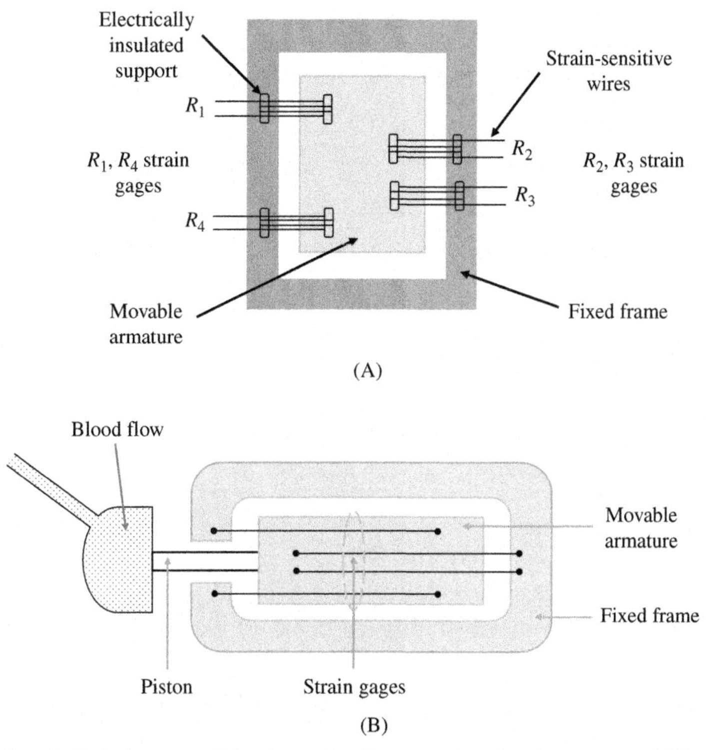

Figure 5.9 Unbonded strain gage: (A) schematic diagram showing its parts and (B) representation of a blood pressure transducer.

connected to the fixed frame and the other to the movable armature. The movable armature is coupled to the specimen and as it is deformed under stress, two wires are submitted to a tensile force while the other two to compressive force, changing their resistances. Figure 5.9B shows a schematic diagram of a direct blood pressure transducer. The flow of blood is in contact with a piston, which moves back and forth by the pressure wave together with the fixed frame of the displacement transducer, varying resistances of wires wrapped between the fixed frame and the moving armature. A pair of wires is compressed and its resistance decreases; the other pair of wires is tensioned and its resistance is increased. The resistance variation information is used for computing the blood pressure (Cobbold, 1974; Webster, 2010).

5.2.1.2.3 Semiconductor strain gages

In the 1950s, scientists at Bell Laboratories discovered the piezoresistive characteristics of Ge and Si. In the 1970s, the first semiconductor strain gages were produced with silicon and germanium crystals of high purity and artificially doped (extrinsic semiconductors). When subjected to an external force, Ge and Si crystals undergo a

Table 5.2 Sensitivity of semiconductor strain gages

Grid material	Sensitivity G
Silicon type P	100 to 170
Silicon type N	−100 to −140
Germanium type P	102
Germanium type N	−150

reorganization of their crystalline domains, allowing more mobility to electronic charges and, beyond physical deformation and variation of electrical resistance, they also exhibit resistivity changing. Equation (5.10) can be rewritten as

$$G = \frac{\Delta R/R}{\Delta L/L} = 1 + 2\upsilon + \frac{\Delta\rho/\rho}{\Delta L/L} = 1 + 2\upsilon + \pi E \tag{5.13}$$

where

π is the piezoresistive coefficient (m^2/N)

E is the Young's modulus or modulus of elasticity (Pa, psi).

In Equation (5.13), the metal strain gage behavior is explained by $(1 + 2\upsilon)$ parcel, the dimensional effect, but to semiconductor strain gages, the piezoresistive parcel, πE, predominates. The change in resistivity has a greater effect on the value of the resistance than the change in geometry. Although semiconductor materials exhibit substantial nonlinear behavior and are temperature sensitive, sensitivity is more than 50 times greater than metal strain gages (Table 5.2) (Cobbold, 1974; OMEGA, 2014a,b).

Semiconductor strain gages are fabricated as loose units, usually of P Silicon, and as inserted units, which are P Silicon regions diffused in a larger N Silicon substrate (wafer) or vice versa. Loose units have different formats as bar (strait and thin strips) and U shape (Figure 5.10A). P diffused regions of inserted units can have the most variable formats, as complex rosettes or simple squares (Figure 5.10B).

Loose semiconductor strain gages are micro machined from a bulk of single grown crystal of P Silicon and they are used isolated or combined to form several configurations of measuring circuits (usually Wheatstone bridges). Inserted/diffused strain gages are obtained from the same diffusion process used in the integrated circuits fabrication. Active diffused regions should coincide with the larger strain areas of the object under test, commonly with one or two areas being used to temperature compensation. Same adhesive types used to bond wire and foil metal gages can be used to bond loose and inserted semiconductor gages. A thin layer of epoxy is commonly used.

Linearity error of loose semiconductor strain gages is in the range 10–20% while inserted gages have linearity error $\approx 1\%$. Table 5.3 resumes some characteristics of metal and semiconductor strain gages (Cobbold, 1974; Dally et al., 1993; Geddes & Baker; 1968; Webster, 2010).

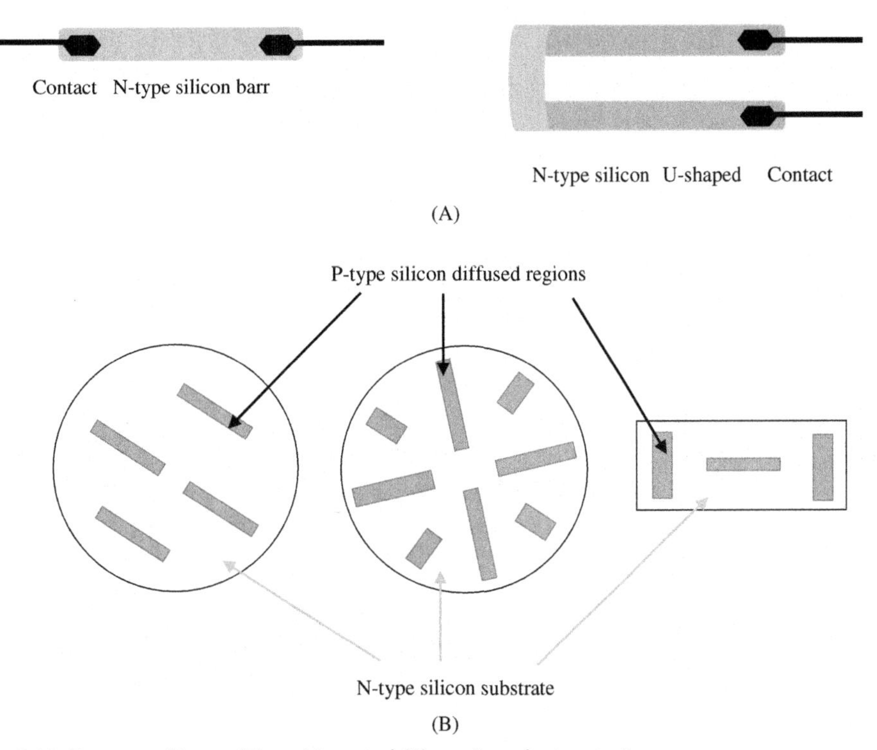

Figure 5.10 Formats of loose (A) and inserted (B) semiconductor strain gages.

Table 5.3 Typical values of metal and semiconductor strain gage characteristics

Strain gage characteristic	Metal	Semiconductor
Strain range ($\varepsilon = \Delta L/L$)	$(1 \times 10^{-1}-40 \times 10^{3}) \times 10^{-6} \times \varepsilon$	$(1 \times 10^{-3}-3 \times 10^{3}) \times 10^{-6} \times \varepsilon$
Sensitivity (G)	2.0–12	100–170
Nominal value (Ω)	120, 350, ... , 5,000, 10,000	1,000–5,000
Resistance tolerance	0.1–0.2%	1–2%
Linearity error	1–5%	10–20%—loose ≈ 1% inserted
Size (mm)	3–6 (smaller and larger sizes available)	1–5 (smaller sizes available)

5.2.1.2.4 Measuring circuits

Wheatstone bridge circuit is ideal to achieve the high accuracy needed for measuring typical small changes in resistance (a fraction of nominal resistance for full-scale displacement) imposed by the elastic limits of strain gage and test specimen materials. Several bridge configurations can be used—quarter, half, or full-bridge—with one to four active strain gages to measure strain through the bridge imbalance with a precision voltmeter. Each configuration results in a different equation to determine the strain

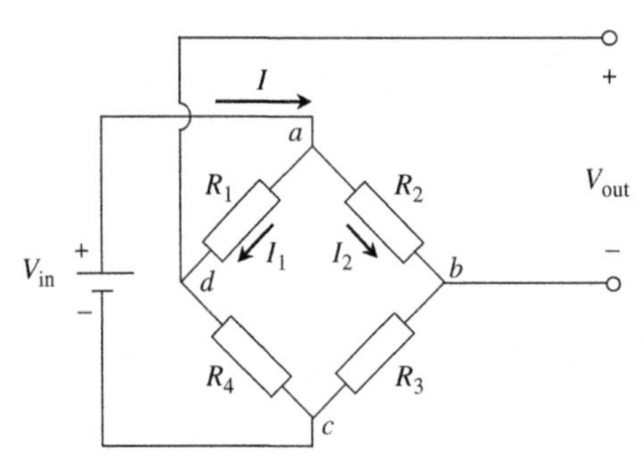

Figure 5.11 Wheatstone bridge circuit.

and thus, the displacement (Cobbold, 1974; Dally et al., 1993; Geddes & Baker, 1968; National Instruments Corporation 1, 2014; OMEGA, 2014a,b). Figure 5.11 shows a generic bridge circuit and below follows the overall solution equation for V_{out} as a function of V_{in} and the values of the resistances in the four arms or the bridge.

When the bridge is balanced: $V_{out} = 0$, $V_{ad} = V_{ab}$, and $V_{dc} = V_{bc}$, the potential drops in the branches adc and abc are equal to V_{in}:

$$I_1 = \frac{V_{in}}{R_1 + R_4} \quad \text{and} \quad I_2 = \frac{V_{in}}{R_2 + R_3} \tag{5.14}$$

$$V_{out} = R_4 I_1 - R_3 I_2 = 0 \tag{5.15}$$

and finally

$$V_{out} = \left(\frac{R_4}{R_1 + R_4} - \frac{R_3}{R_2 + R_3}\right) V_{in} \tag{5.16}$$

Making all resistances in the bridge equal to R and replacing one of them by a strain gage with nominal unstressed resistance also equal to R, for example, R_3, the configuration is called one-quarter bridge (Figure 5.12A). In the balance, the output of the bridge is null. If the strain gage resistance R changes to $(R + \Delta R)$, the voltmeter indicates $V_0 \neq 0$, that is proportional to the strain experienced by the strain gage. Equation (5.16) becomes

$$V_{out} = \left(\frac{R + \Delta R}{2R + \Delta R} - \frac{R}{2R}\right) V_{in} \tag{5.17}$$

or

$$V_{out} = \frac{\Delta R}{2(2R + \Delta R)} V_B \cong \frac{\Delta R}{4R} V_B \tag{5.18}$$

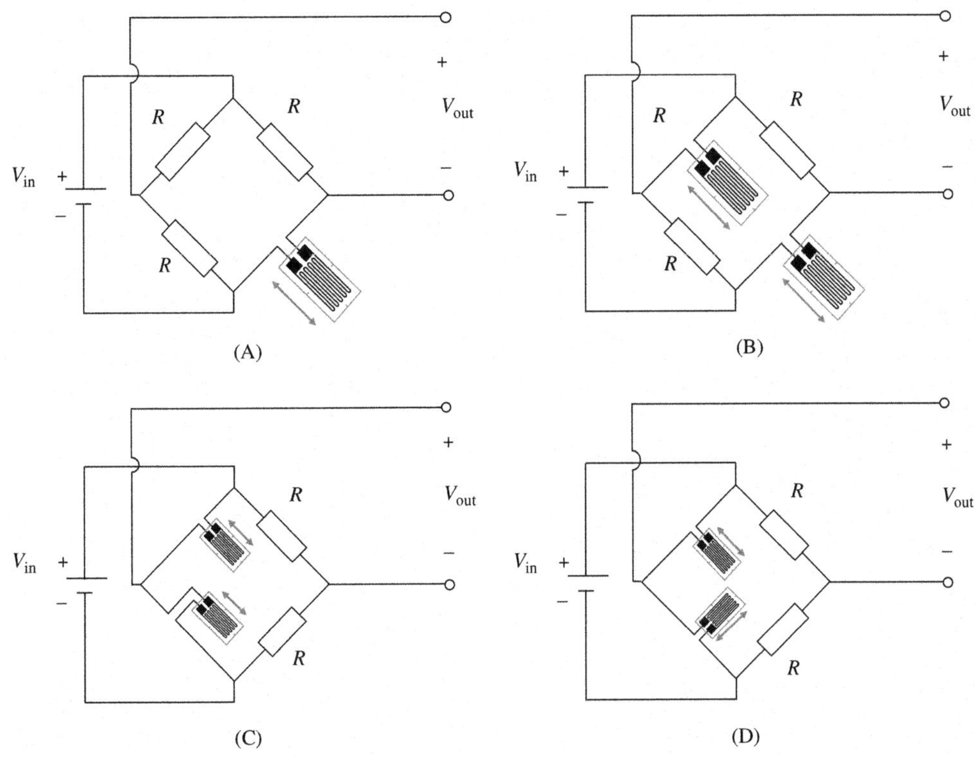

Figure 5.12 Examples of different configurations of Wheatstone bridge circuit: (A) one-quarter bridge and (B–D) half-bridges.

As

$$\varepsilon = \frac{\Delta L}{L} = \frac{\Delta R}{GR} \tag{5.19}$$

replacing Eq. (5.19) in Eq. (5.18), results in

$$V_{out} \cong 0.25 G\varepsilon V_{in} \tag{5.20}$$

Replacing two resistors by strain gages, the configuration is called half-bridge and the resulting equation depends on which resistors are replaced and the direction of sensitivity of the gages. If two resistors are in opposed arms of the bridge, for example, R_1 and R_3, by active strain gages, both sensitive to tension or compression (same direction forces) (Figure 5.12B), the output voltage is calculated by

$$V_{out} = \frac{G\varepsilon}{2 + G\varepsilon} V_{in} \tag{5.21}$$

If active strain gages replace two resistors, but in adjacent arms (R_1 and R_4) (Figure 5.12C), one sensitive to tension and the other to compression (opposite direction forces), the unbalanced output voltage is

$$V_{out} = \frac{G \cdot \varepsilon}{2} V_{in} \tag{5.22}$$

Replacing R_1 and R_4 by active strain gages sensitive to tension or compression, but in perpendicular directions (Figure 5.12D), the unbalanced output voltage is

$$V_{out} = \frac{G\varepsilon(1-\nu)}{2 + G\varepsilon(1-\nu)} V_{in} \tag{5.23}$$

where ν is the Poisson's coefficient: $\nu = -\varepsilon_L/\varepsilon_T$ defined in Eq. (5.5), and ε_L and ε_T are the strains in lateral and longitudinal directions, respectively.

Various combinations can be made with the positions of the strain gages on the bridge, making them active or not, acting in the direction of deformation or opposite to it, or even perpendicular to the deformation being measured, resulting in a different equation and in a different measurement sensitivity. It is easy to notice that Eq. (5.22) has twice the sensitivity of Eq. (5.20). According to Eq. (5.20), for $V_{in} = 5$ V, if the gage resistance changes 1%, results in an output voltage $V_0 = 1.25$ mV; with the same conditions, the output voltage of the half-bridge circuit of Figure 5.12C will be $V_0 = 2.50$ mV. The linear relation between the strain and the output voltage of Eqs. (5.20) and (5.22) is easily noticed while Eqs. (5.21) and (5.23) show nonlinear relations between output voltage and strain.

The biggest sensibilities are obtained with active gages in the four arms of the bridge (Figure 5.13), which is not always easily implemented due to additional space required in the specimen surface. This configuration is called full-bridge and allows several combinations of stressed strain gages in different directions, each one resulting in a particular equation with different sensitivity and output/input linear or nonlinear relation. Ideally, strain gages with the same nominal unstressed resistances should be

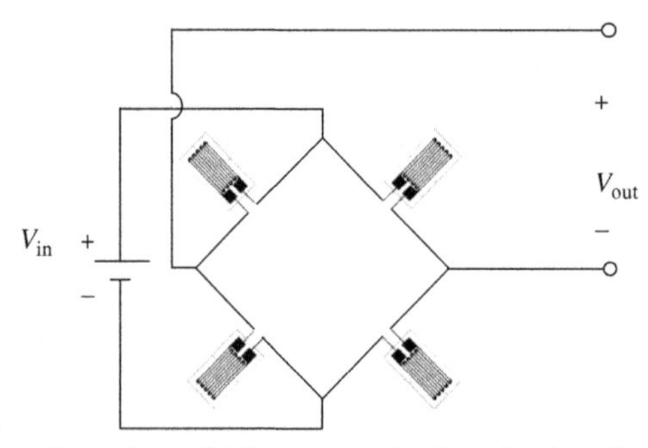

Figure 5.13 Full-bridge configuration of Wheatstone bridge circuit. All gages are stressed (under tensile or compressive forces).

used in the four arms of the bridge, even if only one is active; the other three would act as dummy gages, for compensation, mainly of temperature. Practically, this solution is not always adopted due to its higher cost.

5.2.1.2.5 Influence of the temperature on strain gage performance

The strain gage and the specimen under test are affected by environment condition changings, as for example, electromagnet field, humidity, and temperature. The temperature is the most important factor affecting the measurement of displacement with strain gage. Different materials are present: the grid (metallic or semiconductor), substrate (paper, ceramic, epoxy, semiconductor), adhesive, and the specimen under test; each one is affected by the temperature changing with its own thermal coefficient. In addition to changes in the temperature of the strain gage caused by ambient temperature, the current flowing through it contributes to its heating, and modifies its resistance, giving rise to thermal gradient between the grid and the substrate and the specimen, which creates emf (thermocouple effect). The measuring circuit interprets the resistance modification, caused by temperature modification, as a strain change in the specimen. Different thermal expansion coefficients of grid, substrate, and specimen add strain (traction or compression) to the measurement. The sensitivity factor G also will experience a change because the length of the resistance will change due to temperature variation. These factors should be considered when evaluating the output signals obtained in the measuring circuits. What matters is the material deformation effect and not due to temperature variation.

In order to keep apparent strain due to temperature changes as small as possible, each strain gage is matched during the production to a linear thermal expansion coefficient and are auto compensated to the substrate materials modifying their compositions. In practice, it is possible to minimize the temperature-dependent modification of the gage resistance using a dummy gage, which is exemplified in Figure 5.14A. The dummy gage is equal to the active one and is applied to a separate piece of the same material as the specimen under test, but it is not submitted to strain, only to the same environment conditions. If both gages, active and dummy, are in adjacent arms of the Wheatstone bridge, the resistance variation caused by temperature is canceled. The use of dummy gage also enlarges the sensitivity of the measurement (Dally et al., 1993). The dummy gage can also be applied to the specimen under test, but in a position that does not allow it to be strain sensitive, as shown in Figure 5.14B.

5.2.2 Capacitive transducers

The operating principle of a capacitive transducer is the variation in the nominal capacitance (C) of a capacitor, or two or more interconnected capacitors, due to a nonelectrical quantity, in this case, the displacement. A capacitor consists of a set of two conductive plates separated by a dielectric. Generally, it is possible to change the capacitance varying the distance between the plates of the capacitor, the value of the

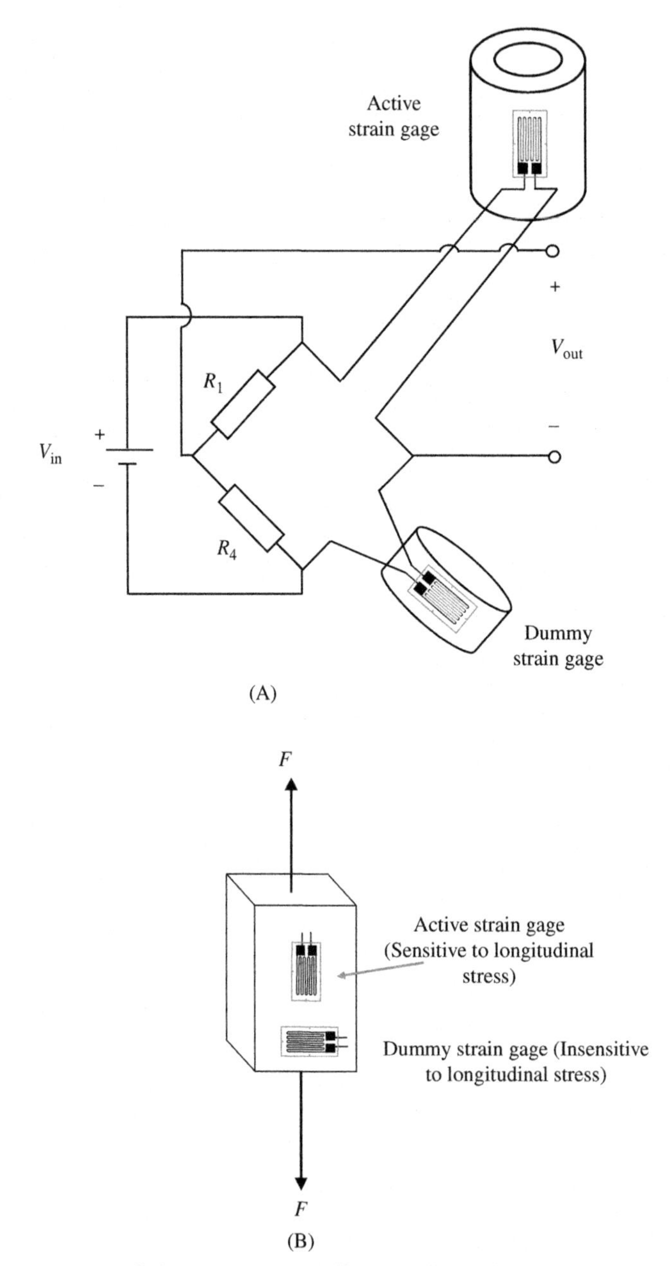

Figure 5.14 Minimization of the temperature effect on the strain gage resistance using dummy gage in the same specimen (B) and in a separate piece of the same material as the specimen (A).

dielectric or the common area of its plates (Figure 5.15). The capacitance of a capacitor with parallel plates is expressed by

$$C = \varepsilon_0 \varepsilon_r \frac{A}{x} \tag{5.24}$$

where

ε_0 is the vacuum permittivity
ε_r is the dielectric constant of the insulating layer between the capacitor plates
A is the plate surface
x is the distance between the plates.

Thus, it is possible to vary any of the parameters of Eq. (5.24) and to use the capacitance variation to calculate the displacement measurement:

$$\Delta C = f(\varepsilon_r, A, x) \tag{5.25}$$

The parallel plate capacitor with variation of the distance between the plates is the simplest and most widely used as a displacement transducer. Deriving Eq. (5.24) with regard to the distance between the plates (x), we obtain an expression for the sensitivity of this type of transducer:

$$S = \frac{\Delta C}{\Delta x} = -\frac{\varepsilon A}{x^2} \tag{5.26}$$

where

$$\varepsilon = \varepsilon_0 \times \varepsilon_r$$

The transducer sensitivity is better to capacitors with little separation between plates and large areas.

Figure 5.15 shows some of the possibilities of varying the parameters of the plane plates capacitor to measure linear displacement. In addition to the distance between the plates, it is also possible to measure linear displacements varying the dielectric, and therefore, E, and the common area between the plates (Cobbold, 1974; Dally et al., 1993; Geddes & Baker, 1968; Webster, 2010).

A blood pressure transducer can be built with a capacitive displacement sensor: a parallel plate capacitor in which one metal plate is fixed and the other plate is a thin, flexible diaphragm. The diaphragm is deformed with the variation of arterial blood pressure by varying the distance between the capacitor plates and thus the capacitance. The variable capacitance is typically used in an electronic circuit with high gain amplifier and powered by sinusoidal voltage with frequency of tens of kHz. The output voltage obtained is directly proportional to the separation of the capacitor plates. This distance varies in a range of lower frequencies (heartbeat) than that of the excitation frequency of the circuit and is determined by demodulation and filtering. Another example of biomedical

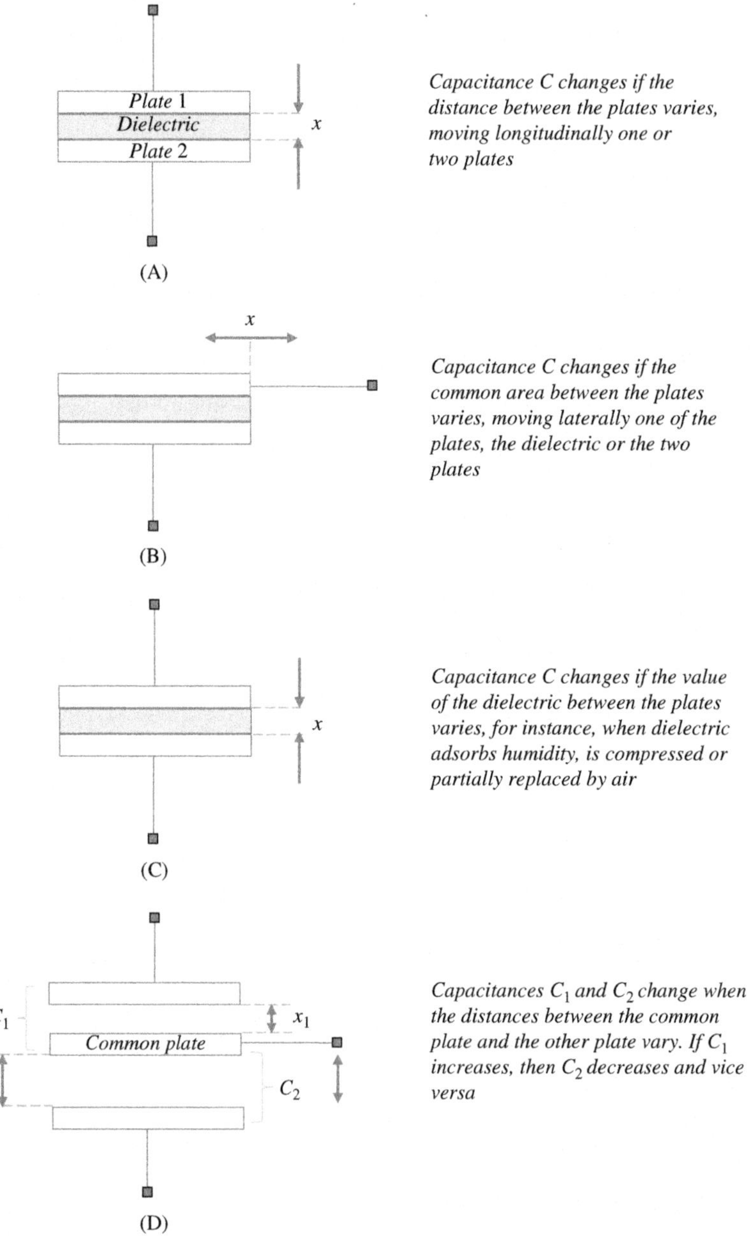

Figure 5.15 Capacitor with parallel plane plates with variable distance between plates (A), with common area variable (B), and with variable dielectric (C). Differential capacitor with plane plates (D).

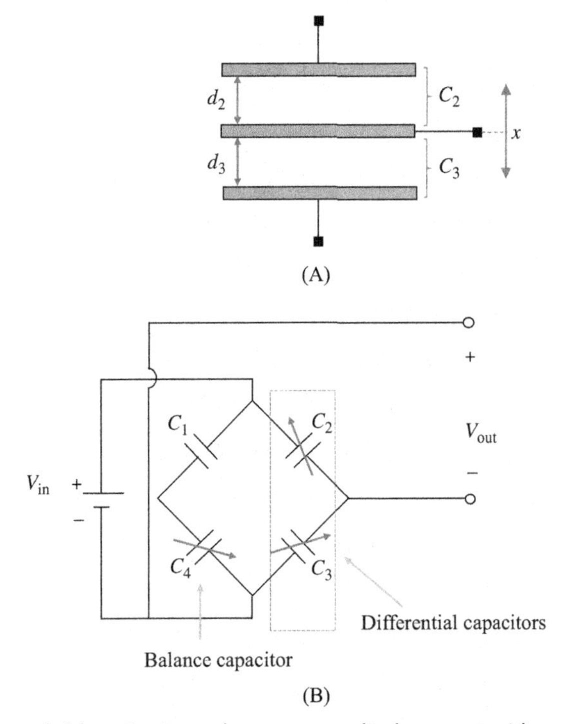

Figure 5.16 Wheatstone bridge circuit used to measure displacement with capacitive transducer.

application of capacitive displacement transducer is the measurement of the wall displacement of the heart or blood vessel, with similar electronic circuit, but with a shielded parallel plate capacitor, in which the movable plate is the conductive surface of the biological tissue (or target plate). Shielding the fixed plate (or sensor head) increases the response linearity (Dally et al., 1993). Commercial versions can measure distances from tens of micrometers to a few centimeters and have flat band pass from DC to 500 Hz.

If differential capacitors are used, then the Wheatstone bridge is the indicated measuring circuit (Figure 5.16), usually with one fixed capacitor, the two variables capacitors of the transducer, and one adjustable capacitor used to balance the bridge (Cobbold, 1974).

The equations describing the operation of the capacitive transducer of Figure 5.16A are shown below. At the balance $C_1 = C_2 = C_3 = C_4$ and $d_2 = d_3 = d$, that is, the distance between the plates of the two differential capacitors is the same. Both capacitors, C_2 and C_3, have the same area, A, and the displacement of the moveable plate is x. When the central plate moves upward, the differential capacitances are

$$C_2 = \frac{[\varepsilon A]}{[d - x]} \tag{5.27}$$

$$C_3 = \frac{[\varepsilon A]}{[d + x]} \tag{5.28}$$

The displacement of the central plate causes a fractional difference of capacitance, which varies linearly with the variation in the plates distance in each capacitor:

$$C_2 - C_3 = \frac{[\varepsilon A]}{[1/(d-x) - 1/(d+x)]} \tag{5.29}$$

$$C_2 - C_3 = \frac{[\varepsilon A]}{[2x/(d^2 - x^2)]} \tag{5.30}$$

And

$$C_2 + C_3 = \frac{[\varepsilon A]}{[1/(d-x) + 1/(d+x)]} \tag{5.31}$$

$$C_2 + C_3 = \frac{[\varepsilon A]}{[2d/(d^2 - x^2)]} \tag{5.32}$$

Dividing Eq. (5.31) by Eq. (5.32) results in

$$\frac{(C_2 - C_3)}{(C_2 + C_3)} = \frac{2x}{2d} = \frac{x}{d} \tag{5.33}$$

The proportionality and linearity between the fractional capacitance change and the displacement x is easily noticed. The output voltage for a displacement x is calculated as

$$V_{\text{out}}(j\omega) = V_{C_4}(j\omega) - V_{C_3}(j\omega) \tag{5.34}$$

The voltage drop in C_4 is

$$V_{C_4}(j\omega) = \frac{(V_{\text{in}}(j\omega)/j\omega C_4)}{[(1/j\omega C_1) + (1/j\omega C_4)]} \tag{5.35}$$

or

$$V_{C_4}(j\omega) = \left[\frac{C_4}{(C_1 + C_4)}\right] V_{\text{in}}(j\omega) \tag{5.36}$$

Similarly, the voltage drop in C_3 is

$$V_{C_3}(j\omega) = \left[\frac{C_3}{(C_2 + C_3)}\right] V_{\text{in}}(j\omega) \tag{5.37}$$

Then

$$V_{\text{out}}(j\omega) = \left\{\left[\frac{C_4}{(C_1 + C_4)}\right] - \left[\frac{C_3}{(C_2 + C_3)}\right]\right\} V_{\text{in}}(j\omega) \tag{5.38}$$

In the balance, C_4 is adjusted to be equal to C_1. Then:

$$V_{out}(j\omega) = \left\{ \frac{1}{2} - \left[\frac{C_3}{(C_2 + C_3)} \right] \right\} V_{in}(j\omega) \tag{5.39}$$

or

$$V_{out}(j\omega) = \frac{(C_2 - C_3)}{2(C_2 + C_3)} V_{in}(j\omega) \tag{5.40}$$

Replacing Eq. (5.33) in Eq. (5.40):

$$V_{out}(j\omega) = \frac{x}{2d} V_{in}(j\omega) \tag{5.41}$$

Equation (5.41) shows that the output differential capacitive transducer is independent of the capacitors area A and dielectric permittivity ε.

Another possibility of obtaining a linear displacement capacitive transducer is to use a capacitor with cylindrical plates, instead of plane plates (Figure 5.17). There are several possibilities of implementing a linear displacement transducer with the differential capacitor shown in Figure 5.17B: moving the dielectric, the common plate or

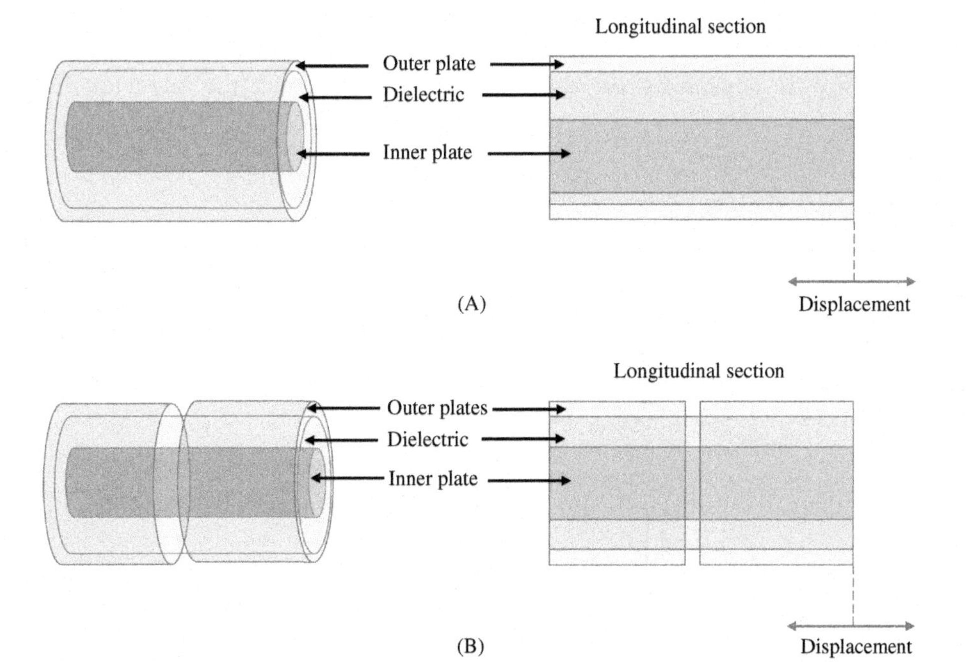

Figure 5.17 Cylindrical plates capacitor used in linear displacement transducer: single unit (A) and differential capacitor (B). Any of the plates or the dielectric can be attached to a moving object to measure its displacement.

each of the outer plates of the two capacitors (Cobbold, 1974; Dally et al., 1993; Geddes & Baker, 1968; Webster, 2010).

Rotational displacement also can be measured with capacitive transducers implemented with plane or cylindrical plates. Usually the rotary object is attached to a moving plate in a way to change the common area of the plates of the capacitor, and the capacitance variation is used to calculate the object displacement.

5.2.3 Inductive transducers

Inductive transducers of displacement show linearity, long life of use, high sensitivity, and good dynamic response. Environment conditions, as humidity and temperature, have little effect on their performance. The principle of operation of the inductive displacement transducer is the variation of the self-inductance or auto-inductance (L) of an inductor or the mutual inductance (M) of two inductors (All about Circuits 2, 2014; Cobbold, 1974; Dally et al., 1993; Geddes & Baker, 1968; Helfrick & Cooper, 1990; Khandpur, 2005; Northrop, 2005; Webster, 2010).

When electric current flows through the inductor, it stores the energy of the moving particles as magnetic field. It is formed basically by a coil with n loops of metal wire, as is shown in Figure 5.18. The wire can be wound around a ferromagnetic material, which enlarges the inductance by concentrating the magnetic flow lines within the loops. Equation (5.42) calculates the magnetic flow density. The magnetic field intensity is dependent on the number of loops and the inductor length (Eq. (5.43)).

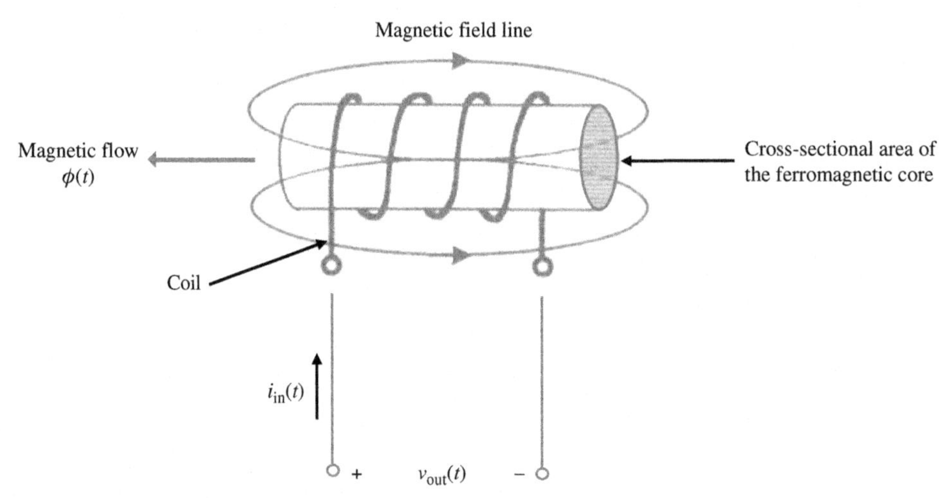

Figure 5.18 Schematic diagram of an inductor. When a current $i_{in}(t)$ flows through the coil, it generates a magnetic field, whose lines are concentrated within the loops of the coil by the presence of the ferromagnetic core, and an output voltage $v_{out}(t)$, which is proportional to the inductance value (L).

$$B = \frac{\phi}{A} \tag{5.42}$$

$$H = \frac{i_{\text{in}}(t)n}{l} \tag{5.43}$$

where

B is the magnetic flux density (Tesla, T)
H is the magnetic field intensity (Ampère/m)
ϕ is the magnetic flux intensity (Weber, Wb)
A is the section area of the core (m^2)
l is the length of the inductor (m)
n is the number of loops of the inductor.

The inductance L is the parameter that relates the input electric current $i_{\text{in}}(t)$ with the magnetic flow $\phi(t)$ and with the output voltage $v_{\text{out}}(t)$:

$$\phi(t) = Li_{\text{in}}(t) \tag{5.44}$$

$$v_{\text{out}}(t) = L\frac{\mathrm{d}i_{\text{in}}(t)}{\mathrm{d}t} \tag{5.45}$$

The inductance of a coil with n loops is given by

$$L = n^2 G\mu \tag{5.46}$$

where

n is the number of loops in the coil
μ is the effective permeability of the medium
G is the geometric factor of the coil ($G = k\pi r^2/l$, k is a fabrication constant, r is the coil radius, and l is the coil length).

Each of these parameters can be modified mechanically. The mutual inductance of two coils also depends only on geometrical parameters that can be modified by mechanical displacement. The SI unit for inductance is the henry (H): $1\ \text{H} = 1\ \text{T} \times \text{m}^2/\text{A}$.

Figure 5.19 shows a few solutions to obtain displacement transducers based on variable inductance. The measurement is accomplished by attaching the movable part of the transducer in the structure, which is displaced, changing some of the factors that determine the inductance of the transducer, and allowing the displacement to be related to the variation of inductance. Usually the inductor is part of an electronic circuit and the voltage or current output signal is processed to obtain the displacement value.

According to examples shown in Figure 5.19, the inductance modification occurs because the displacement x

1. changes the coil geometry (coil length in Figure 5.19A);
2. changes the permeability (or reluctance) due to core displacement (Figure 5.19B) or the air gap variation (Figure 5.19D);

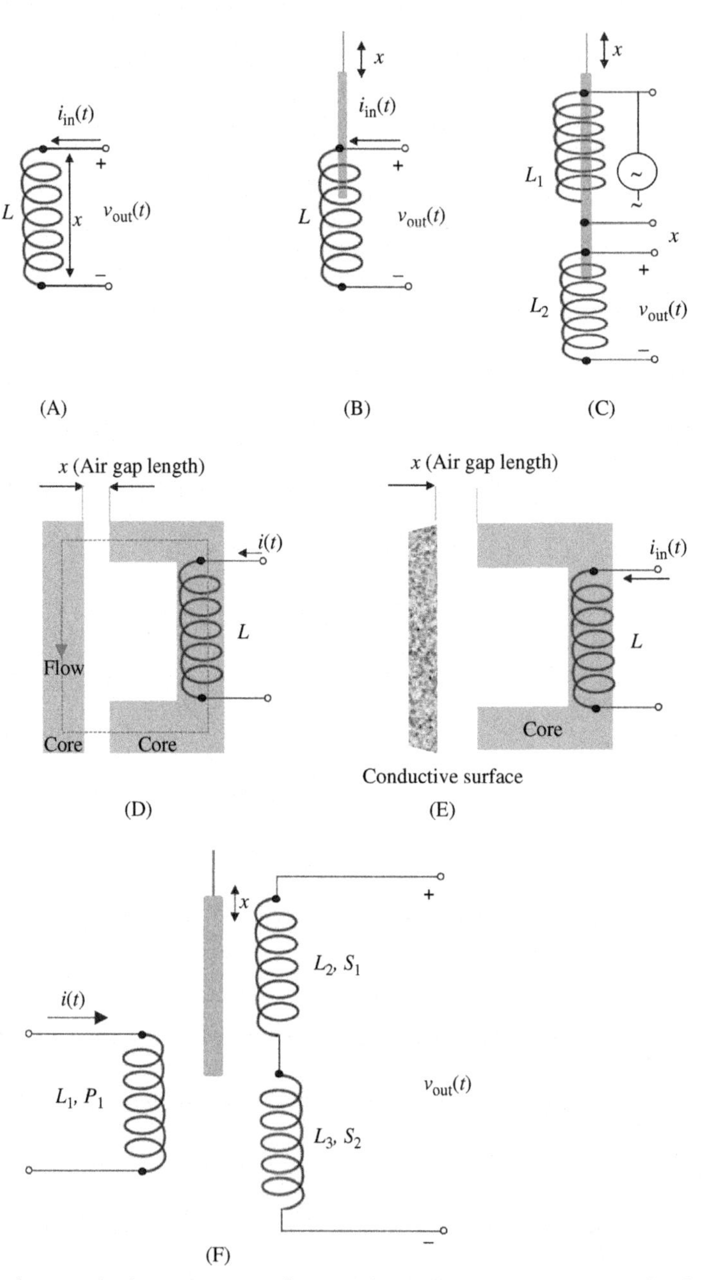

Figure 5.19 Inductive displacement transducers. The inductance L varies with changes in coil geometry (A), permeability of the medium (B) and (D), mutual magnetic coupling (C), distance between a conductive material and the coil's magnetic field (E), and mutual magnetic coupling between the primary and two secondary coils (F).

3. modifies the mutual magnetic coupling between inductors by changing the position of a common core (Figure 5.19C) or the distance between the coils. The mutual inductance is the property of an inductor, in which electric current flows, to induce a voltage in another nearby inductor;
4. changes the distance between a conductive material and the coil's magnetic field, inducing eddy currents on the material (Figure 5.19E);
5. modifies the mutual magnetic coupling between the primary and two secondary coils by the displacement of the common core (Figure 5.19F). This arrangement is known as LVDT (linear variable differential transformer).

An inductive displacement transducer as that shown in Figure 5.19B is used in intravascular pressure transducers. The micromanometer of Allard–Laurens was developed in the early 60s (Allard, 1962; Cobbold, 1974) and its operating principle is used until today in the construction of intravascular pressure transducers. It is placed at the tip of a catheter and is carried to the interior of the heart chambers, allowing the simultaneous capture of the pressure wave and heart sounds. The variable coil is part of an LC oscillating circuit and the movable core is placed between two diaphragms; the first diaphragm moves together with the blood flux, pushing the core against the second diaphragm and changing the inductance value. The output signal frequency changes according to the blood pressure. A low pass filter separates the frequency components of the blood pressure curve and the phonocardiogram is obtained at the output of a high pass filter ($f > 50$ Hz).

There are commercially available dedicated inductive transducer developed with inductive Wheatstone bridge to measure arterial or venous blood pressure in mmHg. Usually contains two constant low resistances and two variable reactive inductances in the bridge circuit. The blood pressure moves a diaphragm that is attached to the armature, common to the two coils (a displacement transducer similar to that shown in Figure 5.19C), changing their inductances. Voltage excitation of the bridge circuit is 5 V_{RMS} at 2,400 Hz, for example, and a variable resistor (1 kΩ) adjusts the output sensitivity (a few tens of μV/V/mmHg).

The inductive displacement transducer shown in Figure 5.19D is a magnetic circuit made from a ferromagnetic core with a coil wound on it, an air gap separating the core with the coil and a movable part of ferromagnetic material. This movable part is usually attached to the moving structure. An electric current flowing in the coil represents a source of magnetomotive force (MMF), which drives the magnetic flux through the magnetic circuit. The air gap causes substantial increase in the reluctance of the circuit, decreasing the magnetic flux. A slight variation in the air gap results in a measurable inductance changing, which affects the output voltage and is used to determine the displacement value.

Figure 5.19E shows a displacement transducer based on the eddy current induced in a conductive material by the magnetic field produced by the active coil wound

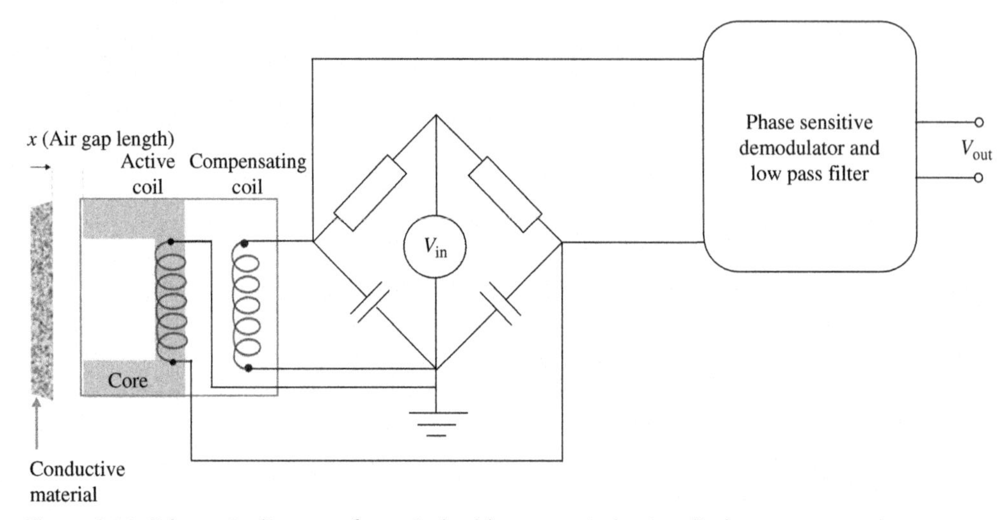

Figure 5.20 Schematic diagram of a typical eddy current inductive displacement transducer.

around a ferromagnetic core. This local electric current induces a magnetic field opposite in sense to the one from the active coil and reduces the inductance in the coil. When the distance between the target and the probe changes, the impedance of the coil changes correspondingly. This change in impedance can be detected by a Wheatstone bridge circuit (excitation signal frequency 50 kHz to 10 MHz) and processed to determine the displacement or position of the conductive material with regard to the core (Figure 5.20). In addition to the active coil, a temperature compensation coil is also included in the circuit. Commercially available eddy current transducer specifications range 0.25–30 mm; 20–40 mm long with 2–75 mm diameter; resolution up to 0.1 μm; and linearity 0.5%.

Most LVDTs are wired as shown in Figure 5.19F, with the secondary windings in opposite directions. The LVDT is one of the most used inductive transducers due to linear relation between the output voltage and the core displacement, which is usually attached to the moving structure. The LVDT is a transducer that converts a linear displacement or position with regard to a mechanical reference (or zero) in a proportional electrical signal, which contains phase (for sense of direction) and amplitude (length or distance information).

The LVDT operation is based on the electromagnetic coupling of the primary and secondary coils and does not require electric contact between the movable part (core or armature) and the transformer windings. A ferromagnetic core, made of high permeability material (NiFe), links the electromagnetic field of the primary coil to the secondary coils. The AC input voltage (typically a few kHz sinusoidal signal) has constant peak-to-peak amplitude. The core displacement changes the coupling between the primary and two secondary coils (Figure 5.21A–C). Since the number of coil

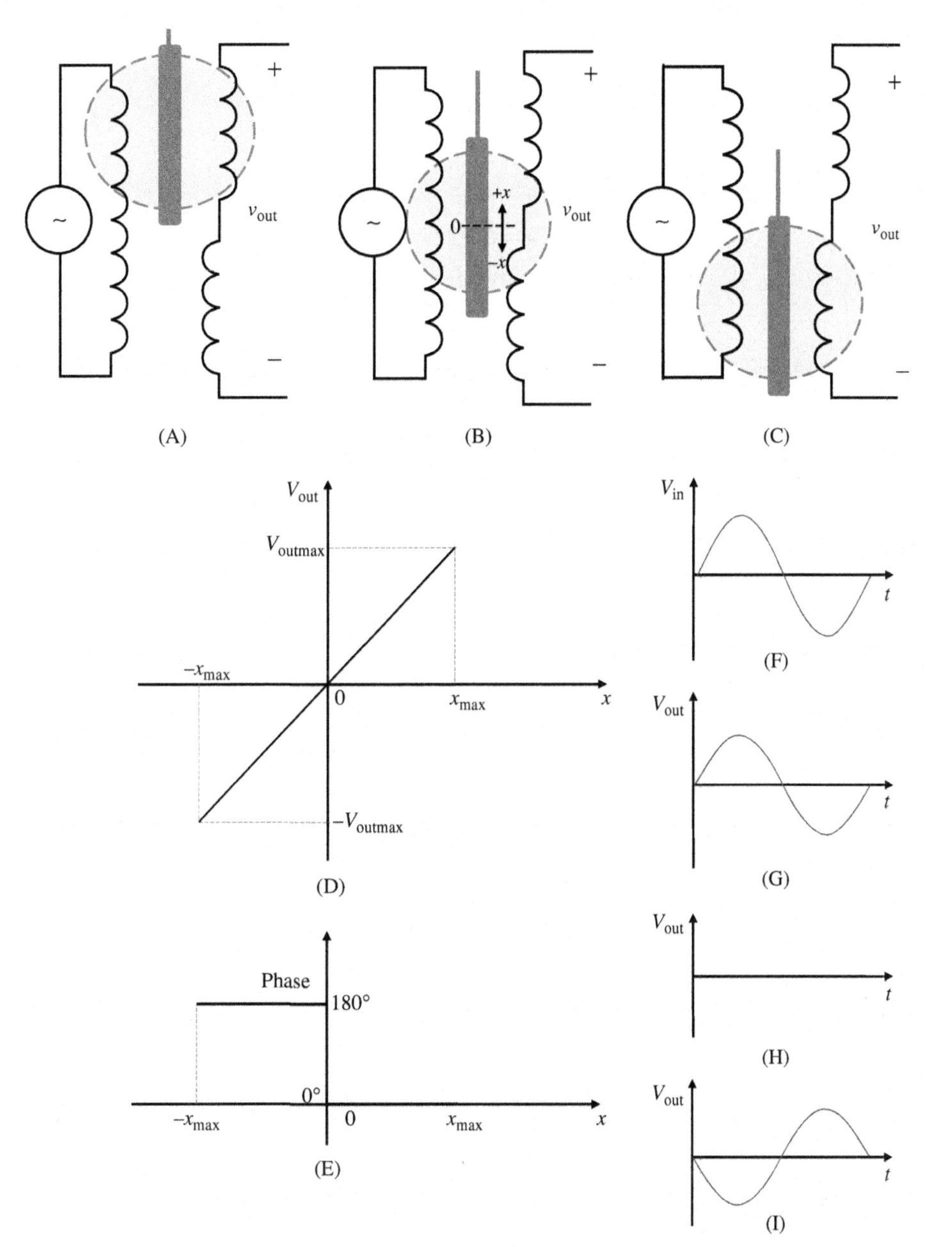

Figure 5.21 LVDT (A) to (C) core excursion from one extremity to other passing through the central position. (D) and (E) amplitude and phase of the displacement in function of time when the core moves from the origin to the end of the working range. (F) Excitation signal. (G) v_{out} is in phase with v_{in}; core excursions from x_{max} to $-x_{max}$. (H) Core is in central position ($x = 0$), $v_{out} = 0$. (I) v_{out} is in counter-phase with v_{in}; core excursions from $-x_{max}$ to x_{max}.

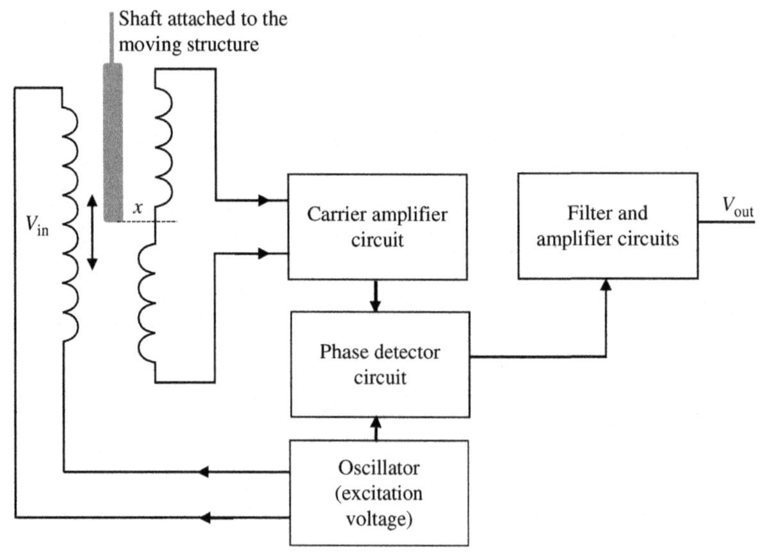

Figure 5.22 Typical electronic circuit for exciting the LVDT and conditioning its output voltage for detecting displacement.

windings is uniformly distributed along the transformer, the voltage output is proportional to the core displacement when it slides through the range and the output voltage varies linearly with the displacement, in function of the input voltage, as is shown in Figure 5.21F–I. The primary and secondary coils are commonly separated by high-density glass and the whole is covered by epoxy resin and an outer layer of stainless steel. Some models of LVDT-based displacement transducers have the conditioning electronic embedded in the same package.

When the primary coupling with the upper secondary is larger than the lower, V_{out} is in phase with V_{in} (Figure 5.21A and G). When the core is in the central position, the primary is equally coupled to both secondary coils, which are connected in series, but wound in opposite directions, and their contributions cancel out: $V_{out} = 0$ (Figure 5.21B and H). When the primary coupling with the lower secondary is larger than the upper, V_{out} is in phase opposition with V_{in} (Figure 5.21C and I). Figure 5.21D and E shows the amplitude and phase of the displacement in function of time when the core moves from the origin, passing through the central position to the end of the displacement range.

Figure 5.22 shows the block diagram of a typical electronic circuit for LVDT exciting and output voltage conditioning for displacement detecting. The oscillator (≈ 2 kHz) generates the excitation voltage to the primary coil and feeds the phase detector circuit. The LVDT output voltage, modulated by the oscillator frequency, is amplified and sent to a phase detector circuit, which compares the primary coil oscillation voltage to the amplified LVDT output voltage. Both voltages will be in phase if the displacement is in one direction or in counter phase if the movement is in the opposite direction. Finally the bipolar output voltage is demodulated (low pass filter) and amplified.

Some typical characteristics of commercial LVDTs are listed below:

Primary excitation: 3–15 V_{RMS}, 50 Hz to 20 kHz (most used: 3 V, 2.5 kHz and 6.3 V, 60 Hz)

Sensitivity: 0.5–20 mV/V/25 μm (0.001″) = 0.5–20 mV for 25 μm displacement to each 1 V of excitation voltage in the coil

Working range: 0.1–250 mm

Linearity: ±0.1–0.5% FS

Accuracy: ±0.25% FS

Temperature sensitivity coefficient: 0.25%/100°F.

A common biomedical application of LVDT-based displacement transducer is in the construction of blood pressure transducer, even intravascular ones for direct and invasive measurements. There are commercially available miniature LVDTs that allow their use in applications where standard size of LVDTs is not suitable, which is the case of most biomedical applications. The Series 230 miniature AC LVDTs (Trans-Tek Incorporated 1, 2014) are designed for high precision measurement of displacements in the range 12.7 μm (0.005″) to 2.54 cm (1.0″). With external diameter <1 cm (0.375″) and nonlinearity error of ±0.25% of FS, they have low mass core to suit to weight sensitive applications or high accelerations. LVDTs are also used in the construction of sophisticated devices for brain surgeries like probe drives used to place and monitor implantable stimulating electrodes in deep brain for Parkinson disease therapy.

LVDT is often chosen to construct displacement transducers due to its advantages, for example, relative low cost; robustness to be used in a wide variety of environments; no friction resistance, since the iron core does not contact the transformer coils, resulting in an infinite (very long) working life; high signal-to-noise ratio and low output impedance; negligible hysteresis; theoretical infinitesimal resolution, but with displacement resolution limited by the resolution of the amplifiers and voltage meters used to process the output signal; and fast response time, but limited by the inertia of the iron core and the rise time of the amplifiers. LVDT is an absolute output device in opposition to the incremental output transducers and it responds only to axial displacements of the core and is generally insensitive to radial displacements caused by misalignment. LVDTs are more sensible than strain gages, but require more sophisticated signal (analog and digital) processing.

It is also possible to list some disadvantages, for example, the core or armature needs to be in direct or indirect contact with the displacing structure, which is not always possible or desirable; and the LVDT dynamic response is limited to 1/10 of its resonance frequency, which most of the times results in frequencies close to a few kHz.

5.3 VELOCITY TRANSDUCERS

Velocity is a vector that consists of a magnitude (speed) and a direction. Linear velocity is defined as the rate of change of the position vector with time at an instant in time. The velocity transducer is an electronic device used to measure the velocity of displacement of an object, linear (m/s) or angular (rotations/min; grades/s) by converting mechanical energy into an electrical output signal (current or voltage) that is proportional to the velocity of the object. The displacement measurement ($x = f(t)$) of the object can be the starting point to determine the velocity. If the object moves from position x_1 to position x_2 in the time interval t_1 to t_2, the average speed is

$$v_{avg} = \frac{x_2 - x_1}{t_2 - t_1} = \frac{\Delta x}{\Delta t} \tag{5.47}$$

If the time interval is very small, the average velocity becomes the instantaneous velocity $v(t)$:

$$v(t) = \lim_{t \to 0} \frac{\Delta x}{\Delta t} = \frac{dx(t)}{dt} \tag{5.48}$$

And acceleration $a(t)$ is obtained through another differentiation operation:

$$a(t) = \frac{dv(t)}{dt} = \frac{dx^2(t)}{dt^2} \tag{5.49}$$

The differentiation is an operation that emphasizes high frequency noise, decreases the signal-to-noise ratio, and makes it difficult the electronic determination of acceleration from the displacement. Other solutions are used to obtain velocity and acceleration transducers. An accelerometer is a device that allows the measurement of acceleration. Its output can be integrated one and two times to get velocity and displacement, respectively:

$$\begin{aligned} v(t) &= v(0) + \int_0^t a(t)dt \\ x(t) &= x(0) + \int_0^t v(t)dt \end{aligned} \tag{5.50}$$

where $v(0)$ and $x(0)$ are the velocity and the displacement at time 0, respectively. Integrals are computed from time 0 to some later time t.

Unlike differentiation, the process of integration decreases the noise and increases the signal-to-noise ratio. Although it is necessary to take care with the DC deviation of the integrator, this solution is more viable to implement with electronic circuits. The output of a micromachined silicon accelerometer can be amplified, filtered, and integrated with discrete electronic circuits, to get the velocity value. Velocity is seldom measured directly, but rather by calculation from measurement of displacement or acceleration.

Examples of biomedical applications of velocity transducers are the measurement of the velocity of blood flow in a vessel or heart chamber (Nichols, Pepine, Conti,

Christie, & Feldman, 1981) and velocity of displacement of a body segment, such as head, arm, finger, and leg for ergonomic studies (Lee, Lee, Dexter, Klein, & Park, 2007), rehabilitation engineering research (Yoon, Novandy, Yoon, & Park, 2010), Parkinson's disease research (Norman, Edwards, & Beuter, 1999), and development of wearable devices (Patel, Park, Bonato, Chan, & Rodgers, 2012). The principle of functioning of some linear and angular velocity transducers is explained below (Cobbold, 1974; Dally et al., 1993; Geddes & Baker, 1968; Pinney & Baker, 2000; Webster, 2010).

5.3.1 Linear velocity transducers

The transducers most commonly used to measure linear velocity in biomedical applications are those that use the Doppler shift (or ultrasonic method) (Anderson & McDicken, 1999; Chemloul, Chaib, & Mostefa, 2012; Doebelin, 2004; Nishimura et al., 1985) and the electromagnetic methods.

5.3.1.1 Ultrasonic (Doppler effect) linear velocity transducer

Ultrasonic transducers have one or more piezoelectric elements made of single crystals of quartz (SiO_2) and ferroelectric materials (ceramics) such as $BaTiO_3$ (barium titanate), $LiNbO_3$ (lithium niobate), $LiTaO_3$ (lithium tantalate), and PZT (zirconate titanate lead). When subjected to intense electrical alternating voltage, they vibrate at the ultrasound frequency ($f > 20$ kHz). The ultrasound propagates through a medium with speed and attenuation that depend on the medium characteristics and ultrasound frequency, interacts with targets, undergoes diffraction, part of its energy is transmitted, reflected, and diffracted.

Doppler velocimeters are used for remote sensing of linear velocity and do not require contact with the moving structure. The radiation (mechanical as ultrasound or electromagnetic as light or microwave) reflected by a moving object has frequency (f_R) different from the radiation transmitted (f_T) by a static source. The frequency difference ($f_T - f_R$) is called Doppler shift (f_D) and its value is proportional to the velocity of the object. Ultrasonic radiation with appropriate chosen frequency, to get good resolution and to minimize attenuation, is used to investigate different biological tissues; then the radiation reflected or transmitted is processed to retrieve information about the displacement velocity of tissues. Ultrasonic Doppler velocimeters are used in several noninvasive biomedical applications, for example, to measure the flow velocity of blood in arteries and veins, and the displacement velocity of heart valves and walls of heart chambers.

The Doppler shift can be obtained with continuous and pulsed ultrasound. In the continuous mode (continuous wave Doppler or CW Doppler), it is necessary to use two transducers, one transmitter and one receiver. Figure 5.23 shows a representation of measurement of a moving target velocity with CW Doppler. Transmitter continuously emits an ultrasound beam, which heats the target and partially reflects back; the receiver transducer continuously collects the reflected beam. If the target is moving away from the transmitted ultrasonic beam, the sound is reflected at a lower frequency

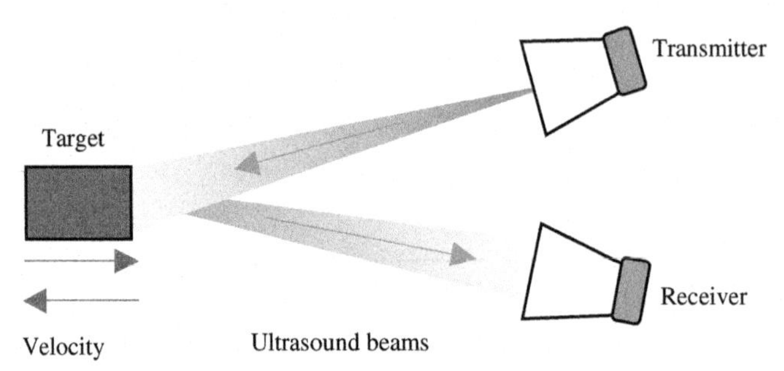

Figure 5.23 Representation of the CW Doppler use for linear velocity measuring.

than it was transmitted (positive Doppler shift). Moreover, if the target is the other direction, that is, it approaches the transmitted ultrasonic beam, the ultrasound is reflected at a frequency higher than the transmitted one (negative Doppler shift).

The Doppler shift is calculated by Eq. (5.51) and the flow velocity by Eq. (5.52):

$$f_D = \frac{2f_T}{c} v \cos\theta \tag{5.51}$$

$$v = \frac{c}{2f_T \cos\theta} f_D \tag{5.52}$$

where

c is the ultrasound velocity in the biological tissue ($\approx$ 1,540 m/s)
f_T is the frequency at which the ultrasound was transmitted (Hz)
f_D is the Doppler shift (Hz)
θ is the angle between incident ultrasound and blood flow directions
v is the blood flow velocity (m/s).

CW Doppler can also be used to measure blood flow velocity. Transmitter and receiver transducers are positioned laterally, on the skin immediately above the structure where the velocity measurement should be made, or transversally, if it is possible, as shown in Figure 5.24. The transmitter emits continuously ultrasound pulses that interact with the medium and moving particles of blood, mainly red blood cells. Part of the ultrasonic energy is transmitted and part is reflected by the cells and collected by the receiver transducer to calculate the fluid velocity.

Figure 5.25A shows the schematic diagram of pulsed Doppler ultrasound velocimetry, the most common method used to measure linear velocity of blood flow. The velocity of a flowing fluid is more difficult to measure than that of a solid object for several reasons, for example, the fluid usually does not move as a solid body, but rather, individual fluid particles move relative to each other; velocity is a function of spatial location within the fluid flow.

In pulsed Doppler ultrasound (Pulsed Wave Doppler or PW Doppler) instead of emitting continuous ultrasonic waves, an emitter sends periodically a short ultrasonic burst and a receiver collects the echoes. One transducer can transmit the burst of ultrasound pulses

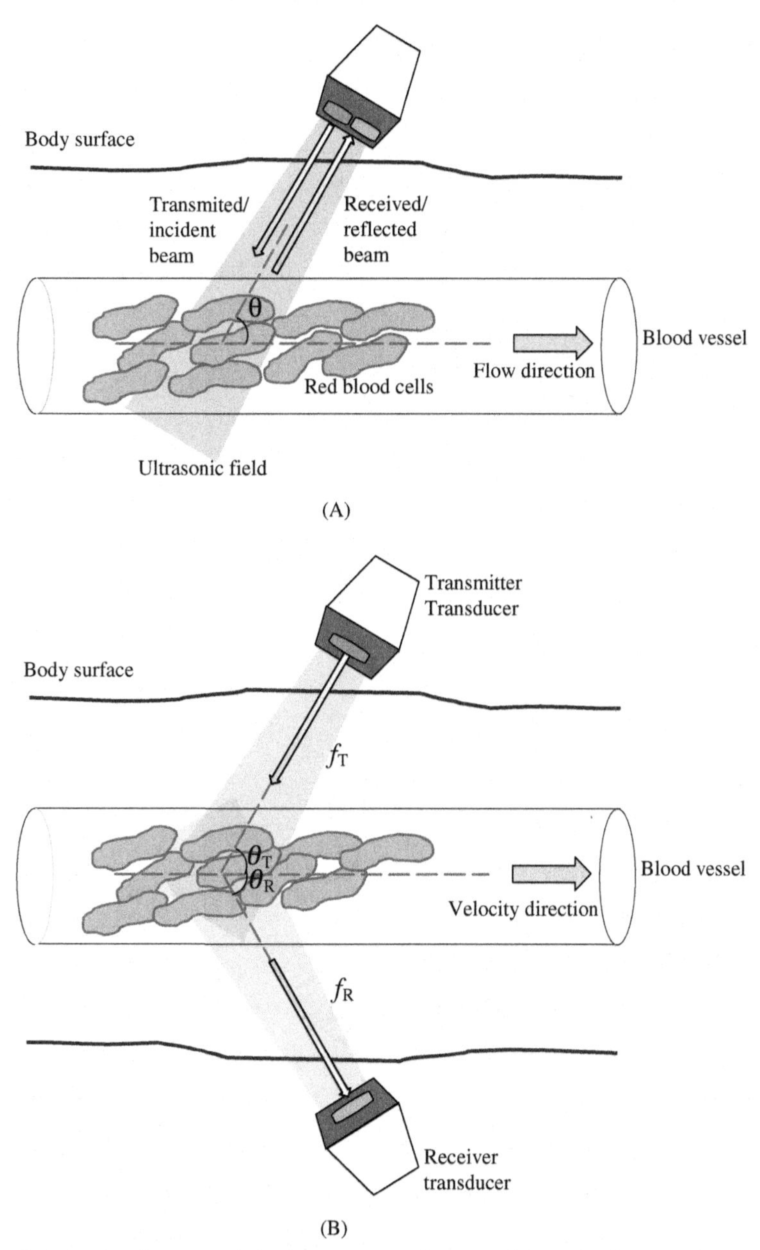

Figure 5.24 Schematic diagram of the continuous ultrasound Doppler linear velocity transducer. Two transducers localized (A) laterally and (B) transversally.

and collect the echoes, alternately. The transmitter is pulsed at the pulse repetition frequency (PRF) which means that one burst is transmitted each $T_{PRF} = 1/PRF$ and this period must be sufficient to all echoes to be collected before another burst is released (Figure 5.25B). The value of PRF depends on the frequency of the transducer and the

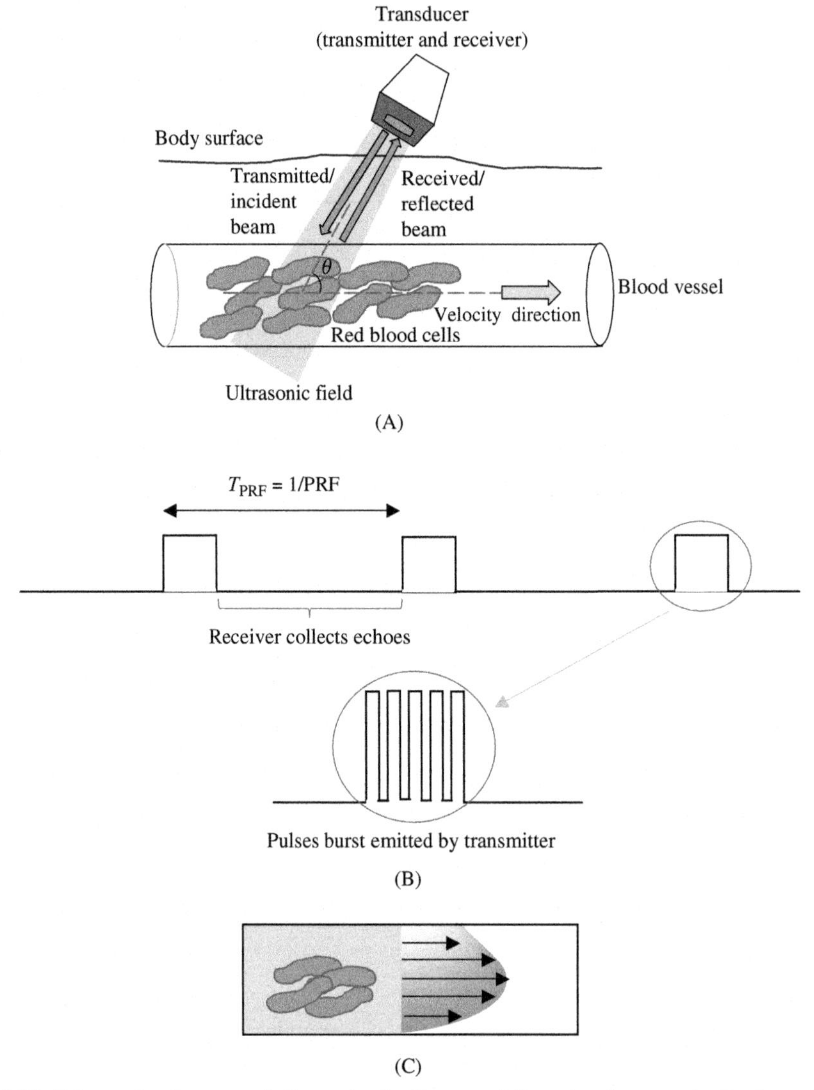

Figure 5.25 Schematic diagram of the pulsed ultrasound Doppler linear velocity transducer (A) and time diagram of transmitter and receiver excitation (B). Velocity profile of reflectors along the blood vessel diameter (C).

distance between the transducer and the reflector ($\text{PRF} < c/2x_{\text{max}}$). The maximum velocity measurable is called Limit Velocity of Nyquist and corresponds to the maximum frequency to which Doppler shift can be measured ($f_{\text{Dmax}} < \text{PRF}/2$). The PRF gives the maximum time allowed to the burst to travel to the reflector and back to the transducer. Increasing the time between pulses (T_{PRF}) increases the maximum measurable depth, x_{max}, but also reduces the maximum velocity that can be measured.

During velocity measurement, the transducer is positioned over the body surface at approximately 30° with regard to the blood flow axial direction. Between transmitter actuations, the receiver continuously collects echoes from all reflectors that may be present in the path of the ultrasonic beam, that is, mainly red blood cells, but also other cells and particles present in the blood plasma. Reflectors in the blood vessel travel according to a velocity profile: particles near the vessel wall have lower velocity than the ones traveling in the center of the vessel (Figure 5.25C). Thus, on the path of the ultrasonic beam the reflectors have different sizes and velocities and are at different depths. The tissues between the transducer and the blood vessel do not interfere with the measurement of blood flow velocity because they are ideally not moving.

One should always assume that the reflectors in the ultrasonic beam path are randomly distributed and the echoes from each reflector are combined in a random fashion, resulting in a random echo. By collecting the incoming echoes at the same time, with regard to the emission of the bursts, the receiver measures shifts of reflectors in different depths. The velocity is measured not by finding the Doppler frequency shift in the received signal, but velocity is derived from shifts in reflector positions between pulses. Considering that, there is only one reflector in the beam path and knowing the delay time (t_{d1}) of its reflected echo to arrive at the receiver, its position (x_1) at the first emission can be calculated as

$$x_1 = \frac{c t_{d1}}{2} \tag{5.53}$$

where c is the sound velocity of the ultrasonic wave in the blood ($\approx$ 1,540 m/s, same as the water).

When the next burst is emitted, after T_{PRF}, the reflector will be at x_2 and its echo will hit the receiver with a time delay t_{d2}:

$$x_2 = \frac{c t_{d2}}{2} \tag{5.54}$$

The reflector is moving at an angle θ with regard to the axis of the ultrasonic beam and its velocity can be measured by calculating the variation of its position between two consecutive emissions:

$$x_2 - x_1 = \frac{c}{2}(t_{d2} - t_{d1}) = v T_{PRF} \cos\theta \tag{5.55}$$

and

$$v = \frac{c}{2\cos\theta\, T_{PRF}}(t_{d2} - t_{d1}) \tag{5.56}$$

The phase shift φ of the received echo is

$$\varphi = 2\pi f_t (t_{d2} - t_{d1}) \tag{5.57}$$

where f_t is the transmitting ultrasound frequency.

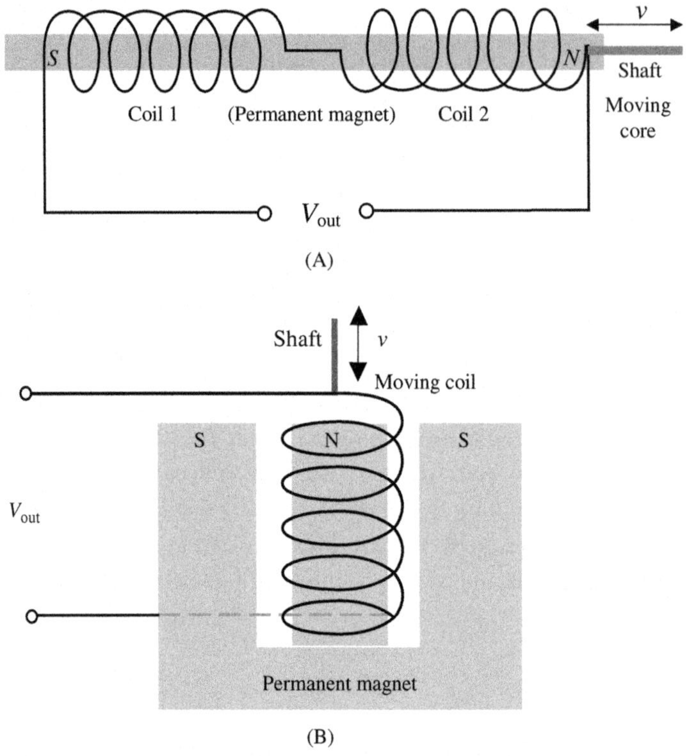

Figure 5.26 Schematic diagram of electromagnetic linear velocity transducer with (A) moving core or (B) moving coil.

Replacing Eq. (5.57) in Eq. (5.56), the reflector velocity is calculated as

$$v = \frac{c\varphi}{4\pi \cos\theta \, T_{PRF}} = \frac{c}{2f_t \cos\theta} f_D \tag{5.58}$$

where f_D is the Doppler frequency shift.

Equation (5.58) gives the same result as Eq. (5.52) developed for Doppler effect, although the phenomena involved is not the same, when measuring blood velocity with PW Doppler (Signal Processing SA, 2014).

5.3.1.2 Electromagnetic linear velocity transducer

Figure 5.26A shows the schematic diagram of a typical electromagnetic linear velocity transducer, usually called LVT. The core, or permanent magnet, moves within the stationary arrangement of two coils in series but with opposed windings. The object whose velocity is to be measured is usually attached to the moving core. No excitation voltage is required and when the object moves, the core displaces together. Since the two coils are wrapped with opposite polarity, and since the magnet also has two poles (north and south), the south pole induces a voltage primarily in coil 1, and the north pole primarily in core 2. Thus, the magnetic field lines passing through the loops of the windings, induce an electromagnetic force, which is proportional to the velocity of the core. The DC output voltage is proportional to the instantaneous velocity of the object displacement (Cobbold, 1974; Dally et al., 1993; Doebelin, 2004; Kazan, 1994; Trans-Tek Incorporated 2, 2014). The DC generated voltage proportional to the velocity of a conductor in a magnetic field can be expressed as

$$V_{\text{out}} = Blv \tag{5.59}$$

where

B is the component of the flux density normal to the velocity
l is the length of the conductor (two coils)
v is the core velocity.

Another possible configuration of electromagnetic linear velocimeter has a static core and moving coils (Figure 5.26B) and similar functioning; the coils are attached to the object whose velocity is measured.

The Series 100 Linear Velocity Transducer (Trans-Tek Incorporated 3, 2014) is an example of commercial electromagnetic linear velocimeters. The displacement of the core through the pair of oppositely wound coils in series provides a DC voltage in the output of the transducer that is proportional to the instantaneous velocity. Transducer working range is 1.27 cm (0.5″) to 61 cm (24″) with sensitivity up to 500 mV/in./s and nonlinearity error of 2.5% FS. This transducer is used in pipette pullers, an application in which the displacement of the heated thin glass tube should be done under controlled velocity.

5.3.2 Angular velocity transducers

Rotating velocimeters are devices that infer velocity by measuring the rotation rate of an object around an axis (such as the angular displacement velocity of a motor shaft or a leg in relation to the knee joint). Such devices do not measure the physical displacement around the axis, but only its rotation. Most of angular velocity measurements are relative ones, that is, the velocity of one rotating object is measured with regard to a stationary object. The measuring technologies most often used to measure relative angular velocity are electromagnetic (variable inductance, DC and AC generating tachometers), variable capacitance, photoelectric, optical, and stroboscopic. Gyroscopic technology is employed to measure absolute angular velocity of inertial objects. Some of the electromagnetic methods are explained below (Cobbold, 1974; Dally et al., 1993; Doebelin, 2004).

5.3.2.1 Electromagnetic angular velocity transducer

Electromagnetic angular velocity transducers utilize the basic electrical generator principle that when there is relative motion between a conductor and the magnetic field,

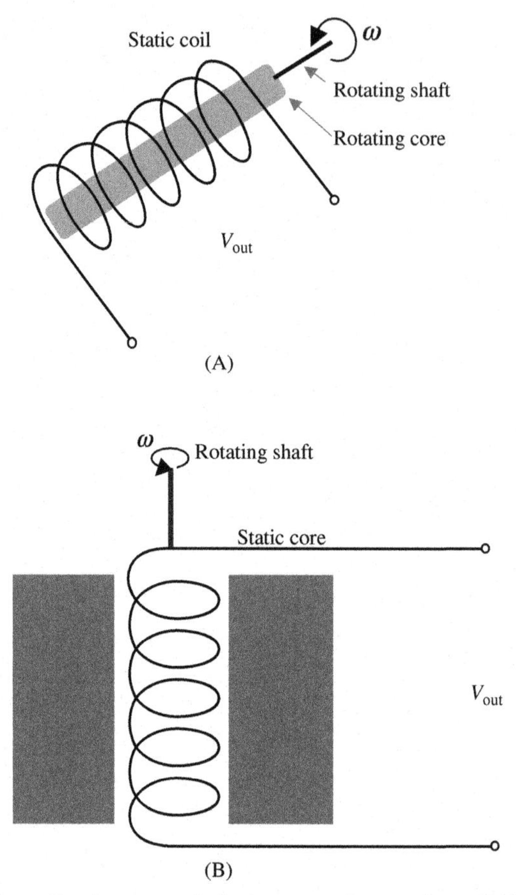

Figure 5.27 Typical schematic diagrams of electromagnetic angular velocity transducers (A) with rotating core and (B) with rotating coil. For circular paths, as usually are the loops of the coil, it follows that the angular velocity $\omega = v/r$, where r is the coil loop radius.

a voltage is induced or generated in the conductor. The relative motion between field and conductor provides changings in the measuring intensity.

Figure 5.27 shows typical schematic diagrams: angular velocimeters with rotating core (A) and rotating coil (B).

A rotating generator transducer produces an output voltage signal proportional to the rotational velocity of the input shaft. Figure 5.27A shows an electromagnetic transducer of angular velocity, which comprises a stationary coil and a movable ferromagnetic core. The coil is connected to the object with angular displacement. When the coil rotates, the magnetic field lines passing through its windings vary, inducing an electromagnetic force, which is proportional to the coil velocity. In Figure 5.27B the moving object is attached to the moving coil, while the ferromagnetic core remains stationary. The same basic Eq. (5.59), relating voltage generated to velocity of a

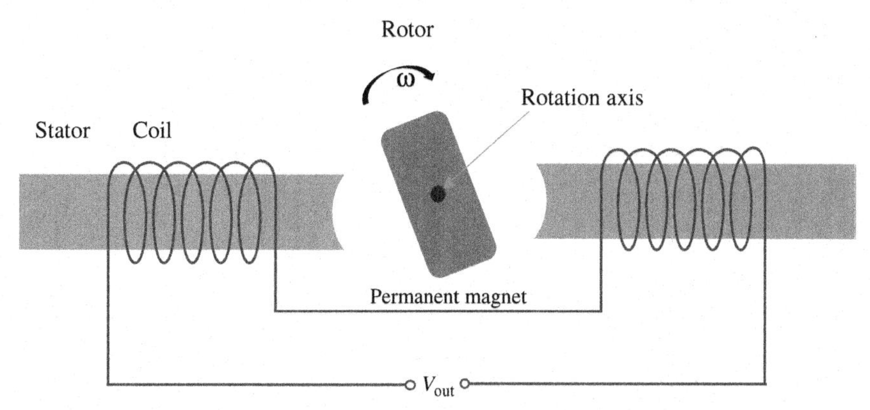

Figure 5.28 Typical schematic diagram of a permanent magnet tachometer generator for angular velocity measurement.

conductor in a magnetic field, is used to compute the rotating object velocity in Figure 5.27A and B. In both cases, the output voltage intensity is proportional to velocity and its polarity indicates the rotation direction.

Figure 5.28 shows a typical schematic diagram of a permanent magnet tachometer generator. The coils are wound around fixed poles of the stator itself and an electromagnet or a permanent magnet rotor produces the magnetic field. The magnetic field rotates together with the object whose velocity is being measured. When the magnet rotor spins within the stator, an emf is induced in the stator windings, which amplitude and frequency are directly proportional to the velocity of rotation. This configuration provides an alternating output signal, which has advantages over a dc voltage, for example, noise and ripple signals can be filtered more readily before further signal amplification, and the calibration can be made in terms of output intensity or frequency.

Figure 5.29 shows the schematic diagrams of a DC generator tachometer and a AC generator tachometer. DC tachometer (Figure 5.29A) is similar in operation to permanent magnet type with the exception of a reversed arrangement of a magnet set on the stator and coils in the rotor. When the rotor spins within the magnetic field of the stator, an electric current is generated in its windings. AC tachometer (Figure 5.29B) has two coils wound in the stator. An AC voltage excites one coil, which induces a voltage in the other coil. The rotor is attached to the moving object and spins within the two coils in the stator, affecting the relationship between the two windings, which in turn, affects the output voltage. The AC output voltage has amplitude and frequency proportional to the stator angular velocity.

By measuring the voltage produced by a tachogenerator, the rotational velocity, usually indicated in RPM, rotations per minute, of whatever it is mechanically attached to can easily be determined. Conditioning circuit can be a simple voltmeter calibrated in RPM, or electronic circuits with amplifier, phase detector, filters, and integrators.

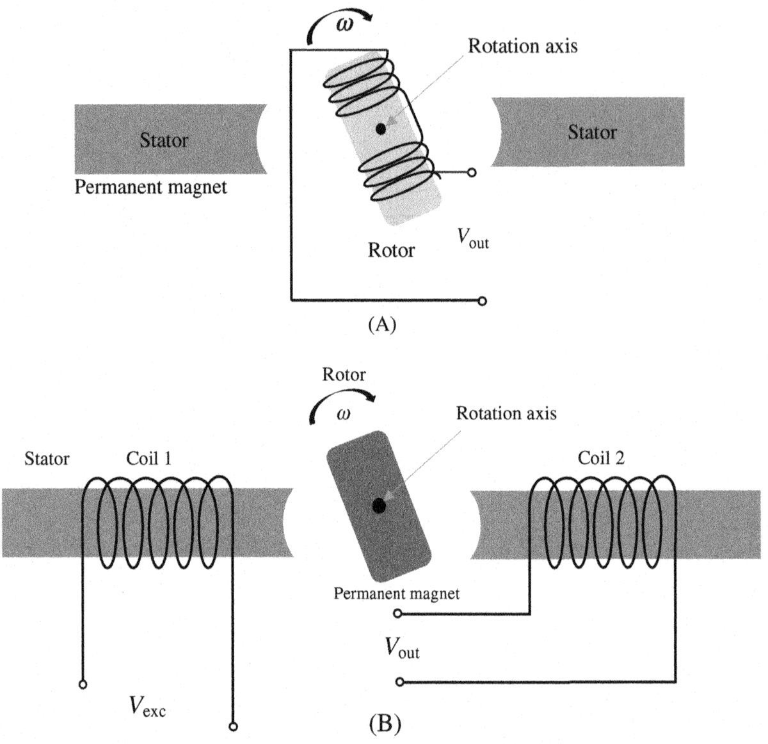

Figure 5.29 Typical schematic diagram of (A) DC and (B) AC tachometer generators for angular velocity measurement.

The output velocity value can be displayed for visualization or used to control the velocity of pumps, engines, machine tools, mixers, fans, conveyor belts, etc.

Typical DC tachogenerators have specifications such as current up to 200 mA, velocities up to 10,000 rpm, and output voltages of 4–200 V per 1,000 RPM and linearity error <1%. The DC voltage output is proportional to the velocity of its mover and is widely used in applications for feedback and display purposes. AC tachogenerators generally are used in applications of display purposes and their typical specifications are velocity up to 4,000 RPM, current up to 50 mA, output voltage of 4–40 V per 1,000 RPM and linearity error <1%. According to the number of poles in the stator design, 2, 8, or 48, the output frequency will be 16.66, 66.66, and 400 Hz, respectively.

5.4 ACCELERATION TRANSDUCERS

Accelerometers are found in many biomedical applications, from the study of human body acceleration and kinematic studies of body extremities tremor to the incorporation of accelerators in implantable medical devices such as drug therapy systems and artificial joints (Bouten, Sauren, Verduin, & Janssen, 1997; Mathie, Coster, Lovell, & Celler, 2004; Mayagoitia, Lotters, Veltink, & Hermens, 2002; Norman et al., 1999). The diversity of areas where accelerometry has been used includes metabolic energy expenditure (which is the standard reference for the measurement of physical activities), physical activity (defining and comparing group of subjects with different activity levels), balance and postural sway assessment, and gait (stability analysis).

The human acceleration has been investigated for many years and an extensive work has already been done with wired and wireless accelerometry. General body motion is measured with a single accelerometer placed close to the pelvis, which is body's center of mass. There are other locations and applications, as thigh or ankle, to study leg movement during walking, wrist, to measure Parkinsonian bradykinesia (slowness of movement, a symptom found in Parkinsonian patients), arm and leg, to study Parkinsonian tremor and chest, to study coughing. Research results of human acceleration have application not only in therapy and rehabilitation of patients but also in monitoring the performance of athletes. Another very promising application of accelerometers is in the detection and prevention of falls of elderly people, which lead to other health problems resulting from fall, disabilities, and reduced quality of life (Bianchi, Redmond, Narayanan, Cerutti, & Lovell, 2010; Menz, Lord, & Fitzpatrick, 2003).

Accelerometers measure the acceleration of objects moving linearly or angularly. In these two types of acceleration, object is subjected to accelerations of up to a few g (g is the gravitational constant $\approx 6.674 \times 10^{-11}$ N(m/kg)^2). Accelerometers measure acceleration, vibration, and shock (intense and abrupt deceleration) and their construction typically involves a seismic mass, a damper or spring, and a rigid encapsulation. The movement of the mass inside the casing is proportional to the force of acceleration on the device. Eventually accelerometers use a displacement transducer (capacitive, resistive, piezoelectric, strain gage, micromachined) for measuring the position of the mass.

Accelerometers measure the inertia force generated when a mass is affected by a change in velocity. Various physical processes are used to build a sensor for measuring acceleration. There are accelerometers developed based on the properties of a rotating mass, but the most common configuration is based on a combination of Newton's law of mass acceleration and Hooke's law, which governs the behavior of spring (Figure 5.30). Newton's law states that if a mass M is under acceleration a, then there must be a force F acting on the mass and is given by

$$F = Ma \tag{5.60}$$

Hooke's law states that if a spring with constant k is stretched from a resting position, through a Δx distance, then there must be a force F acting on the spring and is given by

$$F = k\Delta x \tag{5.61}$$

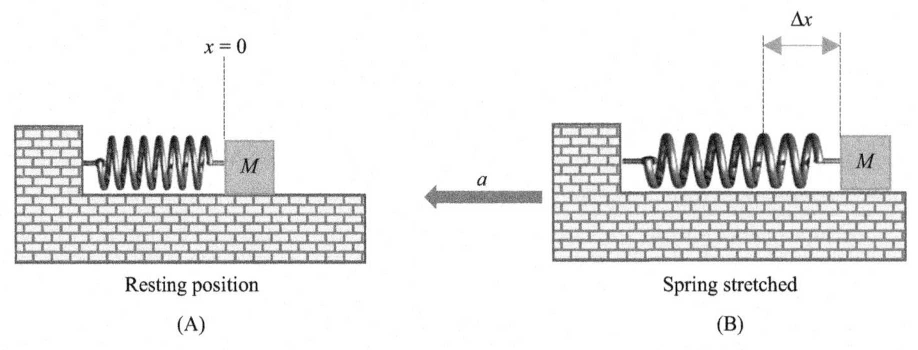

Figure 5.30 Schematic diagram showing the components M, a, and Δx of the system mass-spring: (A) Newton's law and (b) Hooke's law.

where

k is the spring constant (N/m)

Δx is the length of the spring stretching (m)

M is the mass (kg)

a is the acceleration (m/s^2)

According to Newton's and Hooke's laws, the mass in Figure 5.30, connected to the base through a spring, should slide freely on the base, and is under no force during the resting state of the spring (no acceleration). When the entire system is accelerated to the left, the spring extends and applies force on the mass, which is also accelerated. Combining Eqs. (5.60) and (5.61), results in Eq. (5.62), which allows measuring acceleration from linear displacement/stretching of the spring:

$$Ma = k\Delta x \tag{5.62}$$

or

$$a = \frac{k}{M}\Delta x \tag{5.63}$$

If the acceleration is in the opposite direction, the equation remains valid, and the spring is compressed rather than extended. The mass that converts the acceleration into displacement of the spring is called test mass or seismic mass. The spring-mass principle applies to many projects for accelerometers and the various types of accelerometers differ in the way the displacement sensor is implemented. Thus, the measurement of acceleration is reduced to essentially linear displacement measurement.

Vibration is a special type of acceleration characterized by the periodic motion of an object around an equilibrium position. Even when the displacement value is low, very large peak accelerations may result, for example, reaching 100 g or more. It is important to industrial and research environments to determine and monitor

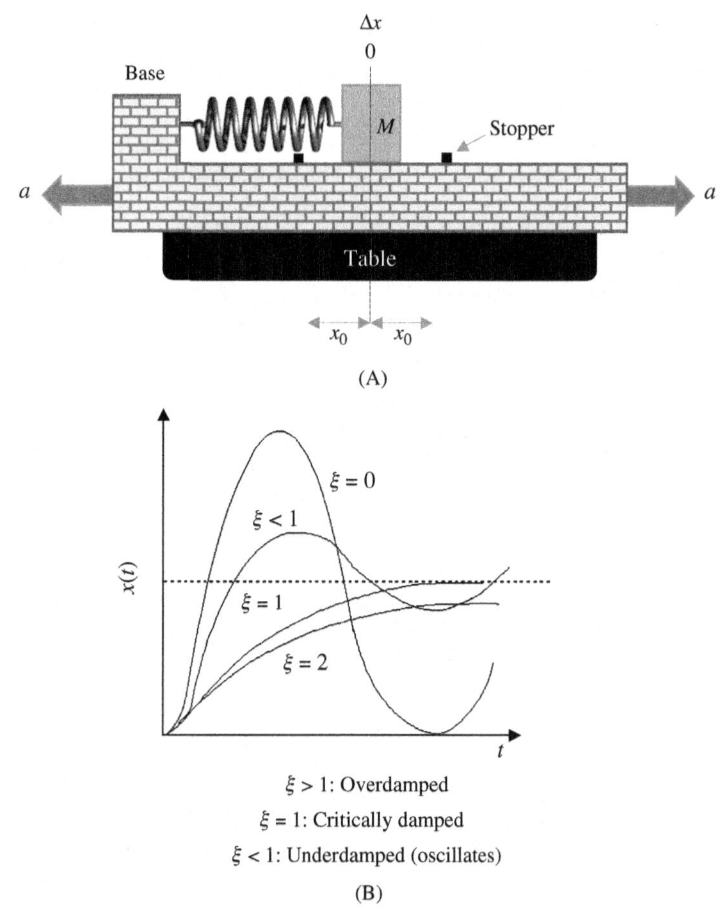

Figure 5.31 Schematic diagram showing the components of the system mass-spring accelerometer used to measure the vibration of a table (A) and effect of the damping factor on the mass displacement (B).

vibrations and the instabilities caused by vibrations of machinery and equipment. Consider the situation shown in Figure 5.31A, at which the mass-spring accelerometer measures the acceleration of a table submitted to longitudinal vibration. The vibration can be modeled as sinusoidal displacement:

$$x(t) = x_0 \sin \omega t \tag{5.64}$$

where

x_0 is the equilibrium position

ω is the angular velocity ($2\pi f$).

The vibration velocity is found deriving Eq. (5.64) with regard to time:

$$v(t) = -\omega x_0 \cos \omega t \tag{5.65}$$

and acceleration is determined deriving the velocity equation with regard to time:

$$a(t) = -\omega^2 x_0 \sin \omega t \tag{5.66}$$

It is easily noticed from Eq. (5.66) that the peak acceleration, $a_{\text{peak}} = \omega^2 x_o$, depends on ω^2, the squared angular frequency, which may result in very large acceleration values, even with little displacements. Vibration of mechanical elements and electronic devices can be destructive; monitoring vibration-type acceleration has importance to prevent adverse events, such as cracks, failures, and damages in equipment and facilities and misinterpretation of device readings.

Replacing Eq. (5.66) in Eq. (5.63) results in Eq. (5.67), which shows that a spring-mass set is a second-order dynamic system, meaning that its response has a natural oscillation frequency without damping expressed by Eq. (5.68). This natural oscillation corresponds to the spring-mass system response to an impulse-like input, even without acceleration. The mass would oscillate back and forth indefinitely, but due to friction between the mass and the base (ideally null), the oscillations are attenuated till the mass stops (Figure 5.31B).

$$\Delta x = -\frac{M x_0}{k} \omega^2 \sin \omega t \tag{5.67}$$

$$f_{\text{n}} = \frac{1}{2\pi} \sqrt{\frac{k}{M}} \tag{5.68}$$

where

f_{n} is the natural oscillation frequency without damping (Hz)

k is the spring constant (N/m)

Δx is the spring extension or mass displacement length (m)

M is the seismic mass (kg)

x_0 is the vibration amplitude.

The natural oscillations are attenuated by a damping factor, expressed by Eq. (5.69):

$$\xi = \frac{1}{2\sqrt{kM}} \tag{5.69}$$

According to ξ value, the response will oscillate or not: if $\xi < 1$, the system I classified as underdamped and will not oscillate; if $\xi = 1$, the system is critically damped (does not oscillate); and if $\xi > 1$, the system is overdumped and also does not oscillate (Figure 5.31B).

When an object in movement is decelerated rapidly, as when a fall or collision occurs, this abrupt slowdown is called shock, a type of linear acceleration, which is also measured with transducers. Shock is characterized by decelerations that occur in milliseconds time interval, with acceleration peak of the order of hundreds of g, a

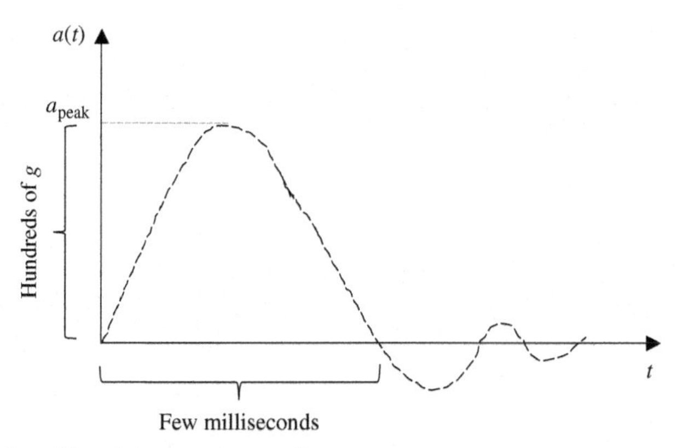

Figure 5.32 Typical profile of the shock waveform.

range of values fair greater than values of linear and angular daily activities (<1 g) and vibration acceleration (up to a few tens of g). The typical waveform of a shock acceleration is shown in Figure 5.32.

Acceleration, vibration, and shock are very fast events and they have a frequency spectrum with high frequency components. Thus, it is important to know the frequency response of the transducer used, compared to the expected frequency of the measured signal. As a rule, the lowest frequency of the accelerometer spectrum should be one-tenth of the lower frequency in the spectrum of the variable to be measured. Its highest frequency should be 10 times larger than the highest frequency in the variable spectrum.

To be able to measure such a rapid event as shock is usually required an accelerometer with a high frequency response and a large working range, around 500 g. As the acceleration signal might only last for 5 ms, it has high frequency spectral components. Piezoelectric transducers, with a 7 kHz band, are suitable for such an application. In order to compare frequency responses, resistive and inductive transducers have a 25 Hz frequency response, LVDT and strain gage devices 150 Hz, and piezoresistive 2 kHz (Taifour, Al-Sharif & Milani, 2008).

Displacement transducers are commonly used as secondary transducer in the measurement of other variables, among them, acceleration. Accelerometers rely on the principle of converting the acceleration to a displacement and then measuring the displacement using a number of different methods. The displacement sensors most commonly used in the construction of accelerometers are resistive (potentiometer), capacitive, inductive (LVDT), piezoresistive (strain gage), piezoelectric and photoelectric elements, with the increasing trend of using micromachining technology. The most important parameters that need to be taken into account when selecting an accelerometer are:

Number of axes—Accelerometers can be uniaxial, biaxial, or triaxial and each of the axes is perpendicular to the others. They are usually referred to as X, Y, and Z, whereby Z is usually the axis in the vertical direction.

Range—The working range of the accelerometer is the effective range that it is able to measure and is usually expressed in multiples of g, for example, 3 g, 50 g, 500 g, etc.
Sensitivity—The amplitude in mV of the accelerometer output per unitary variation of acceleration in m/s^2 ($mV/m/s^2$).
Cross sensitivity—Ideally, an accelerometer axis should show sensitivity only to acceleration at one direction. However, a real accelerometer also shows some response to an acceleration signal that is perpendicular to its axis, which is named cross sensitivity. It is a dimensionless unit, usually expressed as a percentage. Typical range goes from 1% to 5%.
Ressonance frequency—The frequency of the acceleration being measured must be far from the resonant frequency of the accelerometer (Hz) because at this frequency, it responds with large oscillations even to a small driving signal. When damping is small, the resonant frequency is approximately equal to the natural frequency of the system.
Time constant—This represents the speed of response of the device.
Type of output—The output of an accelerometer can be either ratiometric or absolute. A ratiometric output means that the output signal has to be expressed as the ratio of the output voltage divided by the power supply voltage. An absolute output is independent of the value of the power supply voltage.

The functioning of some acceleration transducers is explained below (Cobbold, 1974; Doebelin, 2004; Elwenspoek & Jansen, 1999; Leondes, 2006; Lyshevski, 2002; National Instrument Corporation 2, 2014).

5.4.1 Acceleration transducer with potentiometric displacement sensor

Figure 5.33 shows the representation of a typical potentiometric accelerator. The seismic mass is attached to the potentiometer wiper. The acceleration of the whole

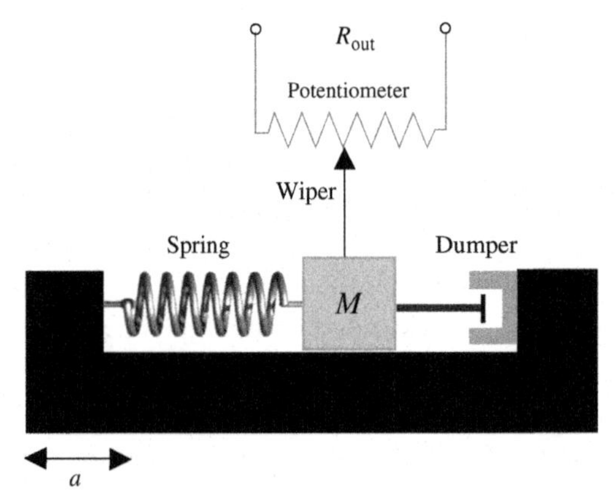

Figure 5.33 Acceleration transducer with potentiometric displacement sensor.

set displaces the seismic mass, which modifies the wiper position and thus, the potentiometer resistance varies. In this accelerometer, the mass position is directly converted into a resistance variation that is used in a conditioning circuit (resistance divider, Wheatstone bridge, etc.) to obtain a voltage or current signal. Additional analog or digital processing gives the acceleration value. Potentiometric or resistive accelerators are suitable for slowly varying accelerations and low frequency vibrations. The natural frequency of these devices is typically <30 Hz, limiting their application to stationary acceleration or low vibration frequency measurements. Typical working range is 0–50 *g* and cross sensitivity and accuracy values are ±1%.

5.4.2 Acceleration transducer with capacitive displacement sensor

Figure 5.34 shows capacitive accelerometers with the seismic mass attached to one of the plates of a capacitor of plane plates (Figure 5.34A) and to the central plate of a differential capacitor (Figure 5.34B). In both examples, the mass is connected to a spring and to a dumper fixed at the accelerometer casing. The mass displacement due to acceleration varies the capacitance, which can be used in different measuring circuits, for instance, a Wheatstone bridge or an LC oscillator, to produce an electrical signal, voltage or current, proportional to acceleration. Capacitive accelerometers have typical working range of 40 *g*, accuracy of ±0.25% FS, resolution of 10^{-4} *g*, and cross sensitivity of 0.5%.

The differential capacitor configuration is used in MEMS (microelectromechanical systems) accelerometers, as the ADXL105, an unidirectional accelerometer, which has nominal capacitance 150 nF, working range ±5 *g*, sensitivity 100 aF ($=10^{-18}$ F) for 1 *g*, bandwidth 10 kHz and 10–22 kHz resonance frequency (Analog Devices, 2014).

Micromachining technology, mainly used to manufacture complex integrated circuits, is also applied to fabricate miniature mechanical devices. Silicon not only has well-established applications due to its electronic properties, but also has some outstanding mechanical characteristics, which make it suitable for producing precision microstructures, as for example, mechanical sensors (Greenwood, 1988). The functioning of this type of sensor is explained from Figure 5.35 that shows the main beam and one of the several parallel cells of the configuration. The main beam is the seismic mass (typically 0.5 μg) and tethers act like a spring. The center plate, that is attached to the main beam (similar to a cantilever), and the fixed outer metallic plates form a capacitive divisor. At the resting condition, with no acceleration, outer plates are equidistant to the center one and both capacitances are equal (Figure 5.35A). Under acceleration (Figure 5.35B), distances between the center and outer plates are modified and thus, C_1 and C_2 capacitance values change. When C_1 increases, C_2 decreases and vice versa. For the measurement of the differential change in capacitance, in each cell, high frequency sine or square waves of same amplitude, but opposite phases feed the outer plates. Without acceleration, the output voltage at center plate is null; under acceleration, the output voltage is no longer

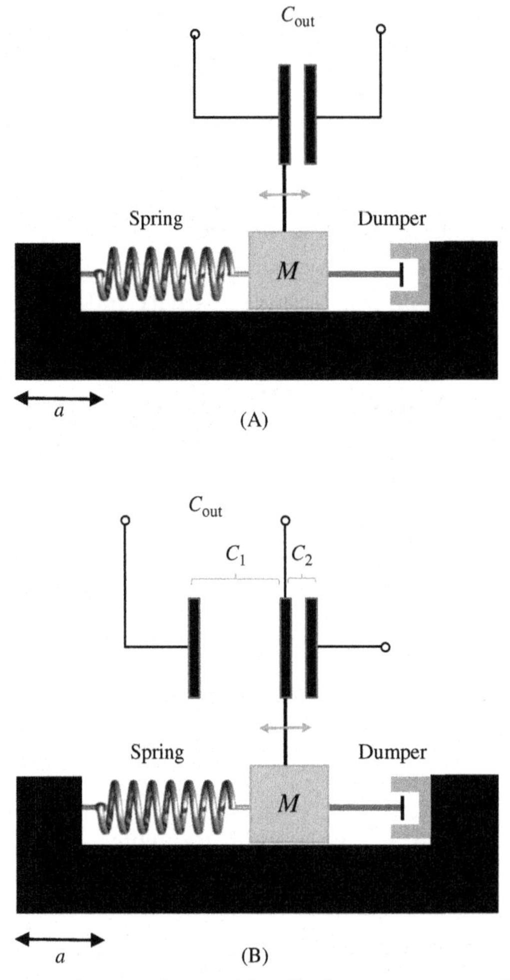

Figure 5.34 Acceleration transducer with capacitive displacement sensor: (A) parallel plates capacitor and (B) differential capacitor.

null. The magnitude of the signal, which is coupled to the center plate, is proportional to the imbalance of capacitance, and its phase indicates the acceleration direction (Kuehnel & Sherman, 1994; Lee et al., 2005). MEMS differential capacitor accelerometer also includes conditioning electronic circuitry. For example, the MMA1200D, fabricated by Freescale, is a silicon capacitive, Z axis sensitivity, surface mount micromachined accelerometer with working range $\pm 250\,g$ for vibration and impact monitoring, which contains housed in its package signal conditioning, a 4-pole low pass filter, temperature compensation and self-test capability to verify the system functionality (Freescale Semiconductor, 2014).

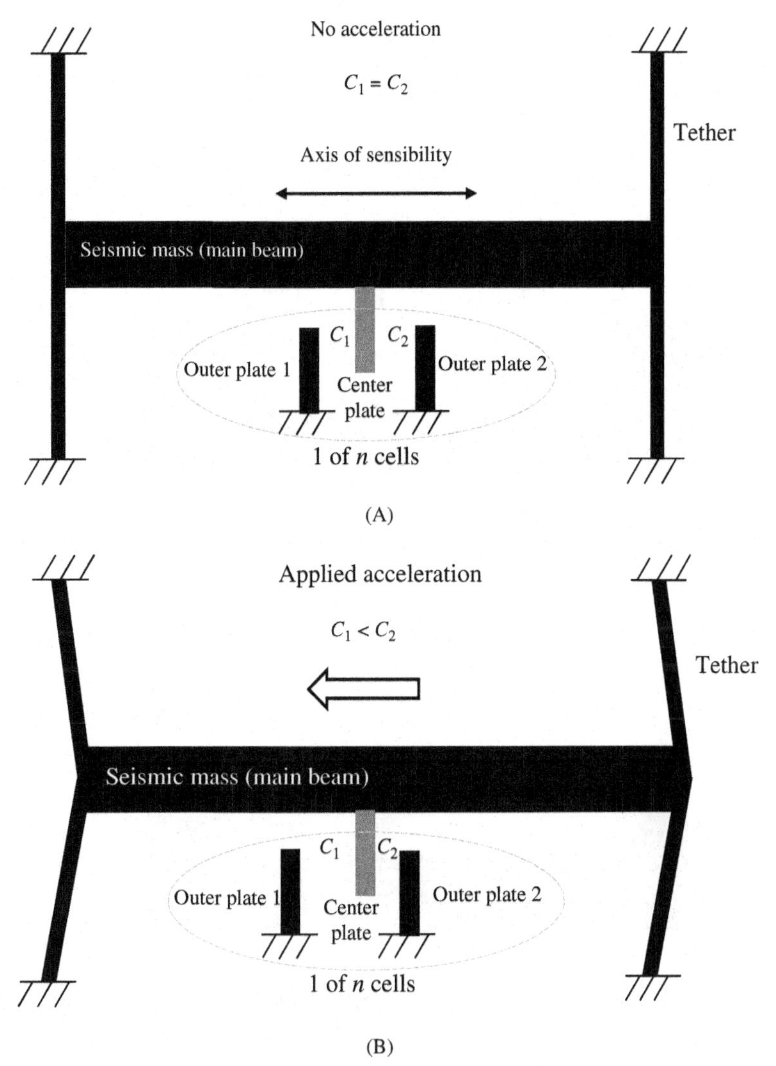

Figure 5.35 Schematic diagram showing 1 of *n* cells of the differential capacitor configuration used in MEMS accelerometer: (A) resting state and (B) under acceleration.

5.4.3 Acceleration transducer with inductive displacement sensor

Several configurations with variable inductance can be used in inductive accelerometer. Figure 5.36 shows two of them. The presence of acceleration can modify mechanically the inductance parameters, due to mass displacement that changes the permeability of the medium, for example, approaching or moving away the two parts of the ferromagnetic core (Figure 5.36A), or varying the number of loops of the coil

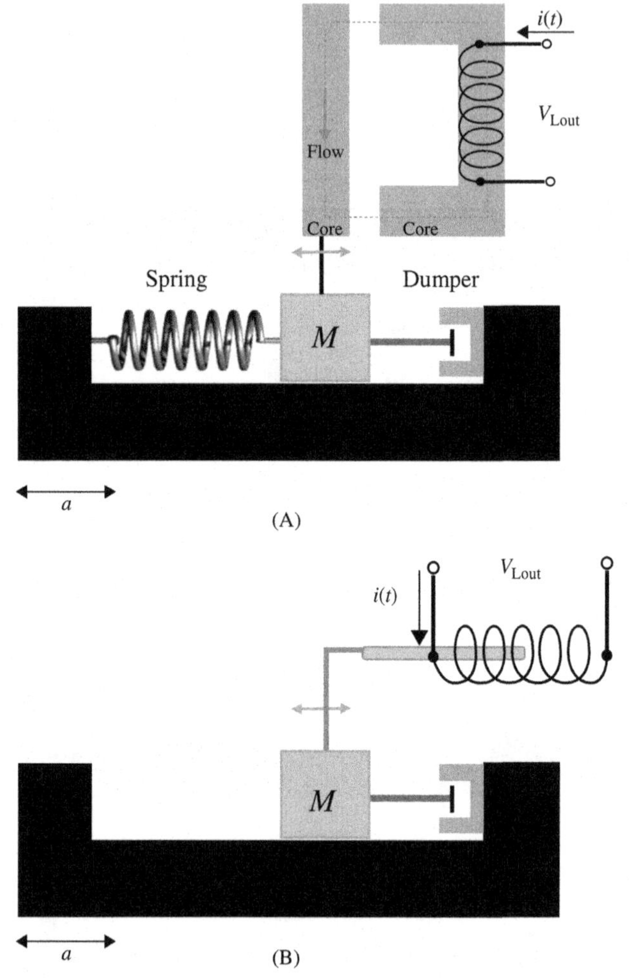

Figure 5.36 Acceleration transducer with inductive displacement sensor. Acceleration changes the permeability of the medium modifying the air gap in the core (A) and the number of loops coupled to the core (B).

that are coupled to the core (Figure 5.36B). The variable inductance is transduced into an acceleration value through measuring the seismic mass displacement. Like capacitive accelerometers, inductive devices have typical working range of 40 *g*, accuracy of $\pm$ 0.25% FS, resolution of 10^{-4} *g* and cross-sensitivity of 0.5%.

5.4.4 Acceleration transducer with LVDT displacement sensor

Figure 5.37 shows an LVDT accelerometer configuration in which the core acts like a seismic mass. Spring steels are attached to the case and to the connection to the core. When the device is submitted to acceleration or vibration, the ferroelectric core

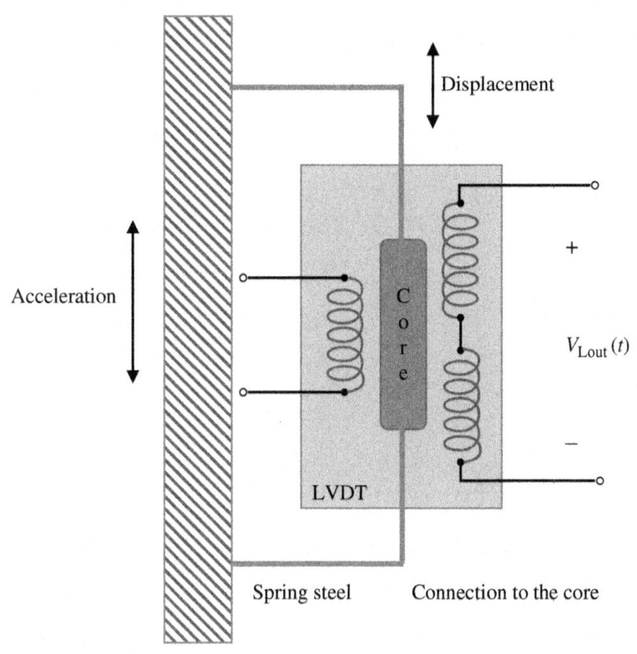

Figure 5.37 LVDT accelerometer.

displaces changing the coupling between primary and secondary coils. The output voltage is directly converted into an AC output voltage linearly proportional to the core displacement.

LVDT has a phase sensitive output voltage and linear relation between its intensity and displacement. The LVDT also does not offer any resistance to movement and is sensitive only to longitudinal core displacement, which in general is advantageous over other types of accelerometers, as for example, resistive potentiometric device. LVDT devices have a working range of 700 g and accuracy of ±1% FS. The spring and the magnet make up a low frequency resonant system and typically natural frequency is <80 Hz. They are commonly used in steady-state acceleration or low-frequency vibration measurements.

5.4.5 Acceleration transducer with piezoresistive (strain gage) displacement sensor

The main components of the piezoresistive accelerometer are the seismic mass (M), a spring (suspension mechanism), and displacement sensor. Figure 5.38A shows a basic piezoresistive accelerometer with cantilever and the displacement sensor, which is formed by four equal strain gages, one pair bonded on the top and the second pair on the bottom of the cantilever. Most used measuring circuit in this case is the

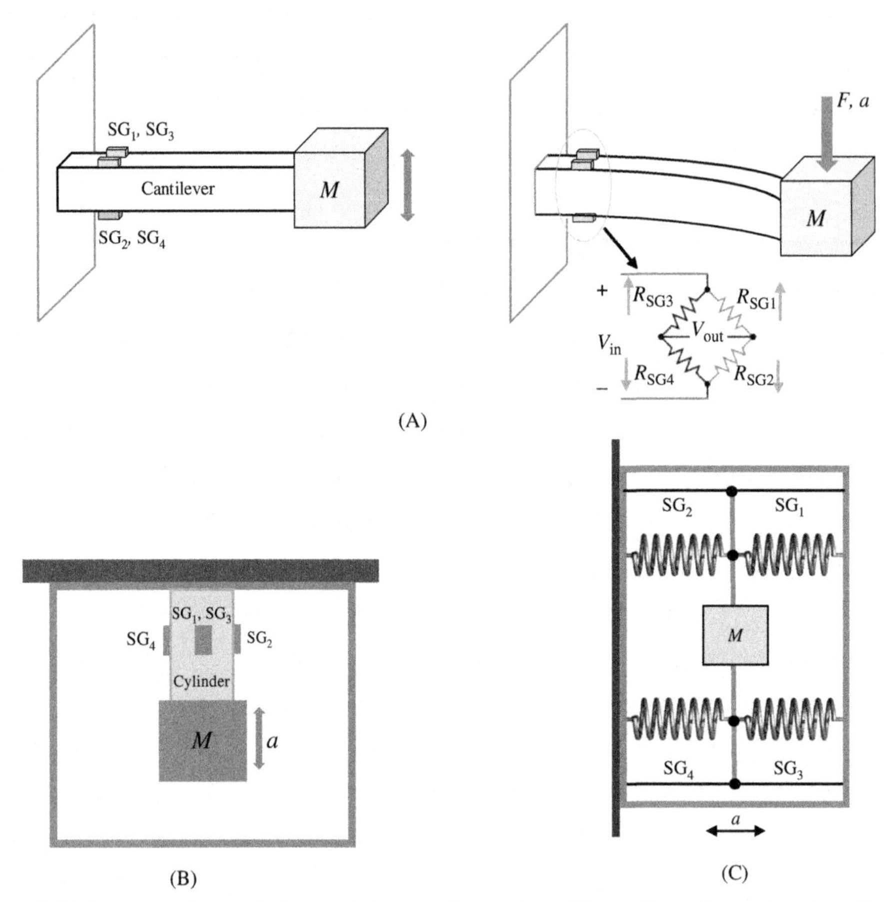

Figure 5.38 Basic structures of piezoresistive accelerometers: (A) cantilever beam type accelerometer with bonded strain gages; (B) cylinder beam type accelerometer with bonded strain gages; and (C) accelerometer with unbonded strain gage.

Wheatstone bridge in full-bridge configuration. Bonded gages used as displacement sensor can be wire, foil, or semiconductor types.

If the device is not under acceleration, both strain gage pairs are in the unstressed state, all four resistances are equal and the bridge circuit is balanced, that is, its output is null. In the presence of acceleration, the seismic mass is displaced upward or downward, bending the cantilever. One pair of gages is tensioned and the resistances increase; the other is compressed and the resistance decreases. The output is no longer null, its magnitude is proportional to the mass displacement and acceleration and its polarity indicates the acceleration direction.

The strain gages are bonded to the cantilever that is connected to the mass and the acceleration is only partially transferred to the cantilever, which causes loss of sensitivity. The cantilever beam type accelerometer has low natural frequency, which limits its application. Filling the case with dumping liquid, which includes a dumper element in the system, helps to increase the natural frequency. The cylinder beam type has higher natural frequency, and its configuration is shown in Figure 5.38B. The solid cylinder acts as a spring and supports the seismic mass. Four strain gages are radially bonded to the cylinder surface to measure its deformation under acceleration. According to the acceleration direction, the cylinder is compressed or stretched and despite of the little resulting deflection, natural frequency is of the order of thousands of kHz. The use of semiconductor gages improves the transducer sensitivity.

Figure 5.38C shows an accelerometer with unbonded strain gage. The gage wires are pretensioned and along with the springs help to support the seismic mass. The transducer case is fixed in the structure submitted to the acceleration. In the resting state, the strain gages are unstressed and all resistances have the same value. If the gages are inserted in a Wheatstone bridge measuring circuit, the output voltage is null. Under acceleration, two strain gages are tensioned (resistance increases) and two are contracted (resistance decreases), unbalancing the bridge. The output voltage magnitude is proportional to the mass displacement and thus, its acceleration. The polarity of the output signal indicates the direction of the acceleration.

Piezoresistive accelerometers have a typical working range of $200\,g$, a resolution $\approx 1 \times 10^{-3}\,g$, accuracy of $\pm 1\%$, and cross sensitivity of $\pm 2\%$. They usually are constructed in smaller sizes and weight than the other types of accelerometers.

Piezoresistive accelerometers can be produced with the MEMS technology. Micromachined accelerometers usually consist of a small mass mounted on a thin silicon membrane and displacement is measured by the use of a strain gage deposited or etched on the membrane. Under the influence of gravity or acceleration, the seismic mass deflects from its neutral position, modifies the strain gage resistance, which is processed by analog or digital circuits.

Figure 5.39 shows the schematic representation of a micromachined piezoresistive accelerometer fabricated using bulk-micromachining (Roylance, 1979). It has a silicon paddle, which acts like a seismic mass, connected to a silicon cantilever beam where an N-type silicon resistor was diffused; silicon beam and paddle stay suspended over an air gap. Under acceleration, the silicon mass bends within the air gap and deflects the cantilever beam, modifying the piezoresistance value. Resting piezoresistance value is $5\,\text{k}\Omega$ and it varies (increases) with acceleration. The resistance variation is directly proportional to deformation, which in turn is directly proportional to the acceleration. The variation of the resistance is measured across the terminals of the device, amplified and processed to provide the acceleration value.

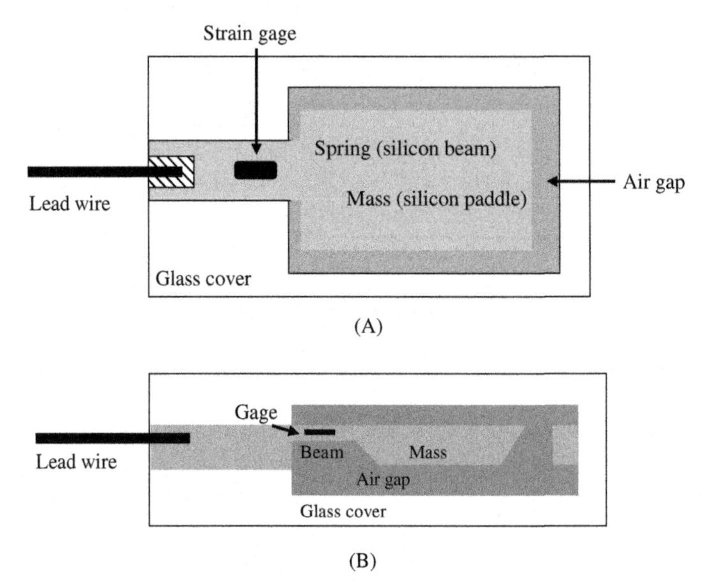

Figure 5.39 Schematic diagram showing the components of a basic structure of micromachined (semiconductor) strain gage (A) top view and (B) cross section.

An alternative configuration has very small cantilever beams, instead of a membrane, supporting seismic masses and strain gages as sensing elements. The strain gages can be directly diffused into the supporting beams, which is a simple and cheap manufacturing process. Under acceleration, the masses deflect and the strain gage resistances change due to the stress induced in the beams.

Most micromachined piezoaccelerometers have low level analog outputs that need amplification and some already have built-in amplifiers for direct connection into external circuitry as, for example, a microcontroller. As semiconductor devices, they have relatively large sensitivity drift with temperature (Chih-Ming, Chuanwei, & Weileun, 2008; Zimmermann, Ebersohl, Hung, Berry, & Baillieu, 1995) and additional strain gages in the piezoaccelerometer structure may be used for temperature compensation and for calibration. Micromachined piezoaccelerometers are available with one, two, or three axis configurations. With three axis, they output acceleration vectors in X, Y, and Z directions (usually Z corresponds to vertical direction).

5.4.6 Acceleration transducer with piezoelectric displacement sensor

A piezoelectric transducer of acceleration has a piezoelectric element that is mounted between a base and a seismic mass inside the casing. Acceleration displaces the seismic mass that develops a force on piezoelectric quartz or ceramic crystal, or on several crystals. The force causes compression, tension, or shear on the piezoelectric material,

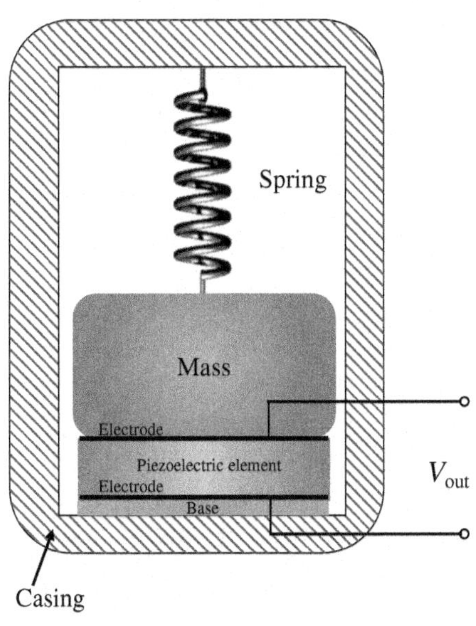

Figure 5.40 Basic structure of a piezoelectric accelerometer.

which produces a charge buildup proportional to acceleration. A spring acts as a dumper and is used to pretension the piezoelectric material. The piezosensing element can be implemented as a thin film of piezoelectric material deposited on the silicon suspension system of the seismic mass. Piezoelectric accelerometers are also constructed as integrated circuits and usually incorporate conditioning electronics in their casing.

Figure 5.40 shows the basic structure of a piezoelectric accelerometer. The piezoelectric element is attached to the seismic mass and to the spring. Under acceleration, the mass displaces and exerts a force ($F = ma = kx$) in the piezoelectric element, which is tensioned or stretched, according to acceleration direction. This mechanical stress causes internal charges redistribution in the piezoelement, which is sensed as a voltage drop measured between the faces of the element. Measurement of the voltage drop, and thus the mass displacement, allows the acceleration determination.

The piezoelectric element output impedance is high and its output signal, typically with amplitude of the order of mV, requires a low noise and high impedance amplifier to avoid loading. It acts as a low pass filter and its natural frequency is usually higher than 5 kHz. Thus, piezoaccelerometers are not suitable for slowly varying or constant accelerations, but are suitable for vibration and shock measurements. Commercial piezoaccelerometers can come with a built-in charge amplifier with high input impedance in the same package, demanding great care to use due to high g values this type of device is subjected. Piezoelectric devices have a long-term stability, resolution of ±0.1%, accuracy of ±1% and a large working range, from 0.03 to 1,000 *g*. Power supply is required only to the units with conditioning electronics incorporated.

The various types of accelerometers described here are open-loop systems. To improve their linearity, electronic circuitry must be added to implement a force balancing structure, obtaining a closed loop operation, which generates opposite forces on the seismic mass to keep it close to its rest position.

5.5 REVIEW THE LEARNING

1. Compare the operating characteristics of the resistive, capacitive, and inductive displacement transducers.
2. Mark with an X in the right answer. The material used in the grid of strain gages must have the following characteristics:
   a. Low sensitivity (G factor), high resistivity, low sensitivity to temperature variations, and low thermal emf when connected to other materials
   b. High sensitivity (G factor), high resistivity, low sensitivity to temperature variations, and low thermal emf when connected to other materials
   c. Low sensitivity (G factor), low resistivity, low sensitivity to temperature variations, and low thermal emf when connected to other materials
   d. High sensitivity (G factor), low resistivity, high sensitivity to temperature variations, and low thermal emf when connected to other materials
   e. Low sensitivity (G factor), high resistivity, low sensitivity to temperature variations, and low thermal emf when connected to other materials.
3. Show the basic structure of an LVDT and the curves of its output voltage for three relative positions of the core and the secondary coils: (i) the core is in the origin ($x = 0$); (ii) the core is in the central position, that is, aligned symmetrically with both secondary coils; and (iii) core is in the maximum excursion. The primary excitation voltage is a sine wave with peak-to-peak constant amplitude and frequency 1 kHz.
4. Show the basic structure of a Doppler ultrasonic velocimeter and explain its operation.
5. Show the basic structure of linear and angular electromagnetic velocimeters and explain their operation.
6. Compare the characteristics (resolution, sensitivity, error of linearity, accuracy, etc.) of ultrasonic and ferromagnetic accelerometers. Suggestion: Assemble a table.
7. Show the basic structure of an accelerometer explaining the function of each component.
8. Consider the operating characteristics of LVDT and piezoelectric accelerometers and choose one to measure vibration-type acceleration and one to shock type acceleration. Justify your answer.

9. Show a drawing with the representation of a micromachined capacitive accelerometer and a measuring circuit. Identify its components and explain its operation.
10. Compare the characteristics (resolution, sensitivity, working range, natural frequency, error of linearity, accuracy, etc.) of piezoelectric, piezoresistive, capacitive, and inductive accelerometers. Suggestion: Assemble a table with the type of accelerometer in the columns and the characteristics in the lines.

REFERENCES

Allard, E. M. (1962). Sound and pressure signals obtained from a single intracardiac transducer. *IRE Transactions on Biomedical Electronics, 9*, 74–79.

All about Circuits 1 (2014). Strain gauges. Volume I—DC, Chapter 9: Electrical instrumentation signals. <www.allaboutcircuits.com/vol_1/chpt_9/7.html> Accessed 18.04.14.

All about Circuits 2 (2014). Strain gauges. Volume I—DC, Chapter 14: Magnetism and electromagnetism. <http://www.allaboutcircuits.com/vol_1/chpt_14/4.html> Accessed 18.04.14.

Analog Devices (2014). ADXL105: ±5 g Single axis high performance accelerometer with analog output. <http://www.analog.com/en/obsolete/adxl105/products/product.html> Accessed 10.06.14.

Anderson, T., & McDicken, W. N. (1999). Measurement of tissue motion. *Proceedings of the Institution of Mechanical Engineers. Part H, Journal of Engineering in Medicine, 213*(3), 181–191.

Barlian, A. A., Park, W.-T., Mallon, J. R., Jr., Rastegar, A. J., & Pruitt, B. L. (2009). Review: Semiconductor piezoresistance for microsystems. *Proceedings of the Institute of Electrical and Electronics Engineers, 97*(3), 513–552.

Bianchi, F., Redmond, S. J., Narayanan, M. R., Cerutti, S., & Lovell, N. H. (2010). Barometric pressure and triaxial accelerometry-based falls event detection. *IEEE Transactions on Neural Systems and Rehabilitation Engineering: A Publication of the IEEE Engineering in Medicine and Biology Society, 18*, 619–627.

Bouten, C. V. C., Sauren, A. A. H., Verduin, M., & Janssen, J. D. (1997). Effects of placement and orientation of body-fixed accelerometers on the assessment of energy expenditure during walking. *Medical and Biological Engineering and Computing, 35*(1), 50–56.

Chan, A. Y. K. (2008). *Biomedical device technology: Principles and design*. Springfield, Illinois: Charles C. Thomas.

Chemloul, N. S., Chaib, K., & Mostefa, K. (2012). In A. A. Santos, Jr. (Ed.), *Application of pulsed ultrasonic Doppler velocimetry to the simultaneous measurement of velocity and concentration profiles in two phase flow. Ultrasonic waves*. InTech. <http://cdn.intechopen.com/pdfs-wm/31682.pdf> Accessed 10.06.14.

Chih-Ming, S., Chuanwei, W., & Weileun, F. (2008). On the sensitivity improvement of CMOS capacitive accelerometer. *Sensors Actuators A Physical, 141*, 347–352.

Cobbold, R. S. C. (1974). *Transducers for biomedical measurements: Principles and applications*. New York: John Wiley & Sons.

Dally, J. W., Riley, W. F., & McConnell, K. G. (1993). *Instrumentation for engineering measurements* (2nd ed.). New York, Chichester: John Wiley & Sons.

Doebelin, E. O. (2004). In M. Hill (Ed.), *Measurements systems—Application and design* (5th ed.). New York: McGraw Hill.

Elwenspoek, M., & Jansen, H. V. (1999). *Silicon micromachining*. Cambridge, U.K.: Cambridge University Press.

Freescale Semiconductor. MMA1200 Technical data surface mount micromachined accelerometer freescale Semiconductor, Inc., 2006. <http://cache.freescale.com/files/sensors/doc/data_sheet/MMA1200D.pdf> Accessed 13.06.14.

Geddes, L. A., & Baker, L. E. (1968). *Principles of applied biomedical instrumentation*. John Wiley & Sons.

Giorgino, T., Tormene, P., Lorussi, F., De Rossi, D., & Quaglini, S. (2009). Sensor evaluation for wearable strain gauges in neurological rehabilitation. *IEEE Transactions on Neural Systems and Rehabilitation Engineering: A Publication of the IEEE Engineering in Medicine and Biology Society, 17*, 409–415.

Greenwood, J. C. (1988). Silicon in mechanical sensors. *Journal of Physics E: Scientific Instruments, 21*, 1114–1128.

Helfrick, A. D., & Cooper, W. D. (1990). *Modern electronic instrumentation and measurement techniques.* Prentice Hall.

Johnson, C. D. (1997). *Process control instrumentation technology.* Prentice Hall.

Kazan, A. (1994). *Transducers and their elements.* Prentice Hall.

Khandpur, R. S. (2005). *Biomedical instrumentation. Technology and applications.* McGraw-Hill.

Kuehnel, W., & Sherman, S. (1994). A surface micromachined silicon accelerometer with on-chip detection circuitry. *Sensors and Actuators A, 45*, 7–16.

Lee, G., Lee, T., Dexter, D., Klein, R., & Park, A. (2007). Methodological infrastructure in surgical ergonomics: A review of tasks, models, and measurement systems. *Surgical Innovation, 14*(3), 153–167.

Lee, I., Yoon, G. H., Park, J., Seok, S., Chun, K., & Lee, K. (2005). Development and analysis of the vertical capacitive accelerometer. *Sensors and Actuators, 119*, 8–18.

Leondes, C. T. (2006). *MEMS/NEMS handbook techniques and applications, Volume 4: Sensors and actuators.* Springer.

Lyshevski, S. E. (2002). *MEMS and NEMS: Systems, devices and structures.* CRC Press.

Mathie, M. J., Coster, A. C. F., Lovell, N. H., & Celler, B. G. (2004). Accelerometry: Providing an integrated, practical method for long-term, ambulatory monitoring of human movement. *Physiological Measurement, 25*(2).

Mayagoitia, R., Lotters, J., Veltink, P., & Hermens, H. (2002). Standing balance evaluation using a triaxial accelerometer. *Gait & Posture, 16*, 55–59.

Menz, H. B., Lord, S. R., & Fitzpatrick, R. C. (2003). Acceleration patterns of the head and pelvis when walking are associated with risk of falling in community-dwelling older people. *Journal of Gerontology: Medical Sciences, 58A*(5), 446–452.

National Instruments Corporation 1. Measuring strain with strain gages. <http://www.ni.com/white-paper/3642/en/> Accessed 20.05.14.

National Instrument Corporation 2. Accelerometers. <http://zone.ni.com/devzone/devzone.nsf/web-categories/4682C4341CAE7FD68625684A004EB0F4> Accessed 10.06.14.

Nichols, W. W., Pepine, C. J., Conti, C. R., Christie, J. G., & Feldman, R. L. (1981). Quantitation of aortic insufficiency using a catheter-tip velocity transducer. *Circulation, 64*, 375–380. Available from: <http://circ.ahajournals.org/content/64/2/375> Accessed 25.05.14.

Nishimura, R. A., Miller, F. A., Jr., Callahan, M. J., Benassi, R. C., Seward, J. B., & Tajik, A. J. (1985). Doppler echocardiography: Theory, instrumentation, technique, and application. *Mayo Clinic Proceedings. Mayo Clinic, 60*(5), 321–343.

Norman, K. E., Edwards, R., & Beuter, A. (1999). The measurement of tremor using a velocity transducer: Comparison to simultaneous recordings using transducers of displacement, acceleration and muscle activity. *Journal of Neuroscience Methods, 92*, 41–54.

Northrop, R. B. (2005). *Introduction to instrumentation and measurements* (2nd ed.). CRC Press.

OMEGA 1 (2014a). *The strain gage.* <http://www.omega.com/literature/transactions/volume3/strain.html> Accessed 25.04.14.

OMEGA 2 (2014b). *Strain gage measurement.* Strain Gage Technical Data. <http://www.omega.com/techref/strain-gage.html> Accessed 30.04.14.

Patel, S., Park, H., Bonato, P., Chan, L., & Rodgers, M. (2012). A review of wearable sensors and systems with application in rehabilitation. *Journal of Neuro Engineering and Rehabilitation, 9*(21), 1–17. Available from: <http://www.jneuroengrehab.com/content/9/1/21> Accessed 10.06.14.

Pinney, C. P., & Baker, W. E. (2000). *Velocity measurement.* CRC Press. <http://www.engnetbase.com> Accessed 10.06.14.

Roylance, L. M. (1979). A batch-fabricated silicon accelerometer. *IEEE Transactions on Electron Devices, 26*(12), 1911–1917.

Signal Processing SA. Background of ultrasonic Doppler velocimetry. <http://www.signal-processing.com/intro_udv.html> Accessed 15.06.14.

Taifour, S., Al-Sharif, L., & Kilani, M. (2008). Modelling & design of a linear variable differential transformer. *Proceedings of the International Conference on Modeling and Simulation* (pp. 18–24). Jordan: Petra.

Trans-Tek Incorporated 1 (2014). Series 230 Miniature AC LVDTs. <http://datasheets.globalspec.com/ds/23/transtek/8385069A-ED9A-42A9-92F9-7F8260C0F5D8> Accessed 10.05.14.

Trans-Tek Incorporated 2 (2014). *Linear velocity transducers (LVTs)* Inductive Technology. <http://www.transtekinc.com/assets/files/Catalog_PDFs_04C/LVTs/LVT_tech04c.pdf> Accessed 25.05.14.

Trans-Tek Incorporated 3 (2014). *Trans-Tek Linear Velocity Transducer Series 100.* <http://www.intertechnology.com/Trans_Tek/TransTek_Series_100.html> Accessed 10.06.14.

Webster, J. (Ed.), (2010). *Medical instrumentation. Application and design* (4th ed.). Wiley & Sons, Inc.

Yoon, J., Novandy, B., Yoon, C.-H., & Park, K.-J. (2010). A 6-DOF gait rehabilitation robot with upper and lower limb connections that allows walking velocity updates on various terrains. *IEEE/ASME Transactions on Mechatronics*, *15*(2), 201–215.

Zimmermann, L., Ebersohl, J. O., Hung, F. L., Berry, J. P., Baillieu, F., et al. (1995). Airbag application: A microsystems including a silicon capacitive accelerometer, CMOS switched capacitor electronics and true self-test capability. *Sensors and Actuators. A, Physical*, *46*, 190–195.

CHAPTER 6

Pressure and Force Transducers

Contents

6.1 PRESSURE TRANSDUCERS

6.1.1 Introduction

Pressure is defined as force applied per unit area and in the International System it is quantified in Newton per square meter (N/m^2) or Pascal (Pa). First devices developed to atmospheric pressure measurement had a water column, later replaced by a mercury column, also used in the initial sphygmomanometers, which led to the common use of mercury millimeters (mmHg) as pressure measurement unit. This unit is also known as Torricelli (Torr), after Evangelista Torricelli, an Italian physicist and mathematician, for his discovery of the principle of the barometer in 1643. 1 mmHg is equal to 133 Pa and 760 mmHg corresponds to 1 atm, which means the atmospheric pressure that supports a column of mercury 760 mm high.

Pressure is measured against a reference, and depending on the type of pressure transducer used, the measured value can be absolute, when the measurement is referenced to vacuum; gage, if the reference is atmospheric pressure; and differential, which means the transducer measures the difference between two pressure values, the unknown and one sealed internal reference pressure.

Pressure transducers are used routinely in clinical practice to identify pathological levels of blood pressure, especially in the diagnosis of hypertension. Hypertension is

Principles of Measurement and Transduction of Biomedical Variables.
DOI: http://dx.doi.org/10.1016/B978-0-12-800774-7.00006-4

the most prevalent major risk factor for cardiovascular and renal diseases. Risk factors for development of hypertension are nowadays well understood, and numerous dietary and personal habits must be addressed to lower population levels of blood pressure in order to prevent diseases resulting from hypertension (Black & Elliot, 2013). In addition to the diagnosis of arterial hypertension, pressure transducers are also used in a wide variety of biomedical applications for control and monitoring purposes. Among them are venous, intraocular (glaucoma) and intracranial hypertension, the monitoring of intra-amniotic pressure, the obtaining of the urethral pressure profile, the continuous or intermittent monitoring of blood pressure in surgical procedures, as well as in the postoperative period, the monitoring of central venous pressure during plasma and blood transfusion and the pressure control of devices such as artificial ventilators and infusion pumps. Pressure transducers support indirect measurement of other biomedical variables such as force, flow (liquid or gas), and velocity.

From the general definition of pressure, it comes that arterial blood pressure is the force, applied by blood, per unit area of the artery wall. It is directly dependent of cardiac output, peripheral resistance of vascular system and blood volume contained in patient's body. The measurement of arterial blood pressure usually provides two values, diastolic and systolic pressures, indicated in mmHg (standard unit). Diastolic is the minimum value detected in the systemic arterial system and it occurs during the diastolic phase of the cardiac cycle. Systolic arterial pressure corresponds to the higher (peak) blood pressure value detected in the arteries during the systolic phase of cardiac cycle.

The arterial pulse, the rhythmic oscillations of arterial blood pressure, is the result of the variation of blood volume in the arterial site, repeated at each cardiac cycle (Figure 6.1A and B). The arterial pulse originates at the aortic root, with each left ventricle systole and propagates along systemic and pulmonary circulation with characteristic profiles (Figure 6.1C). Similar behavior is repeated in the pulmonary circulation from the right ventricle outflow at the entrance of the pulmonary artery, with peak pressure equal to 30 mmHg during the systole, to the pulmonary veins outflow at the entrance of the left atrium, with almost zero pressure.

Desirable values of arterial blood pressure for a health adult are <120 mmHg (systole) and <80 mmHg (diastole) (JNC7, 2003), but blood pressure varies with age, state of health, and clinical situation. At birth, a typical blood pressure is 80/50 mmHg. It rises steadily throughout childhood, so that in a young and healthy adult it is typically 120/80 mmHg. As we get older, blood pressure continues to rise, but at lower speed (Table 6.1).

6.1.2 Methods of measurement of arterial blood pressure

Although the pulsatile nature of blood flow was known since 1500 BC, it was only in 1628 that Sir William Harvey described the blood flow circulation in the human body.

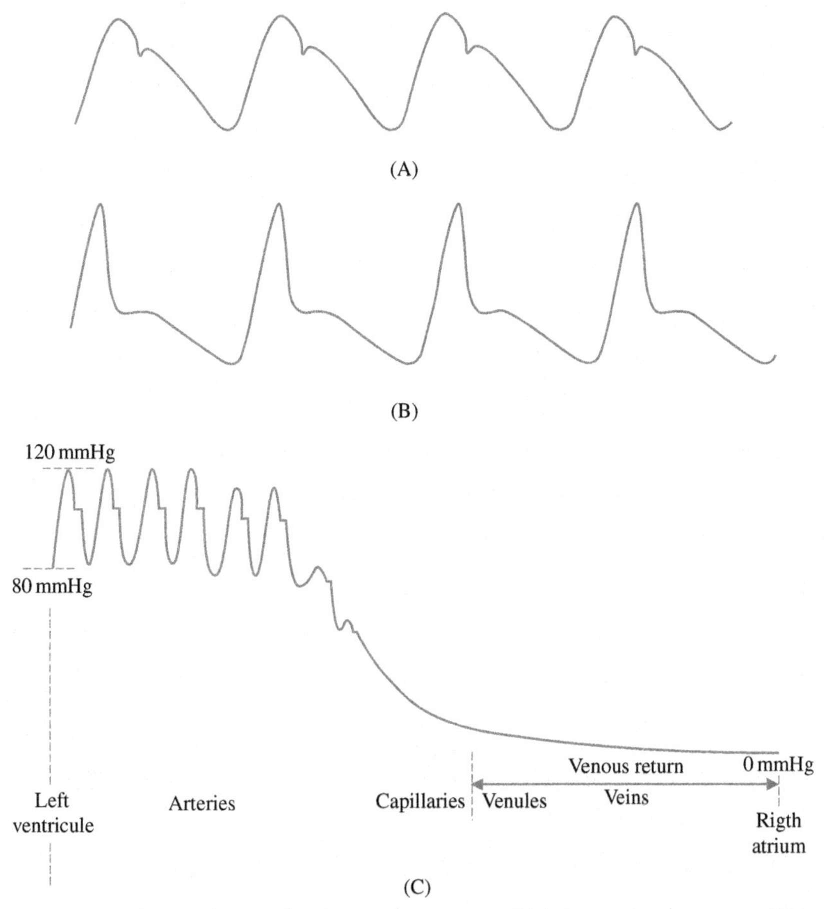

Figure 6.1 Example of typical arterial pulses at (A) aorta and (B) femoral arteries. In addition to the profile changing of the arterial pulse along systemic and pulmonary circulation (C), pressure intensity also changes.

Table 6.1 Arterial blood pressure variation with aging

Age (years)	Arterial pressure (mmHg)
4	85/60
6	95/62
10	100/65
12	108/67
16	118/75
Adulto	120/80
Idoso	140–160/90–100

In 1733, Stephen Hales made the first invasive direct measurement of arterial blood pressure, in a mare, using a graded water column to indicate pressure value. In 1828, Poiseuille, a physicist and physician, enhanced the Hales manometer and developed the hemodynamometer with mercury column instead of water, which reduced the height of the column (mercury density is 13.6 greater than water density). The sphygmomanometer (from Greek *sphygmos*, pulse) of Hérrison (physician) and Gernier (engineer), developed in 1834, allowed a noninvasive blood pressure measurement; the weight of a mercury reservoir with a graded column was placed against the wrist and its weight compressed the artery, which pulse displaced the mercury column. In 1855, Vierordt used an inflatable cuff placed around the arm to constrict the artery and interrupt blood flow. The actual mercury sphygmomanometer was originally idealized in 1896, by Riva-Rocci, an Italian physicist (Riva-Rocci, 1896). This method used a cuff to constrict the blood flow in the arm artery and systolic pressure was determined by palpation (Introcaso, 1996; Parker, 2009; Souza, 2003).

The measuring methods of arterial blood pressure can use indirect (noninvasive, continuous, or intermittent) or direct techniques (invasive, usually continuous). Indirect techniques eliminate the need for surgery, but most of them do not allow obtaining the waveform of the pressure pulse (Chung, Chen, Alexander, & Cannesson, 2013; Souza, 2003). Direct techniques involve the introduction of the sensor element directly in the blood vessel, or an external sensor that is hydraulically coupled to the blood flow, through a catheter filled with isotonic solution, which is inserted into the vessel. Direct techniques allow to detect dynamic changes (waveform) of blood pressure.

6.1.2.1 Techniques of indirect measurement of arterial blood pressure

The techniques of indirect measurement of blood pressure are usually implemented with occlusion device (cuff). Main occlusive techniques are auscultatory (sphygmomanometry), oscillometry, Doppler ultrasound, and tonometry. The photoplethysmography technique (finger arterial pressure technique) also uses a cuff, but it does not occlude the blood flow.

6.1.2.1.1 Occlusive auscultatory technique (sphygmomanometry)

In 1904, Korotkoff (physician) described the auscultatory technique for indirect measurement of arterial blood pressure (Korotkoff, 1905). Auscultatory is the most used technique to measure blood pressure. This method uses a stethoscope and a device known as sphygmomanometer that has a cuff connected to a mercury manometer or to an aneroid gage. The mercury manometer has a mercury column, graded in millimeters, which allows the blood pressure to be directly read in mmHg. The aneroid gage has a metallic pressure-sensing element that flexes elastically under the effect of a pressure difference across the element, displacing a pointer over a graduated scale, usually in mmHg. The cuff, usually placed around the upper arm, is inflated to occlude blood flow and deflated by a manually operated rubber bulb. The stethoscope is placed distally to the occlusion point, over the brachial artery at the elbow, so the operator can hear the sounds of the blood flow (Figure 6.2A).

The value of the blood pressure is determined correlating the sounds heard with the stethoscope placed over the arm's artery and the value read in the manometer's

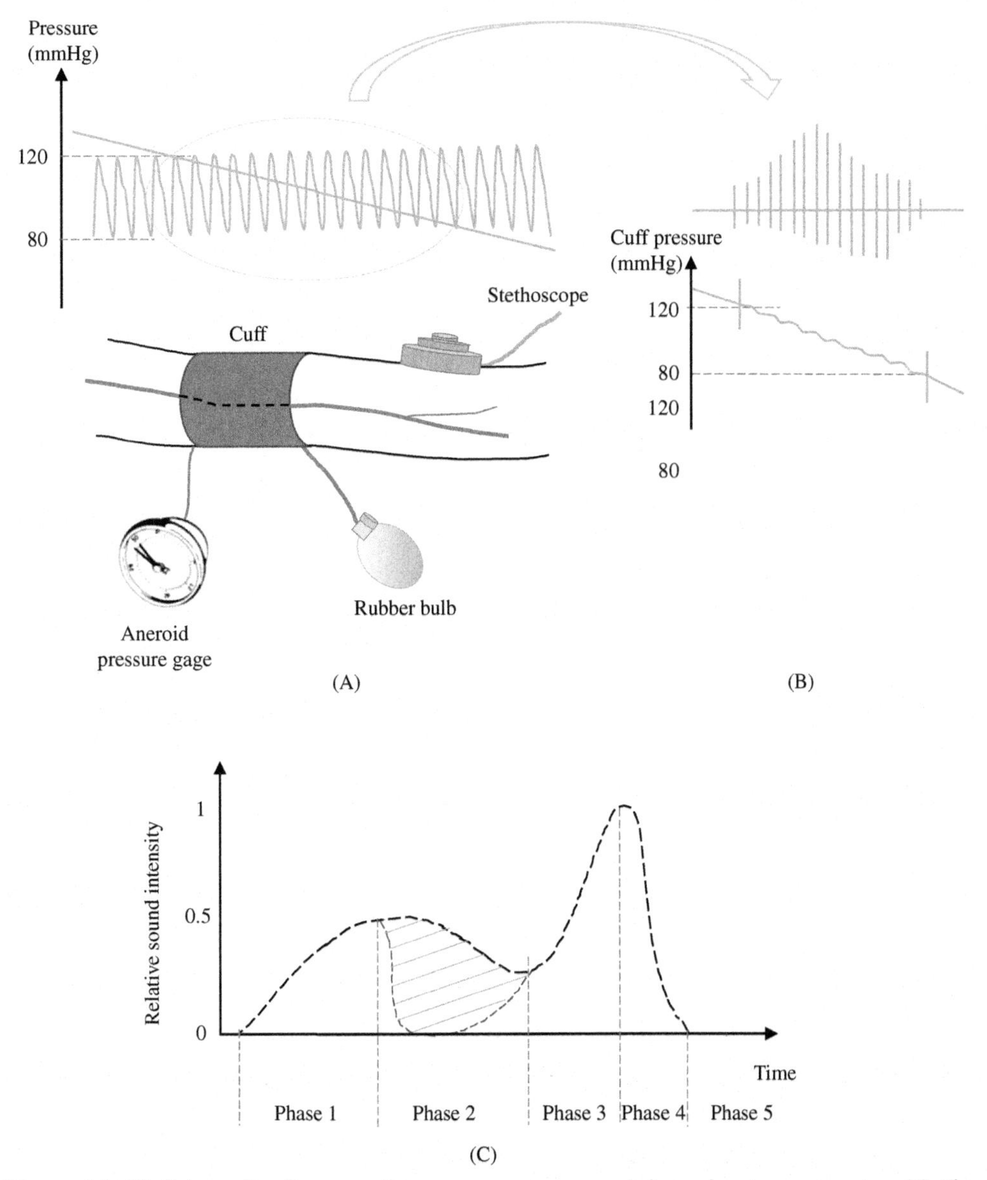

Figure 6.2 (A) Schematic diagram of pressure measurement by sphygmomanometry. (B) The Korotkoff sounds cause fluctuations in the curve of cuff deflation. (C) Phases of Korotkoff sound.

graded scale or other pressure gage. The artery closure and opening during cardiac cycles, while cuff is deflated, causes pressure fluctuations in the cuff (Figure 6.2B) that can be "heard." The sounds that are heard during this procedure are known as Korotkoff's sounds (Figure 6.2C). Auscultatory technique has intermittent character, that is, a new pressure reading demands the repetition of the procedure.

In the schematic diagram of the sphygmomanometry shown in Figure 6.2A, the cuff is inflated to a pressure higher than systolic value, which causes the artery to collapse all over the arterial pulse duration. Then, the cuff pressure is slowly released while operator monitors blood flow with the stethoscope and a pressure gage; when the cuff pressure becomes slightly lower than systolic pressure, the artery opens quite a little and blood starts to flow during the intervals at which blood pressure is greater than the cuff's pressure. The intensity of the sounds of Korotkoff along the pressure measurement is approximately represented in Figure 6.2C. According to the intensity of the sounds, the time interval from sound appearance to its extinction is divided into five phases. The initial phase, when Korotkoff sounds begin to be heard clearly and repetitively, is named Phase 1 and coincides with the palpable identification of the arterial pulse. During Phase 2, sounds are longer and less intense, similar to intermittent murmurs and artery stays open for longer periods than in Phase 1. In Phase 3, sounds become clear and louder again and the artery stays more time open than closed during each pressure pulse. During Phase 4, the sounds become increasingly difficult to distinguish until the cuff pressure equals diastolic pressure and Phase 5 begins. During Phase 5, the cuff pressure is lower than the pressure of diastolic blood, the artery stays permanently open and the sounds disappear. Systolic and diastolic pressures are determined by the operator, which monitors blood flow sounds with a stethoscope ("hears") and a pressure gage ("sees") (mercury column or aneroid display).

The auscultatory gap or *hiatus* is a pressure range during which Korotkoff's sounds may fade away and are not detected, even with the blood pressure lower than cuff's pressure. It usually appears at the end of Phase 1 and may last for up to additional 40 mmHg. The auscultatory gap is one of the motives for measurement of falsely low systolic or elevated diastolic pressures.

The sphygmomanometry technique is highly dependent of training and sensibility of the operator to detect through hearing the beginning and end of sounds. Frequency content of Korotkoff sounds occurs in the audible range from 20 to 300 Hz. There may be differences between measurements made by distinct operators due to differences in their audible sensitivities. In noisy environments, it may be difficult to detect the sounds of opening and closing of the artery. The cuff must be properly adjusted to the size of the patient's arm (skinny, fat, child, adult) without being too tight or too loose, which could cause errors in the measurement of blood pressure. The accuracy of this method is ± 2 mmHg in systolic pressure measurement and ± 4 mmHg in diastolic.

The palpatory and auscultatory occlusive methods experience problems for detecting systolic and diastolic pressures in hypotensive patients, children, or patients that cannot stand still. Furthermore, the perception of change of blood flow from turbulent to laminar depends on the training and sensitivity of the operator. Automatic methods for indirect measurement of blood pressure, oscillometric, Doppler ultrasound, and tonometry overcome these difficulties, reduce the error of manual methods, and also allow obtaining continuous measurement of arterial pressure.

6.1.2.1.2 Occlusive oscillometric automatic technique

The occlusive oscillometric technique is similar to sphygmomanometry, but instead hearing the sounds of blood flow, this method detects the tiny pressure variations in the cuff at each systole/diastole cycle (Figure 6.3). Cuff can be manually inflated and automatically deflated or the whole process can be automatic. When the cuff begins to deflate and its pressure becomes lower than the systolic pressure, blood begins to flow through the constricted artery. The artery wall vibrates because the start of the flow is turbulent, causing fluctuations in the pressure measured by a pressure sensor connected to the cuff. The amplitudes of these oscillations are used to determine systole and diastole pressures. The pressure sensor output is filtered by 0.6 Hz low pass filter to obtain the DC component (cuff pressure) and by a 0.4–6.4 Hz band pass filter to obtain the AC component (pressure fluctuations). Both components, AC and DC, are digitalized and processed. The DC pressure correspondent to the peak of the AC oscillations is the average arterial pressure and complex algorithms, specific from each manufacturer, and experimentally obtained coefficients are used to determine systolic and diastolic pressures.

The oscillometric monitor of blood pressure automatically detects the blood displacement in the brachial artery, determines systole and diastole pressures, and displays

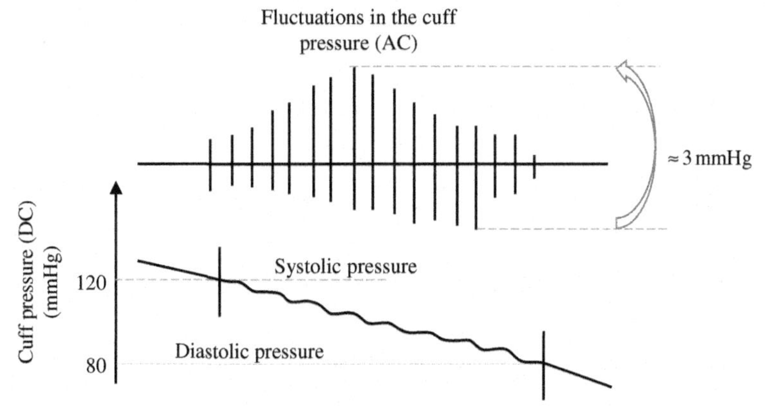

Figure 6.3 Oscillometric technique for indirect measurement of arterial blood pressure.

their values. A stethoscope is no longer necessary, the device evaluates the pressure variations throughout the day and night or smaller periods and can even customize the cuff inflation. Oscillometric technique demands less operator participation in the process of blood pressure measurement, but the oscillometric monitor is more complex and expensive than just a sphygmomanometer. Oscillometric blood pressure monitor usually has microcontrolled circuits, analog circuits, current and voltage supplies, valves and pumps. The microelectronic industry develops dedicated high performance integrated circuits (microcontrollers, operational amplifiers, filters) to supply the demand of automatic devices for blood pressure measurement. Oscillometric technique is also used in the portable wrist blood pressure meters of domestic use (Huang et al., 2009; Ling, Ohara, Orime, Noon, & Takatani, 1995; Mano et al., 2002; Souza, 2003; Stergiou, Lourida, Tzamouranis, & Baibas, 2009).

6.1.2.1.3 Finger arterial pressure automatic technique

The finger arterial pressure technique, or finapres, is a noninvasive automatic method for continuous blood pressure measurement based on a photoplethysmographic system. The finapres technique is applied to the finger and provides beat-to-beat arterial finger blood pressure using the volume clamp technique developed by Peñáz in 1973 (Introcaso, 1996; Peñáz, 1973). Plethysmography allows obtaining blood flow of a leg or arm through the limb volume variation and the resulting waveform is similar to the arterial blood pressure waveform. Figure 6.4 shows the schematic representation of finapres photoplethysmographic or pseudo-photoplethysmographic technique.

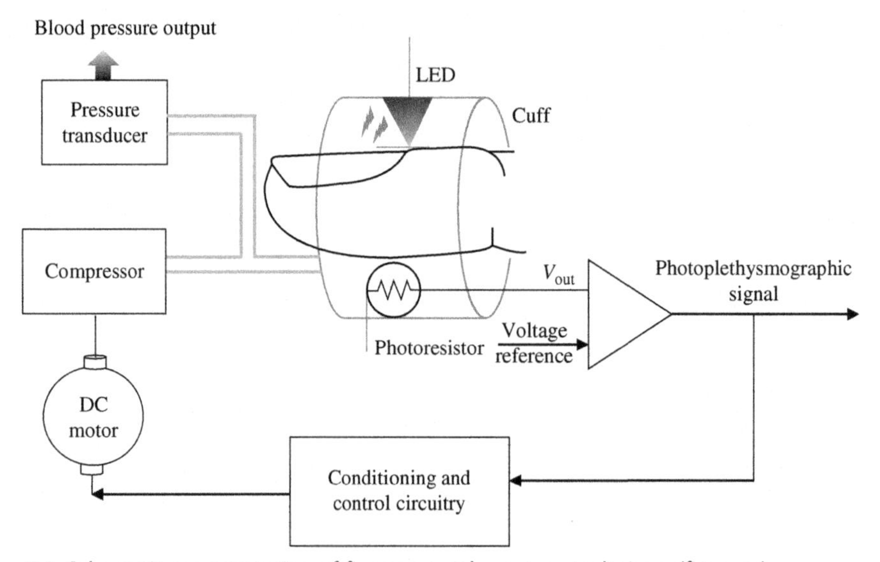

Figure 6.4 Schematic representation of finger arterial pressure technique (finapres).

A cuff is placed around the finger and its pressure is automatically adjusted through pneumatic regulation, to a pressure 5 mmHg below systolic normal pressure, so the cuff compresses the finger, but distal flux is preserved. Inside the cuff, there are an infrared light emitter (LED) and an infrared light detector (photoresistor), transversally opposed, so the infrared light is sent through the finger tissues to the detector (Figure 6.4). Some of the light is reflected by the different tissues and absorbed, mainly by the red blood cells and the sensor detects the light that is transmitted.

When fresh arterial blood comes into the finger during systole, the finger volume increases as does the blood pressure, and then, the cuff pressure is released. When additional blood volume leaves the finger, during diastole, the finger pressure decreases and then the cuff pressure is increased. The light sensor output feeds a servo loop, which controls the compressor and thus the cuff pressure. This way, the pressure in the cuff is constantly adjusted and the artery is kept at the same opening level all over the pulse pressure. Arterial pulse and its blood volume changing modifies blood optical density, and so, the pressure pulse modulates the light intensity that is transmitted through the finger. Constant current feeds the photoresistor and its resistance changings caused by the transmitted light intensity and thus by the blood volume variation are registered in the output voltage (V_{out}). The arterial blood pressure is directly related to the finger blood volume and processing this photoplethysmographic signal (V_{out}) allows the pressure reading (usually in mmHg). Light intensity and wavelength are selected to obtain maximum amplitude of the blood pressure signal.

Finapres output represents the immediate arterial blood pressure variation and allows obtaining continuously the pressure pulse, as do the invasive and direct methods, but without the risks of the invasive and surgical procedures. Since its development, finapres accuracy, compared to invasive continuous methods and noninvasive but intermittent methods, as well as computing algorithms to process the photoplethysmographic signal, has been reported in scientific papers (Friedman, Jensen, Matzen, & Secher, 1990; Kinsella, Whitwam, & Spencer, 2005; Peñáz, Honzikova, & Jurak, 1997; Raamat, Talts, Jacomägi, & Länsimies, 1999; Talts, Raamat, & Jagomägi, 2006). Finapres helps in the diagnosis of pseudo-hypertension, common in elderly patients, which is responsible for overmedication due to wrong measurements of high values of arterial blood pressure with arm occlusive cuff methods. Finapres is a noninvasive alternative to continuously monitoring neonates' arterial pressure (Andriessen et al., 2004; Drouin, Gournay, Calamel, Mouzard, & Rozé, 1997). Automatic continuous noninvasive measurement of blood pressure using finapres offers a valuable aid for monitoring patients during anesthesia (Jensen & Secher, 1989). Jensen and Secher monitored blood pressure of patients, with significant atherosclerosis that were submitted to anesthesia, with oscillometric and finapres techniques and they did not observe significant differences between values recorded using both methods. Imholz, Wieling, van Montfrans, and Wesseling (1998) reviewed the performance of commercial and prototype units of finapres devices published in 43 papers along 15 years. They concluded that finapres has sufficient accuracy and precision to reliable detection of blood pressure changes and that diagnostic accuracy would be achieved with further corrective improvements.

Continuous finger blood pressure measurement provides the ability to measure continuous cardiac output from pulse contour analysis of the finger arterial waveform. Main error sources of finapres technique are the variability of the occlusion cuff pressure (depends on the muscular tonus, which varies from patient to patient) and the increase of systolic pressure due to patient movement. Actual finapres monitors have a hydrostatic height correction unit. Vasoconstriction in fingers and vasospastic conditions have to be prevented, because they affect the peripheral circulation and thus the blood pressure by measurement finapres.

6.1.2.1.4 Occlusive Doppler ultrasound automatic technique

This technique of indirect and noninvasive automatic measurement of blood pressure uses Doppler ultrasound to detect the movement of the blood vessel walls to obtain the systole and diastole pressure values. In Figure 6.5A is schematized the operation of this method. The occlusion cuff has two ultrasound transducers: the first one generates the ultrasonic pulse (e.g., 8 MHz) that is transmitted through the tissues of the arm to a superficial blood vessel, supported by a bone; the second transducer receives the ultrasonic echo reflected by the walls of the artery and blood particles. The occlusion cuff is inflated automatically and continuously, even greater than the systolic pressure and deflated until a lower diastolic blood pressure, while the transmitter and receiver transducers are driven alternately.

During cardiac cycle, the volume and pressure of blood vary in the systemic circulation. The diameter of arteries also varies over the cardiac cycle, which means the distance between the transducer and the wall of the artery (and the blood) changes. Thus, the Doppler shift, the frequency difference between the transmitted signal and the reflected signal by the artery, will change proportionally to the vessel's diameter. During systole, the artery's diameter increases and the blood approaches the ultrasound source (transducer), which generates an increase in the frequency of the signal received by the transducer ($\mathbf{\Delta} \cong 200-500$ Hz). During diastole, the volume of blood in the artery is smaller and the vessel diameter decreases, moving the blood away from the transducer, and therefore, the signal reaching the receiver has a lower frequency than the transmitted signal ($\mathbf{\Delta} \cong 30-100$ Hz).

The cuff shown in Figure 6.5A is adjusted around patient' arm to place ultrasound transducers over a superficial artery, supported by a bone, like brachial artery. The cuff is then automatic and slowly inflated and deflated so several cardiac cycles occur during one cycle of inflation and deflation of the cuff. While the cuff pressure is higher than the blood pressure, the artery remains closed and there is no blood flow in the

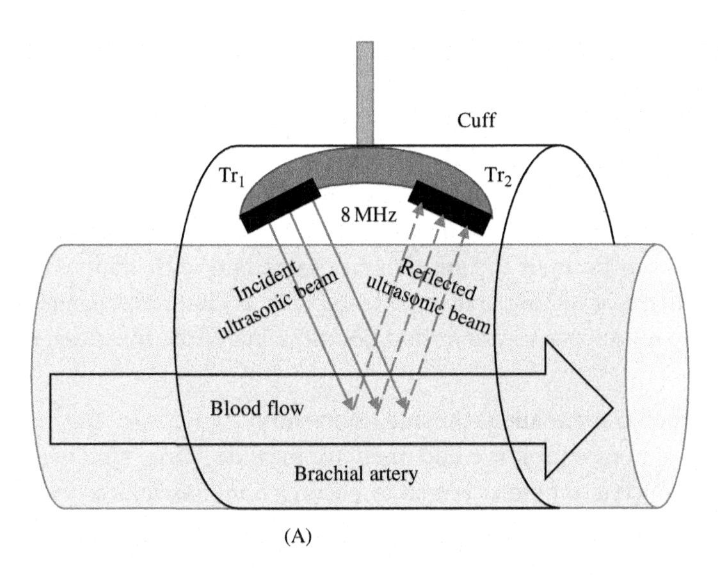

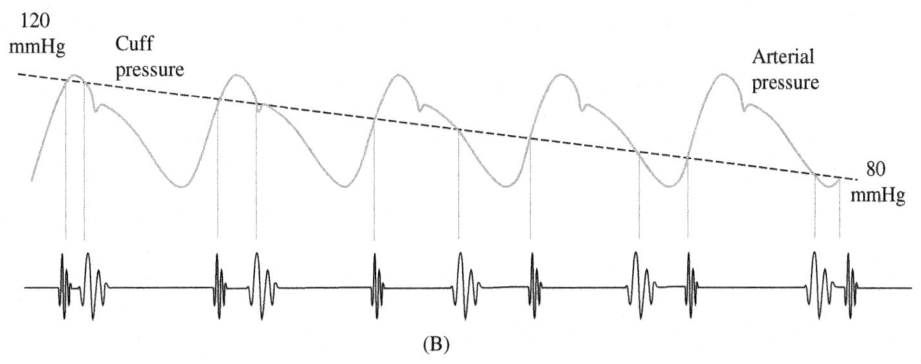

Figure 6.5 (A) Schematic diagram of occlusive Doppler ultrasound automatic technique for blood pressure measurement. (B) Doppler shift variation along deflation of the arm cuff. The sequence of Doppler shifts at the beginning of deflation, when the artery closes (low frequency) after opening (high frequency), is inverted at the end of deflation, when the artery opens (high frequency) after its closure (low frequency).

artery. When the cuff pressure falls below the blood pressure, the artery opens and the blood flows through the artery. Comparing the frequency of transmitted and received (echo) ultrasound signals, the Doppler shift is determined, and its value is higher at the opening of the vessel walls (200–500 Hz) and lower (30–100 Hz) at closing.

The Doppler shifts are measured while the cuff is inflated and deflated, recording the movement of the artery walls in various states of occlusion. The recording of a low frequency Doppler shift immediately after a high frequency (Figure 6.5B) indicates that the artery changed from the open state to the closed and the pressure in the cuff is slightly larger than the systolic pressure. On the other hand, if a high frequency

Doppler shift is detected immediately after a low frequency (also shown in Figure 6.5B) it means that the artery went from closed to open state, and the cuff pressure is slightly lower than the diastolic pressure (Cobbold, 1974; Webster, 2010).

If the cuff pressure is monitored in real time, and the ECG is recorded as reference, the Doppler method, indirect and noninvasive, allows the reconstruction of the pressure pulse and thus, the automation and semicontinuous monitoring of blood pressure. This technique can be used in noisy environment and with hypotensive individuals, but the movements of uncooperative patients, such as children, change the position of the sensor relative to the artery and modifies the value of the measured pressure.

6.1.2.1.5 Tonometric automatic technique (tonometry)

Tonometry is a noninvasive method used to measure static and dynamic pressures. Tonometric automatic technique is used to obtain a noninvasive beat-to-beat blood pressure monitor that displays continuous radial artery waveform as well as systolic, mean and diastolic blood from a pressure sensor directly over the radial artery at the wrist. In addition to blood pressure, it can be used to measure intraocular, intracranial (in newborn), intra-amniotic and intra-abdominal pressures. It is based on the fact that when a vessel under pressure is partially collapsed by an object, the circumferential pressure in the walls of the vessel is removed and external and internal pressures become equal (Figure 6.6A).

Tonometry allows determining pulse pressure curve through balance of forces method. Figure 6.6B shows schematically how it is implemented with a piston mounted in a cylinder, with minimum friction between them; the piston surface is positioned on the body surface, over an artery supported by bone, such as radial artery in the wrist. An external force F is applied to the piston compressing the artery wall until the reaction artery ($F = PA$) is equal to the force applied. Whereas the longitudinal axis of the artery remains parallel to the face of the piston, the planing of the artery wall eliminates the tangential force components, remaining only the perpendicular force components, which are due to pressure pulse of arterial blood. The piston face area (A) is known, as well as the applied external force (F), and thus, from the planing of the wall of the artery, the blood pressure (P) is calculated as

$$P = \frac{F}{A} \tag{6.1}$$

where

A is the piston area
F is the applied force
P is the blood pressure.

Instead of a single piston, multiple sensors (sensor array) can be used to better locate the position of the artery, which ensures that at least one of the sensors will be positioned directly over the artery (Figure 6.6C). The pressure array usually is

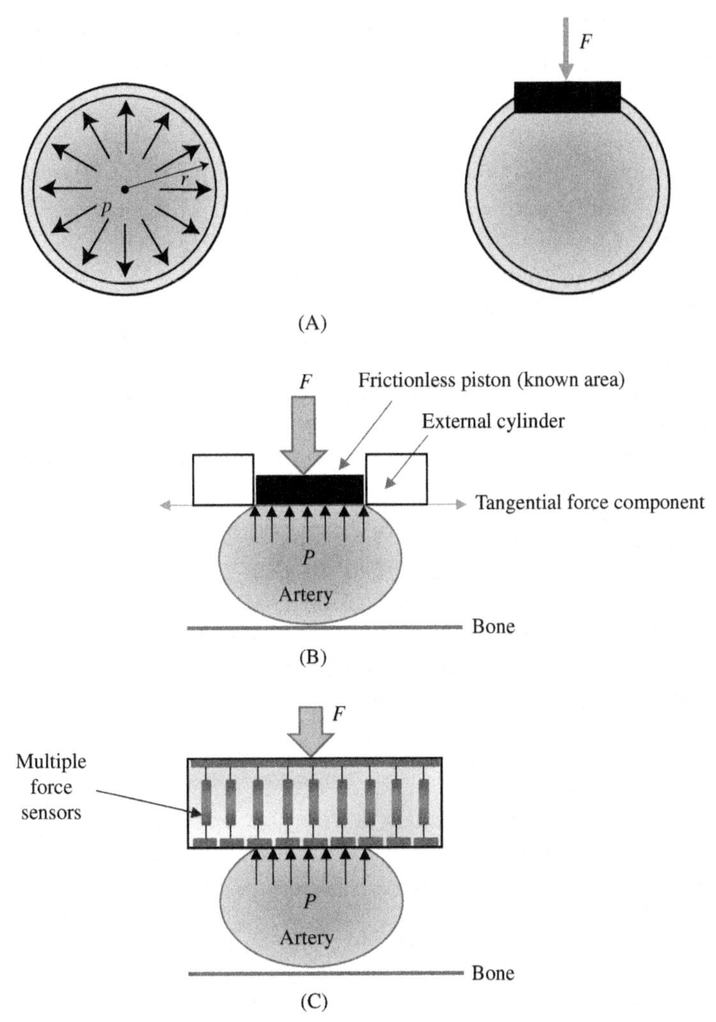

Figure 6.6 Working principle of tonometry (A). Schematic diagram of the tonometry to determine the blood pressure; maintaining the arterial wall flat, tangential components of force are eliminated and perpendicular force components are due to the pulsation of arterial blood (B). Multiple sensors may be used to better locate the position of the artery (C).

constructed with piezoelectric or piezoresistive sensors, linearly arranged, a few tenths of milimeter spaced; the array is housed in a wrist bracelet adjustable to several sizes of patients, infants, and adults. Initially the linear array is zero calibrated to the atmospheric pressure and then is pressed against skin and tissues over the artery by a pump (pneumatic or electronic). A scan is made to locate the optimum sensor position, that is, the site of maximum pressure pulse amplitude. The compression force is continuously increased, according to a artery compression ramp, and measurements are made while the artery wall is flattened: the force sensors detect when the applied pressure equals the pressure of the artery, which is named hold down pressure. With additional compression after artery wall applanation, the artery begins to occlude and the force signal reduces. The tonometric pressure monitor locates the site of maximal radial pulse signal, determines mean blood pressure from maximal pulse waveform amplitude at optimal artery compression, and then derives systolic and diastolic blood pressures (Dueck, Goedje, & Clopton, 2012; Eckerle, 2006; Webster, 2010).

Arterial tonometry technique was developed to be used in noninvasive, indirect, and continuous arterial pressure measurement. Although it can cause some discomfort, its application usually is painless. The movement of the arm, wrist, and tendons results in relatively high errors of pressure measurement. This technique may enable physicians to circumvent arterial cannulation in certain circumstances, such as with low- or intermediate-risk procedures, on patients when beat-to-beat BP measurement is desirable (Dueck et al., 2012; Steiner, Johnston, Salvador, Czosnyka, & Menon, 2003; Weiss, Spahn, Rahmig, Rohling, & Pasch, 1996). Meidert et al. (2014) applied applanation tonometry technology to radial artery for continuous noninvasive measurement of arterial pressure of 24 patients in intensive care unit. They concluded that values of diastolic and average arterial pressure showed acceptable agreement with invasive arterial pressure measurement made with radial arterial catheter, and the precision of systolic measurements needed further improvement to be clinically useful, although they showed good accuracy.

6.1.2.2 Intravascular and extravascular techniques of direct measurement of arterial blood pressure

Occlusive methods of indirect and noninvasive blood pressure measurement presented, using an inflatable cuff to occlude total or partially the blood flow in a limb and assess blood pressure during cuff deflation. The difficulties that may occur during the measurement of blood pressure by occlusive methods are usually caused by inadequate cuff size, wrong placement of the cuff, undetected faults in the cuff and connectors, limb movement, shock and vascular compression proximal to the cuff. Noninvasive tonometry technique provides continuous pressure waveform of the radial artery blood and static values of systolic, mean, and diastolic pressures, but it also presents measurement difficulties with hypotension patients and its use is not completely validated. Measurement techniques developed for noninvasive blood pressure monitoring offer alternatives to continuous blood pressure determinations through arterial cannulation, as for example, Finapres and tonometry; they still do not have comparable accuracy and reliability as direct and invasive methods.

Invasive direct monitoring is able to detect beat-to-beat blood pressure measurement and is the gold standard of blood pressure measurement. The risks inherent to the procedure make it unsuitable for routine blood pressure measurements in asymptomatic individuals, not hospitalized or to general population use, except when this risk is outweighed by the benefits. Due to its invasive nature, the direct method is used almost exclusively in hemodynamic monitoring of critically ill patients, and blood pressure monitoring of patients submitted to surgical interventions under IV anesthesia induction, as during cardiac catheterization, open-chest cardiac surgery, cardiopulmonary bypass and care of polytrauma patients and in intensive care units. Since its introduction in the 1970s, the pulmonary artery catheter was widely used in hemodynamic monitoring providing important information in patients with pulmonary arterial hypertension and right ventricular failure, but there is increasing consensus that the pulmonary catheter should not be routinely used as the primary means of advanced hemodynamic monitoring (Saugel and Reuter, 2014; Vincent et al., 2008). Noninvasive devices for advanced hemodynamic monitoring, including volume clamp method based on the Peñáz principle (Martina et al., 2012; Monnet et al., 2012; Vos et al., 2014), radial artery applanation tonometry (Meidert et al., 2014; Saugel & Reuter, 2013; Steiner et al., 2003), thoracic bioimpedance (Keren, Burkhoff, & Squara, 2007; Raaijmakers, Faes, Scholten, Goovaerts, & Heethaar, 1999), and others (Sokolski et al., 2011), have been developed and their validation and utilization are still under discussion (Chung et al., 2013; Wax, Lin, & Leibowitz, 2011).

While one or more of the new completely noninvasive techniques are validated for advanced management of acute circulatory responses, providing accurate and precise measurements of changes on arterial pulse in pathological and pathophysiological situations, the gold pattern to measure arterial blood pressure is the direct and invasive method.

Direct techniques for measuring blood pressure requires the insertion of a catheter connected to a transducer into an artery with surgical procedures (disinfecting the site, application of local anesthetic, artery dissection, etc.) and have significant risks associated, such as pain, vessel spasm and occlusion, bleeding, and vasovagal syncope.

The cannulation of the radial artery for monitoring of blood pressure is a common procedure in major surgery (such as cardio-thoracic surgery, vascular, and neurosurgery), and in patients admitted to intensive care units. Radial artery is localized in the surface of the arm and rarely occurs ischemia in this artery, because 90% of hand irrigation comes from the ulnar artery. Brachial, femoral, and *dorsalis pedis* arteries are also used. The following text will present some of the concepts addressed in the direct measurement techniques, and therefore in the invasive blood pressure.

The waveform shown in Figure 6.7 is a representation of a typical waveform of arterial pressure. It has a sharp rise correspondent to the beginning of the systole; the peak represents the maximum value of pressure during ventricle ejection. Then the pressure decreases, still during systole phase and after the dicrotic commissure, the pressure continues to decrease, but at a smaller velocity, during the diastolic ramp until reaching the final diastole pressure. The arterial pulse follows the cardiac frequency,

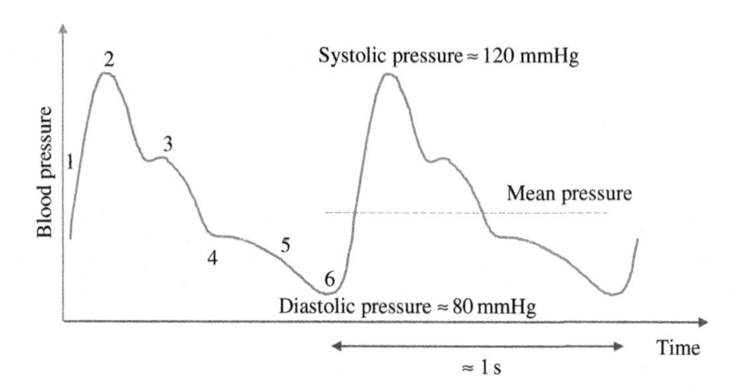

1- Systolic rise
2- Peak systolic pressure
3- Systolic descent
4- Dicrotic commissure
5- Diastolic ramp
6- End diastolic pressure

Figure 6.7 Typical arterial pulse.

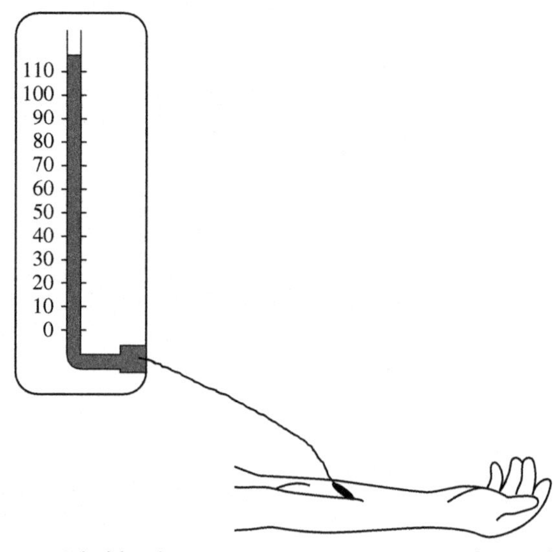

Figure 6.8 Invasive arterial blood pressure measurement with graded mercury column manometer.

typically equal to 60–180 beats per minute, or 1–3 Hz and typical values of arterial pressure are 80 mmHg (diastole) and 120 mmHg (systole). Transducers must be able to detect pressure signals in the range of amplitudes 0–400 mmHg with frequency spectrum 0–50 Hz. Pulse pressure waveform, with all its characteristic details, is obtained only through direct and invasive methods that allow measuring the dynamic behavior of blood pressure (Parker, 2009).

There are two basic modes for intravascular measurement of arterial blood pressure, and both require intravascular access (Cobbold, 1974). In the first, a 0.6- to 2-mm-diameter flexible catheter is filled with sterile liquid and one end is inserted into the artery and remains in contact with the blood flow; the other end of the catheter is connected directly to a graded column of mercury (Figure 6.8). The mercury column manometer has long been considered the most accurate and preferred instrument for obtaining blood pressure measurements. This technique can also be used to measure central venous pressure and spinal fluid pressure. In the second, electronic transducers, intravascular or extravascular are used to measure blood pressure (Figure 6.9). When the intravascular transducer is used, the transducer, connected to the catheter tip, is inserted together with the catheter in the artery and remains in contact with the blood flow (Figure 6.9A). In the extravascular type, a fluid-filled catheter is inserted into the artery and this fluid hydraulically couples the wave of blood pressure to the transducer, which is at the opposite end of the catheter, outside of the artery (Figure 6.9B). The catheter-sensor system should be flushed with heparinized saline solution periodically to prevent the formation of blood clots in the point of vascular access and in the catheter; irrigation can be done manually with a syringe or automatically. The three-way stopcock device allows to irrigate the system, to administer drugs, and to remove blood samples from the same access point to blood flow (Figure 6.9C).

When measuring physiological pressure, the period of the fundamental component of the pulse pressure is equal to the period of the cardiac cycle. Accurate measurements of dynamic pressure require that the measurement system (transducer and conditioning and processing circuits) be able to work with frequencies up to the tenth harmonic of pressure signal, without phase or amplitude distortion. The mercury column manometer, for example, only measures the average pressure (DC level) because its mass acts as a buffer for high frequencies.

When measuring blood pressure with invasive techniques, the electronic components used in the transducers are chosen to meet specific requirements. If the sensor is extravascular, hydraulic coupling and characteristics of the catheter, and of the fluid within the catheter, influence the dynamic response of the measurement. Electronic pressure transducers used in extravascular measurements usually are low cost, lightweight, and disposable. Typical characteristics are sensibility $5\ \mu V/V/1$ mmHg, DC excitation from 2 to 10 V, range from -50 to $+400$ mmHg, nonlinearity and hysteresis $\pm 1-2\%$ of reading, output impedance $<500\ \Omega$, and input impedance $\approx 500\ \Omega$ (require a high input impedance preamplifier). They also have protection against overpressure, for example, from -400 to $+4{,}000$ mmHg. The dynamic response of the measuring system is from DC up to $150-1{,}000$ Hz; the faster the

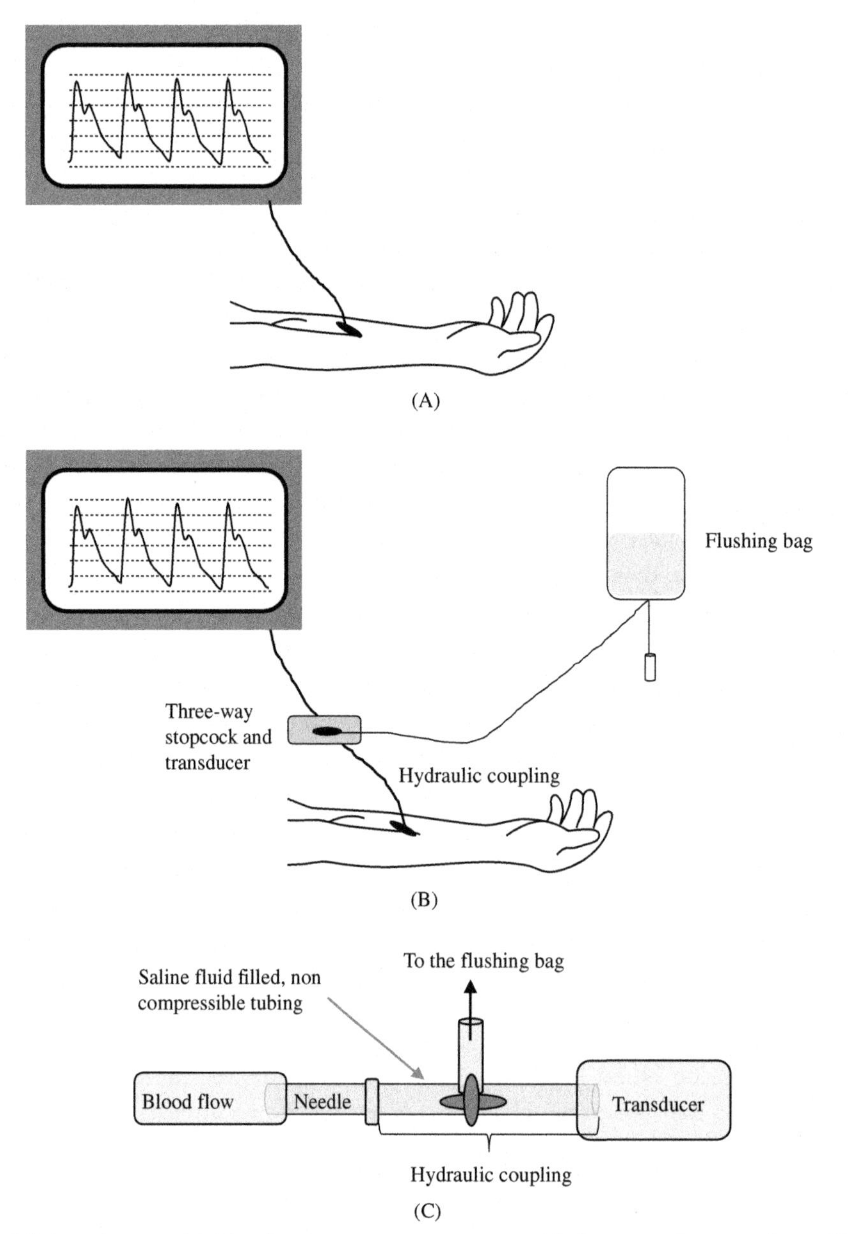

Figure 6.9 Invasive arterial blood pressure measurement with intravascular transducer (A) and extravascular transducer (hydraulic coupling) (B). The three-way stopcock device (C).

heart rate and the steeper the systolic pressure upstroke, the greater will be the dynamic response that is required for the monitoring system. Venous pressure waveforms, which generally do not have steep waves or high frequency components, do not require monitoring systems with such high frequency responses.

6.1.2.2.1 Electronic pressure transducers

Pressure transducers, either intravascular or extravascular type, are mostly primary–secondary type. The primary transducer or sensor is the element that is in contact with the pressure pulse, and generally is a displacement transducer, which transduces the pressure wave into a mechanical displacement. The secondary transducer, also of displacement type, is the one that transduces the mechanical displacement into an electrical signal, which is processed and viewed, for example, in a multiparameter monitor display. The transducers for invasive and direct blood pressure measurement may be introduced directly into the bloodstream (transducer catheter tip), or hydraulically coupled, via fluid-filled catheter, to the blood flow; thus, the electronic pressure transducers are used intravascularly or extravascularly.

6.1.2.2.2 Sources of error in invasive measurement of blood pressure with intra- and extravascular sensors

Direct techniques for measuring blood pressure are able to detect dynamic changes in pressure (waveform) by introducing the sensor element in the flow of blood, or through hydraulic coupling of the sensor with the flow, usually through a catheter filled with solution saline. The catheter filled with fluid is one of the simplest means of direct registration of the pressure curve and one of the most widely used in medicine. In the following, some problems that can arise with direct invasive measurement of blood pressure are discussed.

A very common source of error is the ratio between the diameters of the catheter and the vessel. The external diameter of the catheter used should not be greater than 10% of the internal diameter of the vessel, to avoid reducing significantly the cross-sectional area of the vessel, which would change the pressure measurements. To reduce this error, the diameter of the catheter used must be selected according to the vessel in which the measurement is made and the patient's age.

When using a pressure transducer for intravascular measurements, with the sensor inserted in the vessel, or hydraulically coupled to the blood flow by a catheter, care must be taken to the changes in static pressure due to kinetic and potential energies of the fluid. The Bernoulli equation (Eq. (6.2)) states the conservation of energy in any part of the vessel with fluid flow. The apparent pressure (measured by transducer) is the sum of the static pressure (which is the actual pressure value), the kinetic component (due to the velocity of the blood flow) and the potential component (if there is a fluid column between external sensor and the blood output from the heart). Equation (6.2) determines the apparent pressure:

$$P_a = P_s + \underbrace{\xi g h}_{\substack{\text{Gravitational}\\ \text{potential}\\ \text{energy}}} + \underbrace{\frac{\xi v^2}{2}}_{\substack{\text{Kinetic}\\ \text{energy}}} \tag{6.2}$$

where

P_a is the apparent pressure (measured)
P_s is the static pressure (desired)

ξ is the fluid density (average density of approximately 1,060 kg/m^3 for whole blood)
g is the acceleration of gravity = 9.8 m/s^2
h is the height of the column fluid
v is the velocity of the flow.

When an extravascular sensor is used to measure arterial blood pressure, external sensor should be approximately at the same height as the blood output from the heart (Figure 6.10A); otherwise, a liquid column is formed between them, generating a potential energy difference that will modify the arterial pressure reading. The uncertainty of the height difference of the blood output from heart to the external transducer is responsible for readings higher or lower than the actual. Figure 6.10 shows how this height difference influences the pressure value. When the blood output from the heart is higher than external sensor, apparent pressure is larger than the static pressure (Figure 6.10B) and if the sensor is higher, the pressure reading is smaller (Figure 6.10C). Consider a height difference of 25 cm; the apparent pressure will be

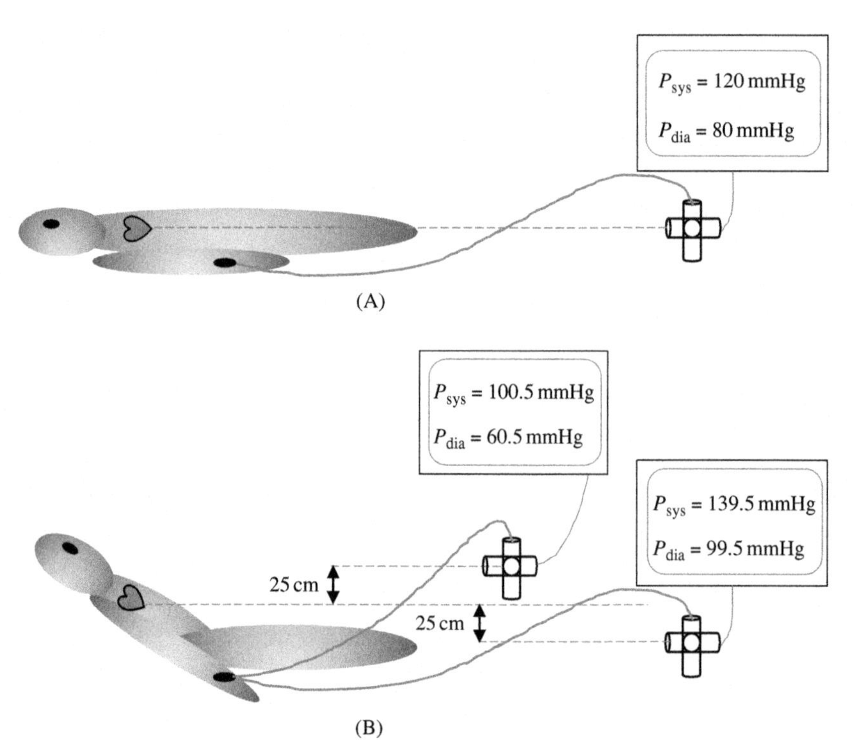

Figure 6.10 When an extravascular sensor is used to measure arterial blood pressure, external sensor should be approximately at the same height as the blood output from the heart (A). A 25 cm difference causes an error of 10.5 mmHg, in both systolic and diastolic pressures, above or below the actual value (B).

approximately 20 mmHg higher than actual (static pressure), due to the potential energy ($P_{\mathrm{PotEnergy}}$) component:

$$P_{\mathrm{PotEnergy}} = \xi g h = 259.7\ \mathrm{kPa} = 19.5\ \mathrm{mmHg} \tag{6.3}$$

Systems for pressure measurement via hydraulic coupling use devices for leveling the pressure transducer in the catheter tip, thereby eliminating the effect of potential energy.

Kinetic energy may represent an important error source to invasive measurement of blood pressure, mainly to venous pressure readings, whose values are lower than arterial. Figure 6.11 shows the influence of the kinetic energy, due to blood flow velocity, in the apparent pressure measured by invasive technique. The ideal situation is the axis of the sensor or catheter positioned perfectly perpendicular to the blood flow axis (Figure 6.11A); in this case, the component of velocity parallel to the axis of the catheter is null, and only the static pressure is measured. Figure 6.11B shows a situation where the catheter is parallel to the flow velocity and the catheter end is at the same direction as the blood flow; the kinetic component is subtracted from the static pressure and the reading is lower than actual. When the catheter is parallel to the flow velocity, but catheter end and flow velocity are at opposite directions, the pressure reading is higher than actual because the kinetic component is added to the static pressure (Figure 6.11C).

The catheter is typically inserted into a peripheral vessel but the pressure is measured in another point in the circulation system, for example, in the pulmonary artery or heart chamber. It is practically impossible to obtain the optimum arrangement with the catheter tip, at the point of pressure measurement, perpendicular to the flow,

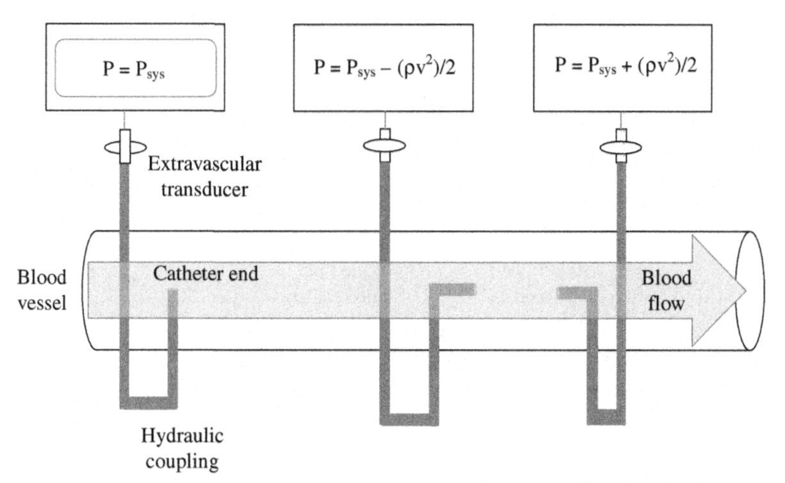

Figure 6.11 Influence of fluid velocity (kinetic component) in the pressure measurement: (A) catheter positioned perfectly perpendicular to the blood flow axis; (B) catheter is parallel to the flow velocity and the catheter end is at the same direction as the blood flow; (C) catheter is parallel to the flow velocity, but catheter end and flow velocity are in opposite directions.

which eliminates the influence of the kinetic component of pressure. According to the pressure measurement site, the kinetic pressure component may represent a quite high error in the pressure reading, particularly in vessels where the blood velocity is high and the static pressure is low. For example, in the vena cava, the blood velocity at rest state is about 30 cm/s and the static pressure is approximately 2 mmHg; kinetic component ($P_{\text{KinEnergy}}$) represents an error of 18% in the invasive measurement:

$$P_{\text{KinEnergy}} = \frac{\xi v^2}{2} = 4.77\ \text{Pa} = 0.36\ \text{mmHg} \tag{6.4}$$

The potential energy affects the measurement of intravascular pressure with hydraulic coupling, while the kinetic factor influences both measurements, intravascular with catheter-tip sensor and extravascular sensor with hydraulic coupling.

In invasive pressure measurements with extravascular sensor, due to the pulsatile nature of the blood flow, there may be reflections of the pressure wave at the catheter tip or in regions of the vessel with constriction to blood flow.

The characteristics of the transmission system of the pressure wave, formed by the fluid-filled catheter and the transducer, can also distort the pressure wave that reaches the primary sensor of the transducer. The catheter—transducer system acts as a transmission line in which the blood pressure is modeled as voltage; the blood flow as electric current; the catheter, fluid and sensor inertances (mass or resistance to acceleration) as inductances; the friction forces between the fluid and the inner wall of the catheter, as resistors; and fluid, catheter and sensor compliances (change in volume due to pressure variations) as capacitances (Chan, 2008; Cobbold, 1974; Webster, 2010). Figure 6.12 shows the simplified model of this system. The resistance R in the model represents the series association of fluid and catheter resistances. The compliance of the sensor (typically a diaphragm) is the most significant capacitance in the model and its value is much higher than the equivalent compliances of the fluid and catheter. The inertance of the sensor

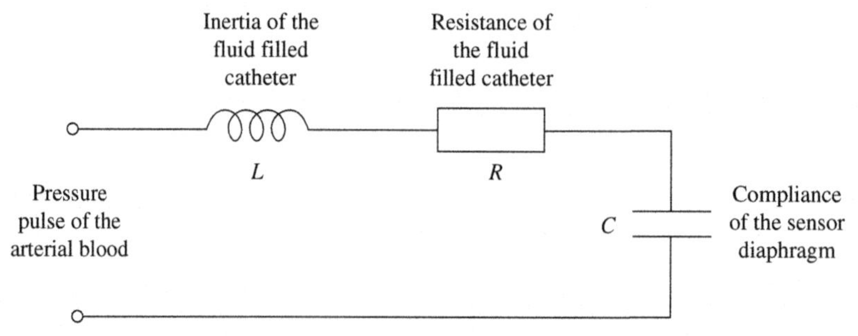

Figure 6.12 Simplified model of the system formed by the transducer and fluid-filled catheter, which behaves as a transmission line.

can be disregarded compared to the values of the catheter and the fluid inertances, which are represented by a single inductor in the model.

The presence of the two energy storage elements in the model of the catheter/transducer system, the inductor and the capacitor, is characteristic of a second-order system, which transfer function has two important parameters: the natural damping frequency f_n and the damping fator ξ. These parameters define the dynamic behavior of the catheter/fluid/sensor system, which can oscillate or not (as seen in Chapter 1). The analysis of the simplified model shows that parameters f_n and ξ are defined by the values of the length and diameter of the catheter, the viscosity and density of the fluid and the displacement coefficient of the effective volume of the system V_e:

$$V_e = V_t + \frac{(V_c + V_f)}{2} \ (\text{mm}^3/100 \text{ mmHg}) \tag{6.5}$$

where

V_t is the coefficient of the volumetric displacement of the transducer

V_c is the coefficient of the volumetric displacement of the catheter

V_f is the coefficient of the volumetric displacement of the fluid.

The catheters (diameter, length, material) and electrical transducers (mainly primary sensor) used in intravascular pressure measurement should be chosen so that the catheter/transducer system presents a stable behavior without oscillations and delay in response. Next, the operation of the main types of eletromechanical pressure transducers is presented. The principles of operation of these primary and secondary transducers were discussed with more details in Chapter 4.

6.1.2.2.3 Types of electronic pressure transducers

6.1.2.2.3.1 Elastic sensors Mechanical and electromechanical pressure transducers usually incorporate an elastic element sensor, which shape changes when pressure is applied to it. The most common elastic sensor elements, the ones that convert the shape change caused by the pressure pulse into displacement, are frequently of the types Bourdon tubes, diaphragm, and bellows (Cobbold, 1974; Dally, Riley, & McConnell, 1993; Geddes & Baker, 1968).

Pressure sensors made with Bourdon tube are hollow elastic material (metal or rubber) tubes with one sealed end that flexes when pressure is applied to the open end. They transduce the elastic deformation of the tube wall (usually with approximately square section) into displacement. In the Bourdon tube shown in Figure 6.13A, the difference between inner and outer pressure causes the rounding of the cross section of the tube (Figure 6.13C) and the translational displacement in the direction indicated. Operation of the transducer type Bourdon tube is simple and reliable, the coefficient of volumetric displacement is typically large (2 mm^3/100 mmHg), and its use is indicated for measuring static pressures.

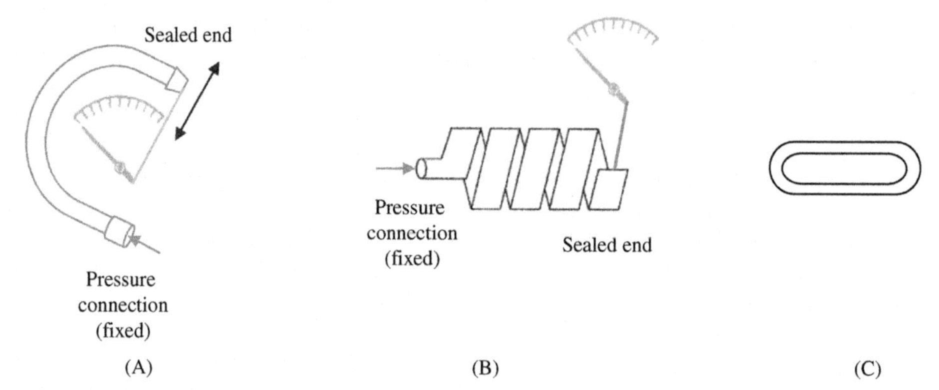

Figure 6.13 Examples of elastic transducer of Bourdon tube type: (A) C-type, (B) helical-type. (C) Most common cross section of Bourdon tubes.

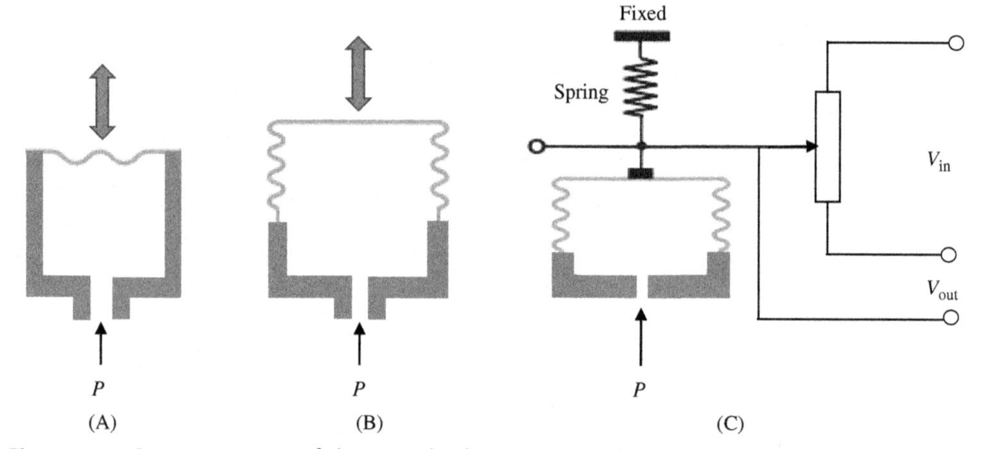

Figure 6.14 Pressure sensors of the type diaphragm (A) and bellows (B). Example of the use of a potentiometer to produce an electrical signal (V_{out}) proportional to the pressure applied to the bellows.

The Bourdon tube is the basis of operation of the Bourdon gage, in which a tube with thin wall of approximately rectangular cross section is manufactured in the form of a curve, according to the example of Figure 6.13C. Under the action of the fluid pressure within the tube, the curve radius of the elastic element changes and this displacement actuates on a gear mechanism with a pointer to indicate the pressure. The model of Bourdon tube is shown in Figure 6.13A (C-type) and Figure 6.13B (helical-type) and is illustrative only. There are many other formats, such as spiral, for greater sensitivity.

Primary sensors of pressure transducers of the type diaphragm or bellows types are shown in Figure 6.14A and B, respectively. Pressure variations displace the diaphragm

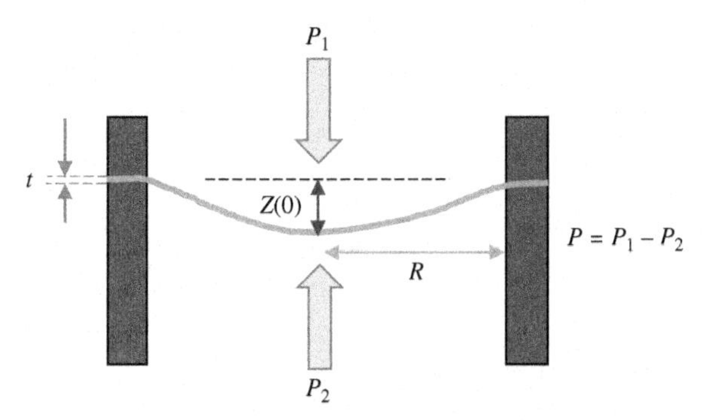

Figure 6.15 Schematic diagram showing the displacement of a diaphragm under a pressure difference P_1-P_2; P_1 is the unknown pressure applied on top face and P_2 is a known pressure (reference) applied on bottom face.

and contract and expand the bellows capsule. The displacement, caused by pressure pulse, can be used to move Bourdon tubes, pointers, wiper of potentiometers (Figure 6.14C), core of LVDT, electrical switches and relays, movable armature of strain gages and other types of eletromechanical elements.

The displacement of the diaphragm is proportional to the pressure difference to which it is subjected (Figure 6.15) and depends on the dimensions and material with which is made. The relationship between the displacement and the physical characteristics of the diaphragm is nonlinear:

$$Z(0) = \frac{3(1-\mu^2)R^4\Delta P}{16Et^3} \tag{6.6}$$

where

μ is the Poisson's coefficient
R is the diaphragm radius
ΔP is the pressure difference (P_1-P_2)
E is the Young's modulus
t is the diaphragm thickness.

The pressure to be measured is applied to one side of the diaphragm or bellows and the resulting displacement in the center of the diaphragm is transmitted to a displacement transducer. Equation (6.6) shows the diaphragm displacement dependence on the fourth power of the radius: diaphragm should not be too small. The same equation also shows the dependence on the inverse of the third power of thickness: thin diaphragm is more sensitive. That is, the best solution is a large and thin diaphragm, two characteristics that are not always possible to meet in the pressure transducer design.

The frequency at which the diaphragm tends to vibrate with when it is somehow disturbed, for example by the pressure pulse, is its natural frequency. For an elastic diaphragm as the one shown in Figure 6.13, the natural frequency f_n is determined by Eq. (6.7):

$$f_n = 2.56 \frac{t}{\pi r^2} \sqrt{\frac{gE}{3\delta(1-\mu^2)}} \tag{6.7}$$

where

μ is the Poisson coefficient
r is the diaphragm radius (m)
g is the acceleration due to gravity (m/s^2)
E is Young's modulus (N/m^2)
t is the diaphragm thickness (m)
γ is the specific weight of the material (N/m^3).

Equation (6.7) shows that to obtain a high natural frequency, in order to avoid vibration and resonance when pressure pulse hits the diaphragm, it should be thick and have a small radius, which would reduce diaphragm sensibility, according to Eq. (6.6). There must be a compromise between the physical characteristics of the diaphragm and the pressure range to be measured, to obtain the desired performance. Diaphragms with natural frequency of about 1 kHz are adequate to most of biomedical applications. Diaphragms made from silicon, instead of silicon rubber and metal, allow to obtain miniaturization, small diameters and thickness of a few tens of μm, in addition to high natural frequencies ($\approx$100 kHz). Semiconductor diaphragms exhibit high natural gage factor but they are temperature sensible; their sensibility decreases 0.25%/°C, which causes the same amount of reduction in the transducer sensibility.

Elastic sensor elements convert the pressure into a displacement, and displacement is then converted into an electrical output by a displacement transduction method. Some of the most common methods, with strain gage, LVDT, variable capacitor, optic, piezoelectric and microelectromechanical elements are presented below.

6.1.2.2.3.2 Strain gages (bonded and unbonded) Strain gage-based pressure transducers normally have a diaphragm-type design that uses strain gages, which are either bonded to, or unbonded, with the strain gages acting as resistive elements. Under the pressure-induced strain, the resistive values change.

Figure 6.16 shows schematic diagrams of pressure transducers where secondary elements are foil bonded (A) and fine wires unbonded (B) strain gages. Pressure transducers with unbonded strain gage use wires stretched around posts attached to the stationary frame and to the movable armature (B). A linkage system, for example, a diaphragm bonded to the movable armature, is designed such that when pressure increases, half of the wires is stretched and the other half is compressed. Pressure pulse distends the diaphragm, which displaces the strain gage armature modifying the wire resistances; the variable resistances, usually mounted in a bridge circuit, are used to

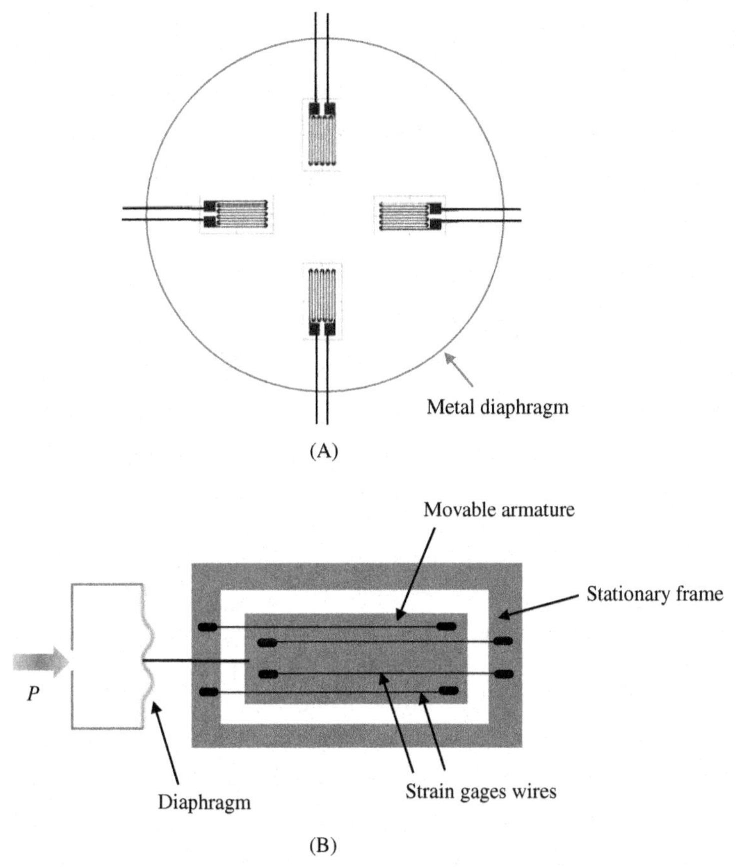

Figure 6.16 Schematic diagrams of pressure transducers where secondary elements are bonded foil (A) and unbonded wires (B) strain gages.

compute the pressure. Metallic unbonded strain gages have a high gage factor ($\approx 2-3$) and no adhesives are required, so they can be used at higher temperatures than bonded gages.

Metal wires or foil strain gages are usually bonded (glued) to the surface of the diaphragm that is submitted to the pressure pulse; typical metal gage factor is ≈ 2 and it provides a resistance variation proportional to the average strain in their active area. High-unstrained resistance are obtained with a significant length of wire or foil area, which does not allow metal strain gages to be made very small.

Metallic strain gages can also be obtained as a film sputtered directly on the surface of a thin metallic diaphragm isolated by a silicon oxide (SiO_2) layer. Format, size, location, and orientation of sputtered gage areas are controlled by masking and gage factors are similar to those of unbonded gauges. The molecular bond created by the sputtering process does not present common problems of bonded gages, as adhesive degradation, between gage and diaphragm, due to strain and temperature. The fabrication process is quite critical, but offers some of the advantages of diffused semiconductor gages, such as high natural frequency and sensibility, as well as the good linearity and temperature characteristics of metal gages.

Pressure transducers with semiconductor diaphragm and diffused semiconductor strain gages can be fabricated using integrated circuit masking and processing techniques. P or N semiconductor regions (strain gages) of several formats and sizes are diffused on a flat semiconductor substrate (diaphragm) of opposite polarity of the gages. The gage factor is dependent on the doping level; high gage factor is related to high resistivity of lightly doped materials. In addition, semiconductor material resistance and gage factor suffer meaningful modifications with temperature. Most of diffused semiconductor pressure transducers are made from doped silicon for gage factor in the 100–200 range, which gives acceptable temperature characteristics. This technique allows extreme miniaturization, precise location, and orientation of the strain gages, which removes the variability resulting from the bonding process, assuring good linearity and high sensitivity; it also reduces production cost and provides high accuracy and repeatability to pressure transducers performance.

The microfabrication techniques used to manufacture microelectromechanical systems (MEMS) allow obtaining semiconductor diaphragms with different design than flat disks of uniform thickness. Anisotropic etching provides precise control of etching directions in the silicon crystal. Complex shapes in extremely small size diaphragms can be manufactured, including shapes with variable thickness across the disc, to achieve optimum arrangements of linearity, sensitivity, and frequency response characteristics.

Semiconductor diaphragms are manufactured with different techniques to allow diverse working ranges, from units of kPa to hundreds of MPa and accuracy from 0.25% to 1% FS. Semiconductor gages do not have the same linear thermal error as foil strain gages and most of electromechanical pressure sensors are electronically processed and have digital compensation that corrects thermal error within the compensated temperature range. Typically, thermal errors of commercial transducers are within the range 0.2–0.5%. All types of strain gages can be used in extravascular blood pressure transducers but miniaturized sizes allow their use at the tip of a catheter to measure blood pressure directly inside a vessel or heart chamber (Cobbold, 1974; Dally et al., 1993; Doebelin, 2004).

6.1.2.2.3.3 LVDT This type of pressure transducers operates on the linear variable differential transformer (LVDT) principle. The LVDT is an electromechanical device which electrical output is linearly proportional to the displacement of a ferromagnetic core. In addition to the core, it has a primary coil and two secondary coils in series, wound in opposite directions. The movable cylindrical magnetic core placed inside

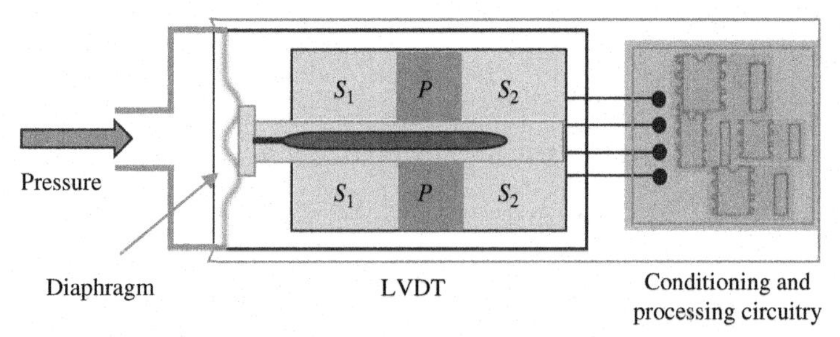

Figure 6.17 Typical LVDT-based pressure transducer with an elastic pressure responsive sensor with integrated electronic circuitry.

the coils provides a path for the magnetic flux linking primary and secondary coils. When alternating current energizes the primary coil, electric voltages are induced in the two secondary coils, with opposite polarities. A movement of the core leads to an increase in magnetic coupling of primary with the coil in the direction of movement, and a reduction of magnetic coupling to the other coil, producing a net output signal from the connected secondaries. A null output signal is produced when the induced voltages are equal in each secondary coil, which occurs when the core is symmetrically disposed between secondary coils.

In the LVDT-based pressure transducer, the blood pulse displacement is transmitted to the LVDT core by an elastic pressure responsive sensor, as for example, a metallic flat diaphragm or capsule-type diaphragm (bellows), which is directly coupled to the core. The transducer shown in Figure 6.17 is an inductive displacement transducer sensitive to the difference of pressure applied between the faces of a capsule-type diaphragm. The pressure pulse stretches the diaphragm, which in turn displaces the LVDT core, modifying the coupling of the primary coil with both secondary coils. The LVDT output tension is linearly proportional to the core displacement and thus, to the blood pressure. Figure 6.17B also shows the conditioning electronic circuits inserted in the same case of the displacement sensor (diaphragm) and transducer (LVDT).

An advantage of using an LVDT-based pressure transducer is that the moving core does not make contact with other electrical components of the assembly, as is the case with other types. This means an LVDT transducer offers high reliability and long life. LVDT-based pressure transducers have good thermal stability, but they are sensitive to magnetic field as well as to vibrations (Cobbold, 1974; Dally et al., 1993; Doebelin, 2004).

6.1.2.2.3.4 Capacitive sensor In the capacitance-based pressure transducer, the sensing element can be comprised of two conductive plates separated by an insulating material (dielectric). Usually a ceramic diaphragm acts as one of the plates or is fixed to one of the plates. The other plate, attached to a rigid substrate (e.g., glass encapsulate ceramic), which is insensitive to pressure changes, works as reference pressure.

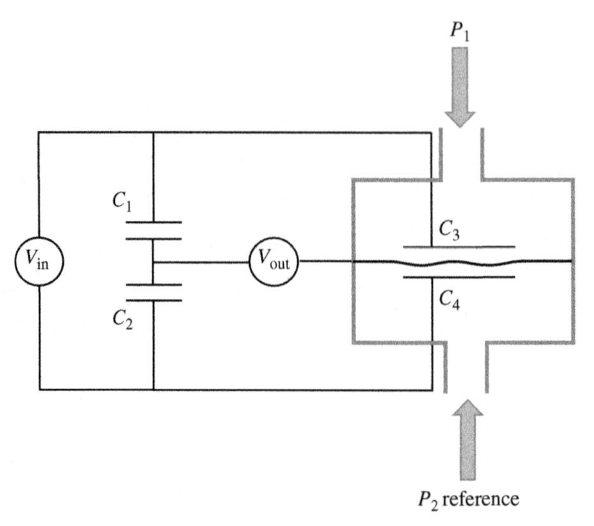

Figure 6.18 Schematic diagram of a differential capacitive pressure transducer.

The reference pressure can be a sealed chamber or a pressure port, so absolute or gage pressures are measured, respectively. The diaphragm is exposed to the process pressure on one side and to a reference pressure on the other. A pressure variation causes it to deflect and the capacitance value changes under pressure-induced displacement. The change may or may not be linear with pressure and is typically a few percent of the total capacitance. This technology is used in industrial and medical applications due to their good price/performance ratio. Pressure transducers are generally very stable and linear, but are sensitive to high temperatures and are more complicated to setup than most pressure sensors. They are used to measure pressures from vacuum to tens of 70 MPa with accuracy within 0.1% of reading or 0.01% of full scale.

Figure 6.18 shows the schematic diagram of a pressure transducer with a diaphragm and a differential capacitor. The differential capacitor is part of a bridge circuit and the diaphragm is the common armature of two serial capacitors. The displacement of the diaphragm, due to pressure variation, results in the increase of one capacitance and decrease of the other, which unbalances the bridge circuit. Usually the output voltage of the bridge circuit feeds an oscillating circuit, which frequency reflects the capacitance and so, the blood pressure value. Actual capacitive pressure transducers have integrated electronic circuits that measure the capacitance variation and convert it into a voltage linearly proportional to the pressure, which is easily converted into a digital signal to be processed and displayed. Integrated circuits can detect very small changes in capacitance due to small diaphragm deflections, with excellent hysteresis and repeatability.

A capacitive pressure transducer is precise, free from self-heating and nondissipative, and therefore free of thermal noise. As with most capacitive sensors, in order to prevent the adverse effects of stray capacitance the signal-conditioning electronics should be kept close to the sensor (Cobbold, 1974; Dally et al., 1993; Doebelin, 2004).

Piezoresistive (strain gage) and capacitive transduction principle have been widely adopted in recent works in the development of micromachined pressure sensor modeling, design, and fabrication (Eaton & Smith, 1997; Eswaran & Malarvizhi, 2013; Nemeth, Jadaan, Palko, Mitchell, & Zorman, 2008; Palasagaram & Ramadoss, 2006). Micromachined pressure sensors are fabricated using bulk and surface micromachining techniques (Eaton, Smith, Monk, O'Brien, & Miller, 1998) and many commercialized MEMS pressure sensors use piezoresistive technique as pressure transduction technique, due to its well-established properties of silicon material and the facilities of existing silicon foundry that can be used for fabrication in batch production. Piezoresistive pressure sensor has high gage factor, but piezoresistivity has high temperature coefficient, which limits the operating temperature and requires temperature compensation circuit. MEMS technology applied to construction of capacitive pressure sensors has been giving rise to micromachined pressure sensors with high sensitivity, low power consumption, temperature insensitive and compatibility with integrated electronic processing. Micromachined pressure transducers has gained importance in biomedical applications due to high sensitivity and good dynamic response (Babbitt, Fuller, & Keller, 1997; Eswaran & Malarvizhi, 2013); instead of silicon and silicon compounds, polymer material is mostly preferred due to biocompatibility. Examples of biomedical applications of pressure sensors manufactured with MEMS capacitive are MEMS-based inhalers, microfluidic chips used in blood gas analyzers, implantable intraocular pressure sensor (Chen et al., 2008), uterine activity monitoring with wireless interface capability (Wu, Young, & Kuo, 2000), pediatric postoperative monitoring application (Seo & Shandas, 2003), and pulmonary function diagnosis (van Putten, van Putten, van Putten, & van Putten, 2002).

6.1.2.2.3.5 Piezoelectric pressure sensors Piezoelectric transducers of pressure use the piezoelectric effect to generate an electrical signal that is proportional to the measured pressure. When an external physical stimulus, as pressure, force, or acceleration, is applied to a piezoelectric material, it is elastically deformed and its internal charge distribution is rearranged so a net charge is developed. This charge results from a flow of electric charge that lasts for few seconds and is proportional to the input stimulus. Unlike static devices, as strain gages and resistors, the electric signal generated by a piezoelectric sensor decays rapidly and this characteristic makes this type of sensor suitable for the measurement of dynamic changing pressures, as is the pressure pulsation of arterial blood and even larger pressures as the ones resultants from blasts and shocks. Piezoelectric sensors can detect pressure modifications that occur within times of the order of a millionth of a second. They can detect pressures between 0.7 kPa and 70 MPa with typical accuracy of 1% full scale (disregarding temperature effect).

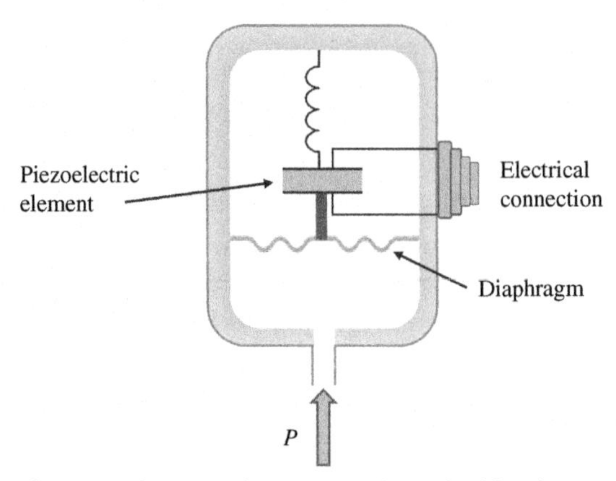

Figure 6.19 Schematic diagram of a piezoelectric transducer for blood pressure measurement.

Most common materials used in piezoelectric pressure sensors are quartz (monocrystalline) and ferroelectric ceramics (polycrystalline). Quartz is a common and naturally occurring mineral, and quartz-based transducers are generally inexpensive. Tourmaline is a naturally occurring semiprecious form of quartz that exhibits submicrosecond responsiveness and is useful in the measurement of very rapid transients. Ferroelectric ceramics are extensively used also in the construction of ultrasound flow and image transducers. Selecting the piezoelectric material properly, the designer can ensure good linearity as well as reduced temperature sensitivity.

Piezoelectric sensors present desirable features as small size, high speed, and self-generated signal, but they are sensitive to temperature variations and require special cabling and amplification. Piezoelectric crystals have high output impedance and require low-noise and very high input impedance amplification. These sensors also provide high-speed responses (natural frequency typically 5 kHz, but can exceed tens of kHz), which makes them ideal for measuring transient phenomena. According to which piezo-characteristic, electrostatic charge, resistivity, or resonant frequency is measured, the piezoelectric sensor is classified as electrostatic, piezoresistive, or resonant. Signals generated by piezoelectric crystals decay rapidly and are detected by electrostatic and piezoresistive sensors. Resonant type sensors are able to do static pressure measurements through detecting and processing the resonant frequency resultant from the pressure applied to the piezoelectric material (Cobbold, 1974; Dally et al., 1993; Doebelin, 2004; Webster, 2010).

Figure 6.19 is a schematic representation of a piezoelectric transducer used for arterial blood measurement.

6.1.2.2.3.6 Optical pressure sensors A typical structure of a fiber optical-based pressure transducer is shown in Figure 6.20A. An opaque vane connected to the diaphragm controls how much of the light intensity emitted by a source (LED) that is

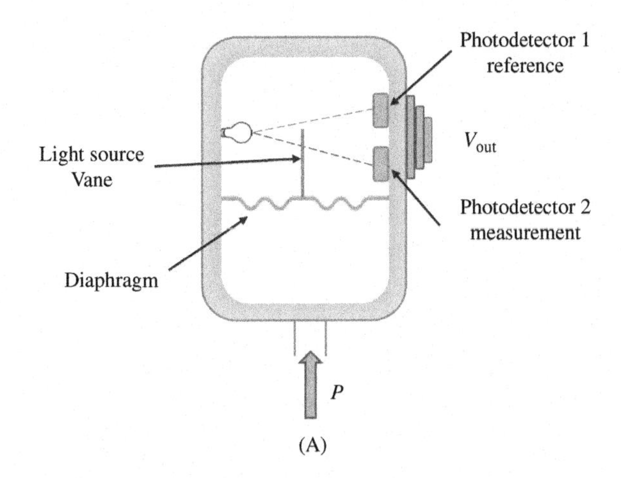

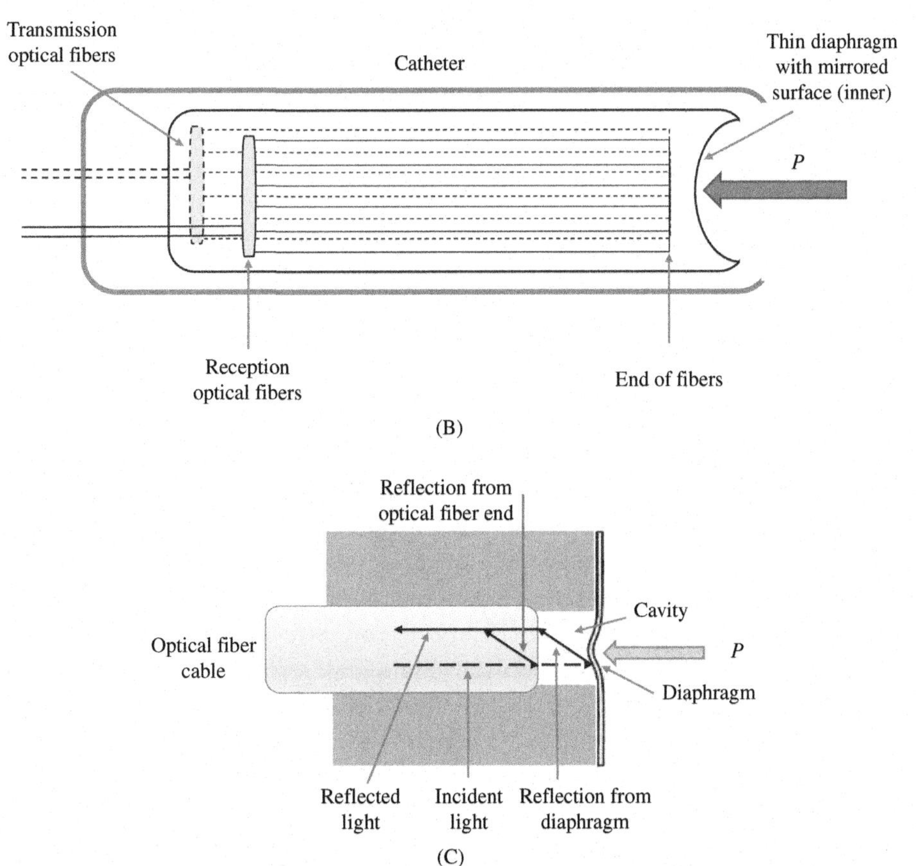

Figure 6.20 Typical schematic diagrams of optical-based pressure transducers: (A) with elastic diaphragm as primary pressure sensor; (B) with optical fiber for light transmission/reception and a diaphragm with reflecting surface as primary pressure sensor; and (C) an optical fiber-based sensor for micropressure reading.

collected by a photodiode. The position of the opaque vane varies according to the position of the diaphragm, which is displaced upward and downward by the pressure wave, letting less or more light to pass, respectively. The photodiode current, modulated by the light passage, feeds an electronic circuit, which output is digitalized and processed to provide pressure value.

Usually, a second photodiode is inserted to work as reference to compensate the variations of the source light intensity that may occur with aging. This type of pressure transducer can be manufactured in small sizes, and shows good thermal stability and its typical working range is 35 kPa to 400 Mpa with accuracy of 0.1% FS.

Figure 6.20B shows a typical structure of an optical pressure transducer with optical fiber for intravascular blood pressure measurement. In this type of device, the measurement of the displacement of the diaphragm due to local pressure is done by two sets of optical fibers, one for transmission and another for reception. A thin diaphragm is attached to the distal end of the intravascular catheter and its inner face is mirrored to receive and transmit light. A broadband light source placed at the proximal end of the catheter illuminates the transmission optical fibers. The light intensity that returns through the reception fibers to light detector is inversely proportional to pressure. The greater the intensity of the pressure, the greater the bending of the diaphragm and less light is reflected. Conversely, if the pressure is low, the surface of the diaphragm remains almost flat and the intensity of reflected light is close to the maximum value. The bundle of fibers is PVC coated and typical diameters are <1 mm. The main advantage of this system is its small size and the total absence of electrical voltage within the catheter. Its main disadvantage is the complexity of construction (Cobbold, 1974; Webster, 2010).

In 2002, Sondergaard et al. described a micropressure transducer for pediatric intensive care use. They investigated the feasibility of using an optical fiber-based pressure transducer for direct measurement and monitoring of tracheal pressure in pediatric intubated patients. They mounted a silicon micromachined sensor at the tip of a very small dimension optic fiber for medical pressure measurements (0.25 mm diameter). The micromachined sensor uses a microcavity for sensing the pressure. It is based on the interferometry principle (Fabry–Perot), which states that the deflection of the microcavity membrane by pressure results in a change in the reflected light intensity when the interference conditions inside the cavity are modified (Xiao, 1996; Yu & Zhou, 2011). The proximal endotracheal pressure measurements made with the optical sensor were compared with measurements taken with a commercial intravascular pressure sensor inserted in the distal portion of the endotracheal tube. The presence of both pressure transducers did not influence pressure drop or airway resistance across the endotracheal tube. They concluded that the fiber optic transducer developed was suitable for monitoring of tracheal pressure in neonatal and pediatric intubated patients; the device provided correct tracheal pressure readings even in the presence of kinking and secretions in the endotracheal tube.

Miniature fiber optic-based pressure sensors that are compatible with single-point entry into the body can be used to complement minimally invasive interventions where the entry point is along a body duct, such as the arterial system or urethra. Typically, the fabrication of these devices involves inserting a single-mode fiber of 125 μm diameter into a sensor body that is sealed by a diaphragm to give sensitivity to external pressure (Figure 6.20C). A halogen bulb provides a broadband light source, which illuminates the optical fiber. The pressure causes the diaphragm to flex. Pressure is measured by tracking the effective cavity length, which is determined from light fringes formed by interference between reflections from the diaphragm and the fiber end. Similar result could be achieved using multiple narrowband lasers, but at prohibitive cost for clinical use (McCartney et al., 2006; Towers et al., 2006).

6.2 FORCE TRANSDUCERS

6.2.1 Introduction

Force transducers are used in many biomedical applications, such as characterization of biological tissues to study mechanical properties of bones, muscles, and tendons; *in vivo* measurements of muscle contraction force with implanted sensors in muscles and tendons; in the force monitoring and control of orthopedic devices, joint implants (knee and hip) and artificial limbs; and in physiological experiments to study muscle activity. The force of muscle contraction of athletes is evaluated through the measurement of the variables of the ground reaction force during leaps and races. The measurement of the force exerted on the teeth while chewing is used in orthodontics and orthopedics studies of the rotation and translation of the teeth and in the analysis of the formation and maxillofacial growth. Other examples are the physiotherapeutic follow of patients during motor rehabilitation and patient monitoring during MRI tests to detect loss of strength/awareness. The force, while biological variable, shows wide variation in amplitude, since μN (fibers and muscle cells) to kN (big muscles and teeth). The contraction force of an isolated myocyte is approximately a few tens of μN causing a cell shortening of a few units of μm and of a myofibril is units of μm (Fearn, Bartoo, Myers, & Pollack, 1993). The isometric flexion force of the elbow is 360 N (McDonagh, Hayward, & Davies, 1981) and of the knee is 700 N (Murray, Gardner, Mollinger, & Sepic, 1980). The vertical component of chewing force over teeth varies from a hundreds to thousands of N while the lateral component is approximately 20 N; in normal human dentition, byte force is 569 ± 80 N in the canine region and 723 ± 138 N at the second molar region (Brunski, Puleo, & Nanci, 2000; van Eijden, 1991). The measurement of the force developed by large muscles,

Table 6.2 Types and characteristics of force transducers

Type of load cell	Working range (N)	Accuracy (% FS)	Thermal sensitivity (% FS/°C)
Thin film strain gage	0.1–100	±0.02–1	0.02[a]
Foil strain gage	$5–50 \times 10^6$	±0.2–1	0.0015[a]
Semiconductor strain gage	$1–10 \times 10^3$	±0.2–1	0.02–0.5[a]
Piezoelectric	$1.5 \times 10^{-3}–120 \times 10^6$	0.3–1	0.02[b]
Hydraulic	$500–500 \times 10^3$	0.25–5	0.02–0.1[c]
Electromagnetic (LVDT)	$10 \times 10^{-3}–1 \times 10^6$	0.5–2	0.02–0.5[c]
Capacitive	$10 \times 10^{-3}–1 \times 10^6$	0.5–2	0.02–0.5[c]

[a] −40°C to +80°C.
[b] −190°C to +200°C.
[c] +5°C to +40°C.

teeth, and muscle fiber cells requires specific transducers, in general of complex construction, and adequate conditioning by electronic circuitry. Table 6.2 summarizes types and characteristics of force transducers or load cells (OMEGA, 2014).

The measurement of physiological forces average amplitude (up to 50 N), such as myocardial contraction, flexion of the fingers, or the gastrointestinal system activity, requires less complex transducers. Piezoresistive load cell with strain gages are the most suitable for measuring the force developed by tendons, which is of the order of several hundreds of N with displacement that can reach up to 5% of the resting length, depending on the elasticity of the tissue.

The unit of force is in the International System Newton (N), which is defined as the force required to accelerate a mass of 1 kilogram per second at 1 meter per second ($kg\ m/s^2$). Mass and force are related through Newton's second law. The second law states that the acceleration of an object is dependent upon two variables—the net force acting upon the object and the mass of the object. The acceleration of an object depends directly upon the net force acting upon the object, and inversely upon the mass of the object. As the force acting upon an object is increased, the acceleration of the object is increased. As the mass of an object is increased, the acceleration of the object is decreased:

$$F = Ma \tag{6.8}$$

where

F is a vector quantity necessary to change the amount of motion of a mass; F is not a fundamental quantity

M is an inertial property, the measure of amount of matter in a body; M is a fundamental quantity

a is the acceleration, is obtained from the length and time, two fundamental quantities.

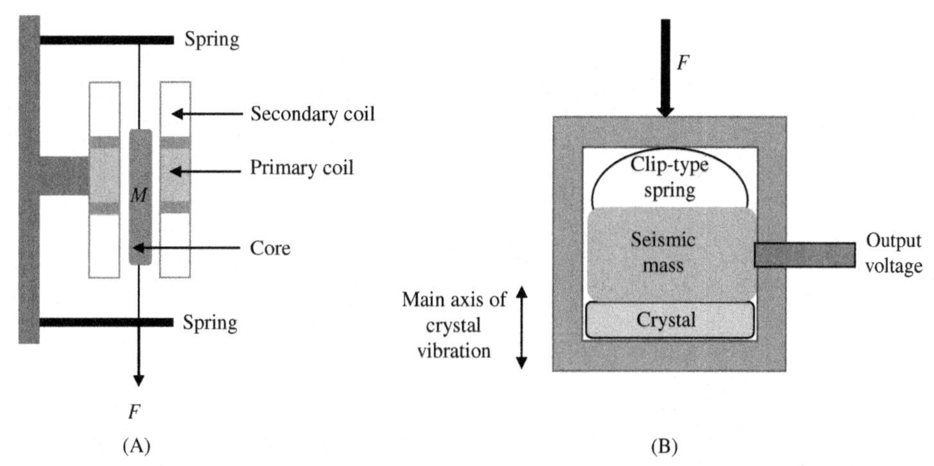

Figure 6.21 Schematic diagrams of accelerometer-based force transducers (A) with LVDT and (B) with piezoelectric crystal.

6.2.2 Methods for measuring force

There are several methods to measure force, using Eq. (6.2) (Newton second law) or Eq. (6.1) (force is pressure times area). Most of them use displacement or pressure transducers. A few techniques are described below.

6.2.2.1 Accelerometer

This technique uses an accelerometer to measure the acceleration (a) to which a known mass (M) is subjected due to the unknown applied force (F) (Eq. (6.8)). The principle of operation of the accelerometer is to measure the force exerted by a seismic mass that is supported by an elastic sensor element. The elastic element can be a piezoelectric crystal, which produces a voltage proportional to the force, a metal spring with strain gage, which electrical resistance reflects the deformation produced by the force, or any other type of displacement sensor (ref).

The type of accelerometer used should be chosen according to the natural frequency required to measure the force. Figure 6.21A shows an accelerometer-based force transducer with an LVDT working as elastic member. In this type of accelerometer, the core of LVDT works as the seismic mass. The displacement of the core is directly converted to AC voltage, which is linearly proportional to the displacement of the core and the unknown force. Typical natural frequency of this kind of accelerometers is lower than 80 Hz and they are commonly used to measure accelerations of the type of low frequency vibration. Figure 6.21B shows an accelerometer-based force transducer that uses a piezoelectric crystal as elastic sensor. The crystal is connected to seismic mass and spring. The applied force accelerates the mass that deforms the

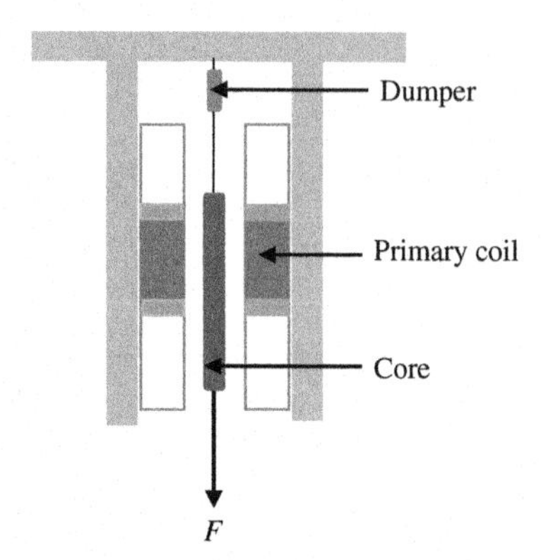

Figure 6.22 Schematic diagram of a force transducer that uses the electromagnetically force developed by an LVDT (displacement transducer) to balance the unknown force.

crystal, generating voltage difference across the crystal. The measurement of this electrical voltage brings information on the mass displacement and allows obtaining the acceleration value. The natural frequency of the crystal can be larger than 5 kHz, and this device is suitable to measure forces that produces high frequency vibrations.

The accelerometer-based force transducer has many biomedical applications, for example, in the evaluation of the muscular force developed by patients, workers, and athletes, to help in physiotherapeutic treatment, ergonomic studies, and improvement of training, respectively. Another example of application is the measurement of the ground reaction force, for example, in jumps and races, once more to help physical training of athletes and also to calibrate orthopedic devices.

6.2.2.2 Force balance

In this method, the unknown force is balanced with a known force. In Figure 6.22, the unknown force is measured by balancing the applied force F against a force electromagnetically developed in the LVDT. F causes the displacement of the LVDT core modifying the coupling between primary and secondary coils. The LVDT output voltage is linearly proportional to the core displacement, and so, to the intensity of the applied force F. Due to LVDT characteristics, the output voltage has practically infinite resolution, and the core frictionless displacement assures long life to this device (ref).

6.2.2.3 Hydraulic load cell

The hydraulic load cell converts the unknown force into a pressure, which is applied to a fluid and then, the resulting pressure is measured. The area where the force is applied is known, so the force can be determined by Eq. (6.1) ($F = PA$).

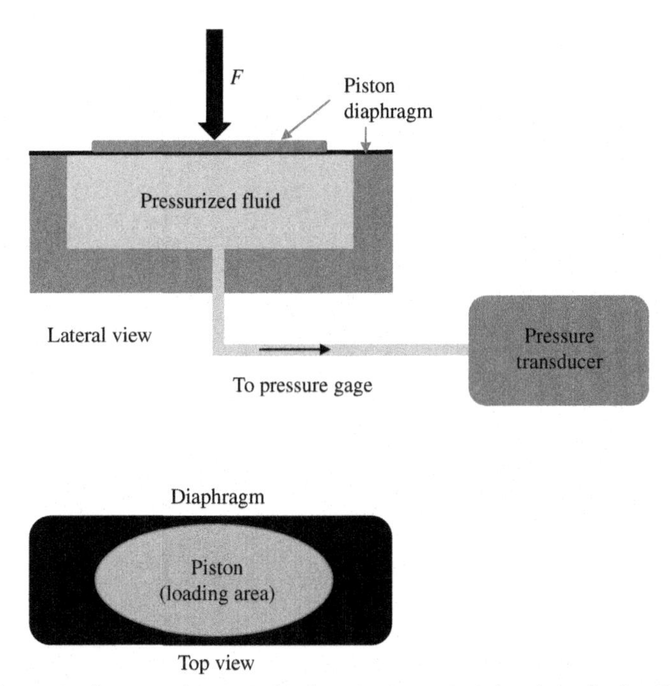

Figure 6.23 Schematic diagram showing the functioning principle of the hydraulic load cell technique to measure force.

The hydraulic load cell is a device filled with a fluid, usually oil, subjected to an initial pressure of known value. It has a known area, named loading area, where the force is applied. The unknown force is applied to the loading area, increasing the fluid pressure, which is measured by a pressure transducer. Figure 6.23 shows the principle of functioning of the use of a hydraulic load cell to measure force.

Hydraulic load cells usually have zero adjustment, measure forces ranging from 500 N to 500 kN with accuracy 0.5–1% FS; they deflect in maximum conditions about 0.05 mm. Hydraulic cells are temperature sensitive and temperature coefficients are typically in the range 0.02–0.1%/°C.

6.2.2.4 Elastic force

This technique measures the strain produced in an elastic material by the unknown force. The application of the force in the elastic element causes it to deflect; then a secondary transducer senses the deflection and converts displacement into a measurable output. This technique is the most used in physiological measurements, for example, in muscle activity study. Examples of devices that use this measurement method are shown in Figure 6.24, with spring dynamometer (A), strain gage load cell (B) and with other types of displacement transducers (C) and (D).

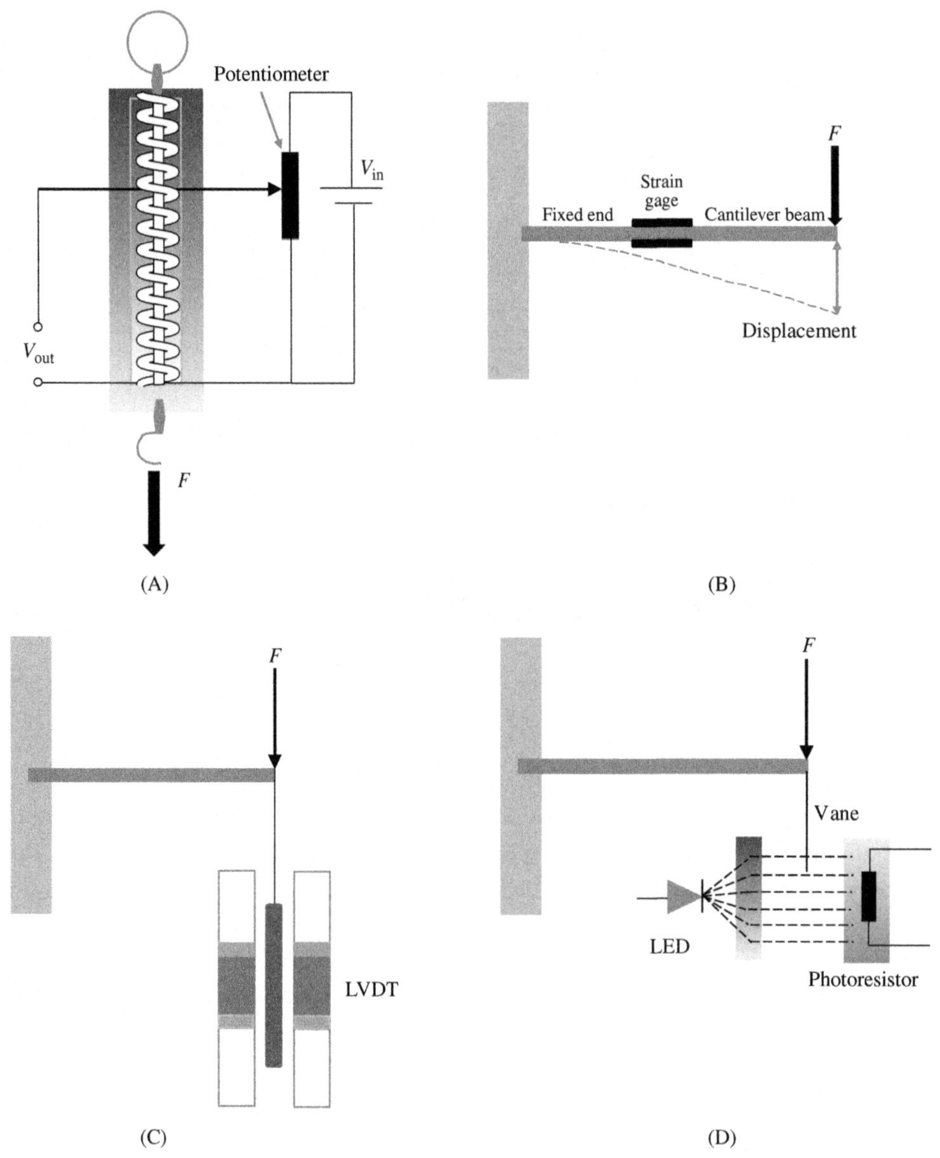

Figure 6.24 Examples of elastic force technique for pressure measurement with different displacement transducers: (A) spring dynamometer; (B) strain gages; (C) LVDT; and (D) optical sensor.

The output of the spring dynamometer (Figure 6.24A) is the force value and it can be read in N on a graded scale, as the spring displacement is directly proportional to the applied force:

$$F = kx \tag{6.9}$$

where

F is the applied force (N)

x is the spring displacement (m)

k is the spring constant (kg/s^2).

The output of the spring dynamometer can be used to generate an electrical signal proportional to the applied force, coupling its output to a passive displacement transducer such as a potentiometer mounted on an electronic circuit (also shown in Figure 6.24A).

The cantilever beam load cell shown in Figure 6.24B has one strain gage bonded on the top face of the beam and one gage on the bottom face. When force F is applied to the beam in the direction indicated, the cantilever bends, top gage is in tension and bottom gage is in compression. The gage resistances are modified due to the cantilever displacement under the force action.

The core of the LVDT shown in Figure 6.24C is displaced according to force F applied to the cantilever beam. The output voltage of the transformer is linearly related to the core displacement and to the force applied. In Figure 6.24D, the vane is displaced together with the cantilever that bends under the applied force F. According to the vane position, more or less light emitted from the LED reaches the photoresistor.

Most used materials in the elastic element are stainless steel, aluminum, metal alloys like copper and beryllium, and semiconductor. Whatever the chosen material, it must have a linear relationship between stress (applied force) and strain (displacement output), with low hysteresis in working range.

Several formats of load cell can be used in the elastic force technique, as cantilever beam, link beam, ring beam, S-beam, cylinder, tube, diaphragm, etc. Some of them are shown in Figure 6.25. Each format is designed to preferably measure the forces along the main axis of the load cell, without interference of force components in other directions, for example, lateral, in the measurement result. The displacement sensors, usually strain gages, are distributed on the surface of the load cell according to the type of force that the transducer should measure. Figure 6.25D shows an example of traction force measurement with a cylinder-type load cell. The ring beam load cell shown in Figure 6.25C has an LVDT mounted inside the ring beam and can be used to measure traction and compression forces (Dally et al., 1993; Doebelin, 2004).

Most of load cells use strain gage as displacement sensor (as in Figure 6.24B) and the Wheatstone bridge is the most common electronic circuit used to measure the resistance variation of strain gages. Bridge circuit is preferred due to its sensitivity and versatility of montage. The number of strain gages in the Wheatstone bridge typically ranges from 1 to 4, with at least one active sensor, that is, at least one strain gage is subjected to deformation caused by the force being measured. Some load cells use 8, 16, 32, or more gages to increase the sensitivity and to measure force in more than one direction. The precise location of the gages, the assembly and the materials used

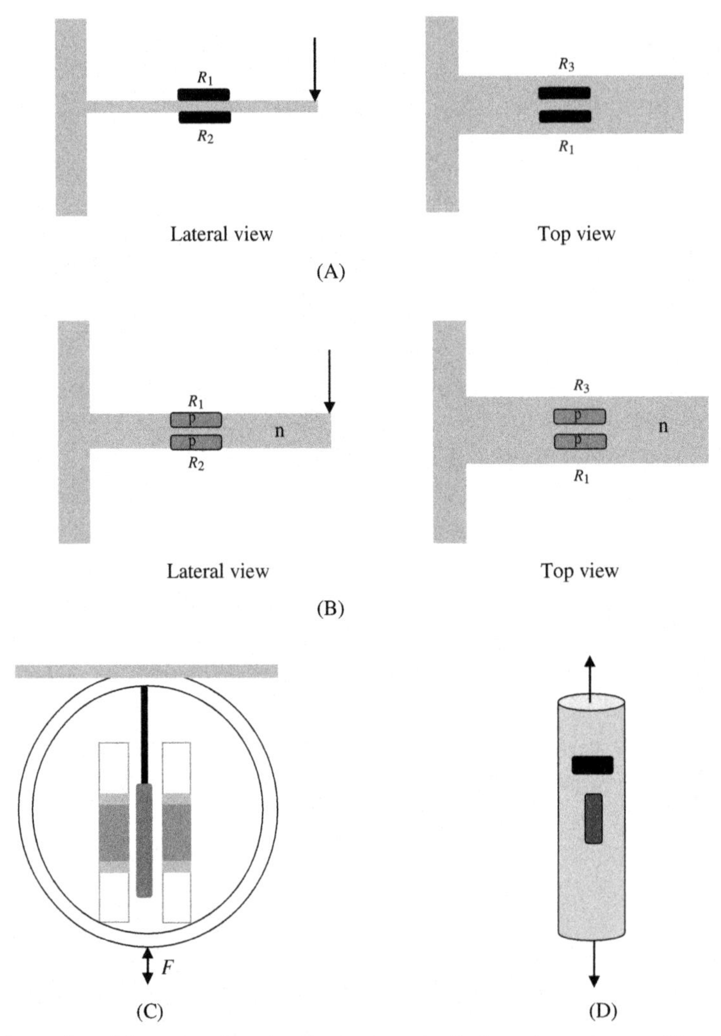

Figure 6.25 Examples of formats of load cells used as elastic force transducers: (A) cantilever beam with four metal foil strain gages bonded on the beam surface; (B) cantilever beam with four semiconductor strain gages (four p regions diffused on an n substrate); (C) ring beam; and (D) cylinder-type load cells.

define the performance of the load cell. The analog output of the transducer, that is, from the bridge circuit, is usually electronically conditioned, and then digitized and digitally processed for visualization of the value of the force; other variables can be obtained from strain measurement, e.g., displacement, pressure, and torque.

In the circuit shown in Figure 6.26A, the cantilever beam-type load cell is used to measure the strain caused by the force F applied on the surface of the beam. Four foil strain gages with equal nominal resistances were bonded on the beam surface, two on the top and

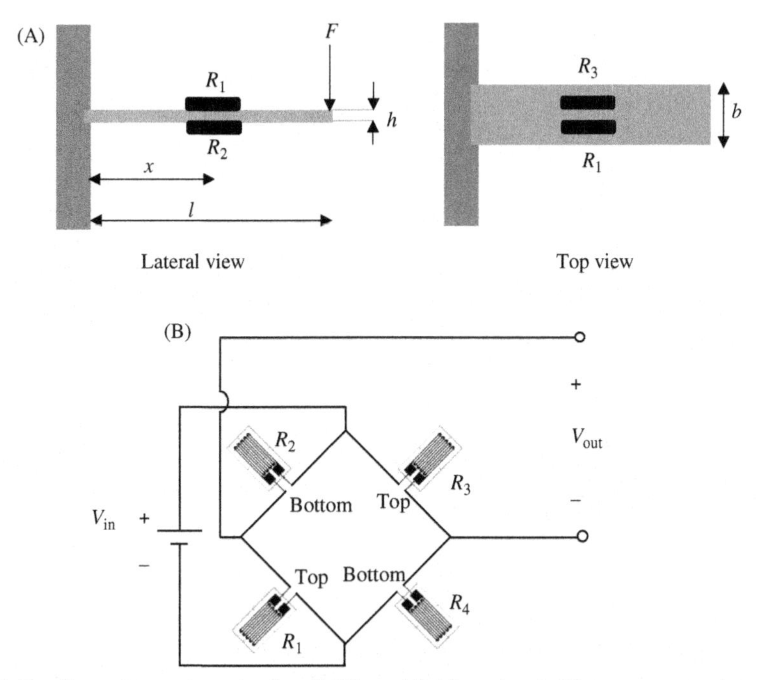

Figure 6.26 Cantilever beam-type load cell (A) and bridge circuit (B) to measure the variation of the strain gage resistances due to axial deformation of the cantilever beam caused by force *F*.

two on the bottom. The four gages work as a displacement transducer, whose resistance varies proportionally to the deformation of the cantilever beam subjected to the unknown force. The gages are mounted in a full bridge configuration circuit (Figure 6.26B), whose output voltage registers the variation of the gage resistances. When the beam is subjected to a force in the direction indicated in Figure 6.26A, the length of the top gages increases and the length of the bottom gages decreases, with correspondent variation of their resistances. The output voltage V_{out} depends of the sensibility G of the beam-type load cell and the force F applied in the cantilever beam.

The open-circuit voltage at the output of the bridge circuit in Figure 6.26B is

$$V_{out} = V_{in} \cdot G \cdot \varepsilon \tag{6.10}$$

where

G is the gage sensibility or gage factor

V_{in} is the input voltage in the bridge circuit

ε is the strain.

And

$$\varepsilon = \frac{\Delta L}{L} = \frac{\Delta R}{GR} \tag{6.11}$$

where

L is the length of the cantilever beam
ΔL is the length variation
R is the nominal resistance of the gages
ΔR is the variation of the gages resistance.

The stress σ/strain ε ratio is equal to the Young modulus of elasticity:

$$\frac{\sigma}{\varepsilon} = E \tag{6.12}$$

The stress in the surface of the cantilever beam is

$$\sigma = M_{\mathrm{d}} \cdot \frac{y}{I} = \frac{6M_{\mathrm{d}}}{b \cdot h^2} \tag{6.13}$$

where

M_{d} is the moment of deflection
$I = L \cdot b \cdot h^3/12$ is the moment of inertia of the area for a rectangular solid
b is the width of the cantilever beam
h is the thickness of the cantilever beam
$y = h/2$ and L is the length of the cantilever beam.

The moment of deflection of the cantilever beam is

$$M_{\mathrm{d}} = F \cdot I \tag{6.14}$$

And

$$\frac{V_{\mathrm{out}}}{V_{\mathrm{in}}} = G \cdot \varepsilon = \frac{6G \cdot (L - x) \cdot F}{E \cdot b \cdot h^2} \tag{6.15}$$

where

x is the distance from the fixed end of the cantilever to the middle length of the gages.

The sensitivity S of the cantilever beam-type load cell is the output voltage to input force ratio:

$$S = \frac{V_{\mathrm{out}}}{F} = \frac{6G \cdot (L - x) \cdot V_{\mathrm{in}}}{E \cdot b \cdot h^2} \tag{6.16}$$

Equation (6.16) shows that S depends on the modulus of elasticity E and of the transversal section $(b \cdot h)$ of the cantilever, the distance over the cantilever from its fixed end to the central point where the gages are bonded (x), the gage factor of the strain gages (G), and the bridge supply voltage (V_{in}). Finally, the force is calculated as

$$F = \frac{V_{\mathrm{out}}}{S} = \frac{E \cdot b \cdot h^2}{6G \cdot (l - x) \cdot V_{\mathrm{in}}} \tag{6.17}$$

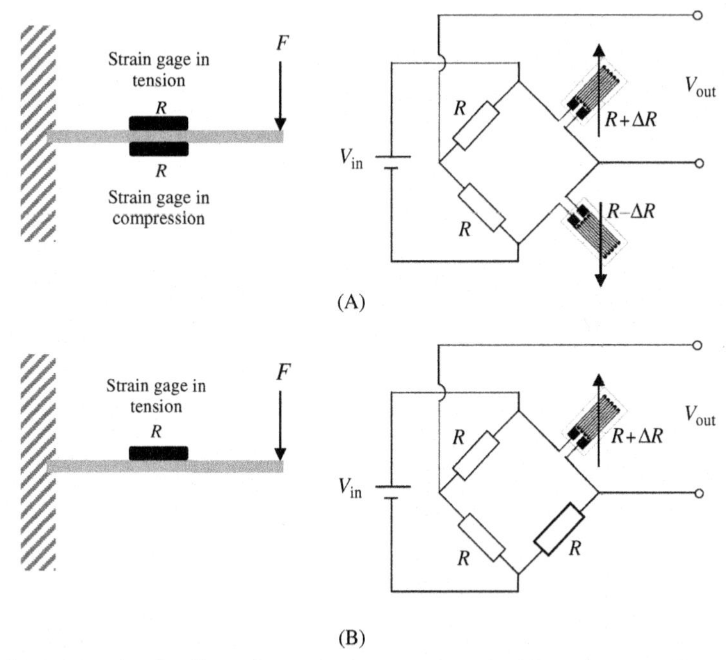

Figure 6.27 Beam-type load cells with two active strain gages (A) and one active strain gage (B) and respective bridge circuits.

Figure 6.27A shows a cantilever beam-type load cell with two active strain gages, one in tension (top) and one in compression (bottom); the bridge circuit is also shown. Nominal resistances of the gages and resistors have the same value. Equations of load cell sensitivity and force F are

$$S = \frac{V_{\text{out}}}{F} = \frac{V_{\text{in}} G \varepsilon}{2} \tag{6.18}$$

$$\frac{V_{\text{out}}}{V_{\text{in}}} = \frac{F G \varepsilon}{2} \tag{6.19}$$

$$F = \frac{2 V_{\text{out}}}{V_{\text{in}} G \varepsilon} \tag{6.20}$$

Figure 6.27B shows a cantilever beam-type load cell with one active strain gage in tension and the bridge circuit. The three resistors are equal and the strain gage nominal resistance has the same value as the resistors. The equation to calculate the force F is

$$V_{\text{out}} = \frac{V_{\text{in}} \cdot F \cdot G \cdot \varepsilon}{4\left(1/1 + G \cdot F \cdot \varepsilon/2\right)} \tag{6.21}$$

The bonded strain gages used the cantilever beam load cell are of foil (120−5 kΩ), thin film (≈10 kΩ), wire grid (60−350 Ω), and semiconductor (120−5 kΩ) types. The semiconductor type has gage factor G much times larger than foil type, are almost hysteresis-free, allows to obtain very small size transducers (with gages diffused in the cantilever), but is temperature sensitive and its output (resistance variation) does not vary linearly with input (strain).

6.3 REVIEW THE LEARNING

1. How does the occlusive method (sphygmomanometry) function for indirect arterial blood measurement? Show diagrams, curves, drawings, etc. to enrich your answer.
2. Which are the differences, vantages, and advantages between sphygmomanometry and oscillometry. How does oscillometry works?
3. Finapres is semiocclusive and indirect method for blood pressure measurement. Explain its principle of functioning and discuss main differences to oscillometric method. Show figures to complement your answer.
4. Doppler ultrasound can be used to measure blood pressure. This method is non-invasive, indirect, and also occlusive. Present its schematic diagram, explain its principle of operation, and discuss its vantages and advantages comparing its functioning to oscillometric and Finapres methods.
5. To the direct and invasive method of blood pressure measurement, with intravascular electronic transducer, provide what is asked:
   a. Describe the principle of functioning. Add schematic diagrams and curves to enrich the answer
   b. Choose two among capacitive and piezoelectric-based electronic transducers and explain their functioning.
6. The dynamic behavior of blood pressure is obtained through direct measurement methods and therefore invasive, in which the pressure transducer is located inside (intravascular) or outside (extravascular) the artery or vessel. Design an extravascular electronic pressure transducer (sensor with primary and secondary sensors) to obtain directly the wave of blood pressure. Present the schematic diagram of the project, identifying all transducer components; suggest an adequate electronic circuit to detect the output signal of the transducer; and justify the choice of the components (primary and secondary sensors) of the transducer (characteristics, material, sensitivity, frequency response, dimensions, general functioning, etc.).
7. Explain which are the main error sources of the invasive methods of blood pressure measurements and how they are minimized.
8. Show the schematic diagram of an optical transducer for intravascular blood pressure measurement and discuss its advantages and disadvantages.

9. Show the schematic diagram of a beam-type load transducer used to measure force. Choose a secondary displacement transducer among strain gages and LVDT and show the electronic measurement circuit.

10. Show the schematic diagram of a force transducer with accelerometer and explain its functioning.

REFERENCES

Andriessen, P., Schoffelen, R. L., Berendsen, R. C., de Beer, N. A., Oei, S. G., Wijn, P. F., et al. (2004). Noninvasive assessment of blood pressure variability in preterm infants. *Pediatric Research, 55*, 220–223.

Babbitt, K. E., Fuller, L., & Keller, B. (1997). A surface micromachined capacitive pressure sensor for biomedical applications. In *Proceedings of the twelfth Biennial University/Government/Industry Microelectronics symposium* (pp. 150–153).

Black, H. R., & Elliott, W. J. (2013). *Hypertension: A companion to Braunwald's heart disease* (2nd ed.). Philadelphia: Elsevier Saunders.

Brunski, J. B., Puleo, D. A., & Nanci, A. (2000). Biomaterials and biomechanics of oral and maxillofacial implants: Current status and future developments. *The International Journal of Oral & Maxillofacial Implants, 15*(1), 15–46.

Chan, A. Y. K. (2008). *Biomedical device technology: Principles and design*. Springfield, Illinois: Charles C. Thomas.

Chen, Po-J., Rodger, D. C., Saati, S., Humayun, M. S., & Tai, Yu-C. (2008). Microfabricated implantable Parylene-based wireless passive intraocular pressure sensors. *Journal of Microelectromechanical Systems, 17*(6), 1342–1351.

Chung, E., Chen, G., Alexander, B., & Cannesson, M. (2013). Non-invasive continuous blood pressure monitoring: A review of current applications. *Frontiers of Medicine*, 7(1), 91–101.

Cobbold, R. S. C. (1974). *Transducers for biomedical measurements: Principles and applications.* New York: John Wiley & Sons.

Dally, J. W., Riley, W. F., & McConnell, K. G. (1993). *Instrumentation for engineering measurements* (2nd ed.). New York, Chichester: John Wiley & Sons.

Doebelin, E. O. (2004). *Measurements systems—application and design* (5th ed.). New York: McGraw Hill.

Drouin, E., Gournay, V., Calamel, J., Mouzard, A., & Rozé, J. C. (1997). Feasibility of using finger arterial pressure in neonates. *Archives of Diseases in Childhood Fetal & Neonatal Edition*, 77(2), F139–F140.

Dueck, R., Goedje, O., & Clopton, P. (2012). Noninvasive continuous beat-to-beat radial artery pressure via TL-200 applanation tonometry. *Journal of Clinical Monitoring and Computing, 26*(2), 75–83.

Eaton, W. P., & Smith, J. H. (1997). Micromachined pressure sensors: Review and recent developments. *Smart Materials and Structures, 6*, 530–539.

Eaton, W. P., Smith, J. H., Monk, D. J., O'Brien, G., & Miller, T. F. (1998). Comparison of bulk- and surface-micromachined pressure sensors micromachined devices and components. *Proceedings of SPIE, 3514*, 431–438.

Eckerle, J. D. (2006). Tonometry, arterial. In J. G. Webster (Ed.), *Encyclopedia of medical devices* (Vol. 6, 2nd ed., pp. 402–410). New York: Wiley.

Eswaran, P., & Malarvizhi, S. (2013). MEMS capacitive pressure sensors: A review on recent development and prospective. *International Journal of Engineering and Technology, 5*(3), 2734–2746.

Fearn, L. A., Bartoo, M. L., Myers, J. A., & Pollack, G. H. (1993). An optical fiber transducer for single myofibril force measurement. *IEEE Transactions on Biomedical Engineering, 40*, 1127–1132.

Friedman, D. B., Jensen, F. B., Matzen, S., & Secher, N. H. (1990). Non-invasive blood pressure monitoring during head-up tilt using the Peñáz principle. *Acta Anaesthesiologica Scandinavica, 34*(7), 519–522.

Geddes, L. A., & Baker, L. E. (1968). *Principles of applied biomedical instrumentation.* John Wiley & Sons.

Huang, Q.-F., Sheng, C.-S., Zhang, Y., Wang, J., Li, Y., & Wang, J.-G. (2009). Accuracy of automated oscillometric blood pressure monitors in the detection of cardiac arrhythmias. *Blood Pressure Monitoring*, *14*(2), 91–92.

Imholz, B. P. M., Wieling, W., van Montfrans, G. A., & Wesseling, K. H. (1998). Fifteen years experience with finger arterial pressure monitoring: Assessment of the technology. *Cardiovascular Research*, *38*, 605–616.

Introcaso, L. (1996). História da medida da pressão arterial: 100 anos do esfigmomanômetro. *Arquivos Brasileiros de Cardiologia*, *67*(5), 305–311.

Jensen, F. B., & Secher, N. H. (1989). Continuous non-invasive measurement of blood pressure. *Ugeskr Laeger*, *151*(51), 3487–3490.

JNC7 (2003). The seventh report of the joint national committee on prevention: Detection, evaluation, and treatment of high blood pressure: The JNC 7 Report. *Journal of the American Medical Association*, *289*, 2560–2571. Available from: <http://www.ncbi.nlm.nih.gov/pubmed/12748199>.

Keren, H., Burkhoff, D., & Squara, P. (2007). Evaluation of a noninvasive continuous cardiac output monitoring system based on thoracic bioreactance. *American Journal of Physiology Heart Circulation Physiology*, *293*, H583–589.

Kinsella, S. M., Whitwam, J. G., & Spencer, J. A. D. (2005). Aortic compression by the uterus: Identification with the Finapres digital arterial pressure instrument. *International Journal of Obstetrics & Gynaecology*, *97*(8), 700–705.

Korotkoff, J. S. (1905). On the subject of methods of measuring blood pressure. *Bulletin of the Imperial Military Medical Academy of St. Petersburg*, *11*, 365–367.

Ling, J., Ohara, Y., Orime, Y., Noon, G. P., & Takatani, S. (1995). Clinical evaluation of the oscillometric blood pressure monitor in adults and children based on the 1992 AAMI SP-10 standards. *Journal of Clinical Monitoring and Computing*, *11*(2), 23–30.

Mano, G. M. P., Souza, V. F., Pierin, A. M. G., Lima, J. C., Ignes, E. C., Ortega, K. C., et al. (2002). Assessment of the DIXTAL DX-2710 automated oscillometric device for blood pressure measurement with the validation protocols of the british hypertension society (BHS) and the association for the advancement of medical instrumentation (AAMI). *Arquivos Brasileiros de Cardiologia*, *79*(6), 606–610.

Martina, J. R., Westerhof, B. E., van Goudoever, J., de Beaumont, E. M., Truijen, J., Kim, Y. S., et al. (2012). Noninvasive continuous arterial blood pressure monitoring with Nexfin(R). *Anaesthesiology*, *116*, 1092–1103.

McCartney, A. J., Bialkowski, M., Barton, J. S., Stewart, L., Towers, C. E., MacPherson, W. N., et al. (2006). Interferometric sensors for application in the bladder and the lower urinary tract. *Proceedings of the Society of Photo-optical Instrumentation Engineers (SPIE)*, *6293*, L2930–L2937.

McDonagh, M. J. B., Hayward, C. M., & Davies, C. T. M. (1981). Isometric training in human elbow flexor muscles. *The Journal of Bone and Joint Surgery*, *65-B*(3), 355–358.

Meidert, A. S., Huber, W., Müller, J. N., Schöfthaler, M., Hapfelmeier, A., Langwieser, N., et al. (2014). Radial artery applanation tonometry for continuous non-invasive arterial pressure monitoring in intensive care unit patients: Comparison with invasively assessed radial arterial pressure. *British Journal of Anaesthesia*, *112*(3), 521–528.

Monnet, X., Picard, F., Lidzborski, E., Mesnil, M., Duranteau, J., Richard, C., et al. (2012). The estimation of cardiac output by the Nexfin device is of poor reliability for tracking the effects of a fluid challenge. *Critical Care*, *16*(5), R212.

Murray, M. P., Gardner, G. M., Mollinger, L. A., & Sepic, S. B. (1980). Strength of isometric and isokinetic contractions: Knee muscles of men aged 20 to 86. *Physical Therapy*, *60*, 412–419.

Nemeth, N. N., Jadaan, O., Palko, J. L., Mitchell, J. S., & Zorman, C. A. (2008). Structural modeling and probabilistic characterization of MEMS pressure sensor membranes. *Journal of Microelectromechanical Systems*, *17*(2), 453–458.

OMEGA (2014). *Load cell design*. <http://www.omega.com/literature/transactions/volume3/load.html#oppri> Accessed September 2014.

Palasagaram, J. N., & Ramadoss, R. (2006). MEMS-capacitive pressure sensor fabricated using printed-circuit-processing techniques. *IEEE Sensors Journal*, *6*(6), 1374–1375.

Parker, K. H. (2009). A brief history of arterial wave mechanics. *Medical & Biological Engineering & Computing*, *47*, 111–118.

Peňáz, J. (1973). Photoelectric measurement of blood pressure volume and flow in the finger. In *Digest of the international conference on medicine and biological engineering*, Dresden (p. 104).

Peňáz, J., Honzikova, N., & Jurak, P. (1997). Vibration plethysmography: A method for studying the visco-elastic properties of finger arteries. *Medical & Biological Engineering & Computing, 35*(6), 633–637.

Raaijmakers, E., Faes, T. J., Scholten, R. J., Goovaerts, H. G., & Heethaar, R. M. (1999). A meta-analysis of three decades of validating thoracic impedance cardiography. *Critical Care Medicine, 27*, 1203–1213.

Raamat, R., Talts, J., Jacomägi, K., & Länsimies, G. (1999). Mathematical modelling of non-invasive oscillometric finger mean blood pressure measurement by maximum oscillation criterion. *Medical & Biological Engineering & Computing, 37*, 784–788.

Riva-Rocci, S. (1896). Un nuovo sfigmomanometro. *Gazzetta Medica di Torino, 47*, 981–986.

Saugel, B., & Reuter, D. A., III (2013). Are we ready for the age of non-invasive haemodynamic monitoring? *British Journal of Anaesthesiology, 113*(3), 340–343.

Saugel, B., & Reuter, D. A. (2014). III. Are we ready for the age of non-invasive haemodynamic monitoring? *British Journal of Anaesthesia, 113*(3), 340–343.

Seo, D.-B., Shandas, R. (2003). Design and simulation of a MEMS-based comb-drive pressure sensor for pediatic post-operative monitoring applications. In *Proceedings of 2003 summer bioengineering conference* (pp. 1239–1240).

Sokolski, M., Rydlewska, A., Krakowiak, B., Biegus, J., Zymlinski, R., Banasiak, W., et al. (2011). Comparison of invasive and non-invasive measurements of haemodynamic parameters in patients with advanced heart failure. *Journal of Cardiovascular Medicine, 12*(11), 773–778.

Souza, F. M. C. (2003). Métodos de medida da pressão arterial—passado, presente e futuro. *Revista Brasileira de Hipertensão, 10*(3), 189–193.

Steiner, L. A., Johnston, A. J., Salvador, R., Czosnyka, M., & Menon, D. K. (2003). Validation of a tonometric noninvasive arterial blood pressure monitor in the intensive care setting. *Anaesthesia, 58* (5), 448–454.

Stergiou, G. S., Lourida, P., Tzamouranis, D., & Baibas, N. M. (2009). Unreliable oscillometric blood pressure measurement: Prevalence, repeatability and characteristics of the phenomenon. *Journal of Human Hypertension Advance, 23*(2), 794–800.

Talts, J., Raamat, R., & Jagomägi, K. (2006). Asymmetric time-dependent model for the dynamic finger arterial pressure: Volume relationship. *Medical & Biological Engineering & Computing, 44*, 829–834.

Towers, D., McCartney, A., Bialkowski, M., James, B., Stewart, L., & Towers, C., et al. (2006). Fiber pressure sensors find application in urology. SPIE News room. <http://spie.org/x8547.xml> Accessed 20.10.14.

Van Eijden, T. M. G. J. (1991). Three-dimensional analyses of human bite-force magnitude and moment. *Archives of Oral Biology, 36*, 535–539.

van Putten, A. F. P., van Putten, M. J. A. M., van Putten, M. H. P. M., & van Putten, P. F. A. M. (2002). Multisensor microsystem for pulmonary function diagnostics. *IEEE Sensors Journal, 2*(6), 636–641.

Vincent, J. L., Pinsky, M. R., Sprung, C. L., Levy, M., Marini, J. J., Payen, D., et al. (2008). The pulmonary artery catheter: In medio virtus. *Critical Care Medicine, 36*(11), 3093–3096.

Vos, J. J., Poterman, M., Mooyaart, E. A. Q., Weening, M., Struys, M. M., Scheeren, T. W., et al. (2014). Comparison of continuous noninvasive finger blood pressure monitoring with conventional intermittent automated arm blood pressure measurement in patients under general anaesthesia. *British Journal of Anaesthesia, 113*(1), 67–74.

Wax, D. B., Lin, H., & Leibowitz, A. B. (2011). Invasive and concomitant noninvasive intraoperative blood pressure monitoring: Observed differences in measurements and associated therapeutic interventions. *Anesthesiology, 115*(5), 973–978.

Webster, J. (Ed.), (2010). *Medical instrumentation: Application and design* (4th ed.). Wiley & Sons, Inc.

Weiss, B. M., Spahn, D. R., Rahmig, H., Rohling, R., & Pasch, T. (1996). Radial artery tonometry: Moderately accurate but unpredictable technique of continuous non-invasive arterial pressure measurement. *British Journal of Anaesthesia, 76*, 405–411.

Wu, H.-C., Young, S.-T., & Kuo, T.-S. (2000). A low-cost pressure sensor for maternal uterine activity monitoring. In *Proceedings of the 17th IEEE instrumentation and measurement technology conference* (Vol. 2, pp. 707–709).

Xiao, Z. (1996). *Applications of artificial microcavities in wafer bonded silicon. Technical Report No. 285* (pp. 1–41). Gothenburg: Department of Solid State Electronics, Chalmers University of Technology.

Yu, Q., & Zhou, X. (2011). Pressure sensor based on the fiber-optic extrinsic fabry-perot interferometer. *Photonic Sensors*, *1*(1), 72–83.

CHAPTER 7

Flow Transducers

Contents

7.1 INTRODUCTION

The measurement of physiological flows is important both to study the functioning of the various systems of the human body and for clinical diagnosis of pathological conditions. Flow transducers are used in various biomedical applications such as gas flow measurement for natural ventilation monitoring, artificial ventilation (ventilators, anesthesia systems) controlling and hospital gas lines supply, gas analyzers, nebulizers and apnea monitor, in addition to liquid flow measurement of peripheral venous and arterial blood flow and extracorporeal blood flow during hemodialysis and surgeries with heart–lung bypass.

The fluid may be gaseous, liquid, or present multiple phases, with flow of liquids, gases, and solids all together. The flow can be relatively simple as an intravenous saline solution or biochemically active as the blood, which is a non-Newtonian fluid, that is, its viscosity varies with the degree of deformation suffered. To explain the principle of operation of the various types of flow transducers, in this text, the fluid will always be blood.

Principles of Measurement and Transduction of Biomedical Variables.
DOI: http://dx.doi.org/10.1016/B978-0-12-800774-7.00007-6

The measurement of the concentration of O_2 and other nutrients in the cells is an important source of information for diagnosing many types of diseases, among which, those that involve the heart. However, direct measurement is usually very difficult to be taken and measurements of other quantities that are, somehow, related to the concentration of nutrient use. One of the most used is the magnitude of blood flow. Measurement of blood flow in veins and arteries is important to assess the functioning of heart valves, and cardiovascular prostheses, as well as to detect air embolism, atherosclerosis, thrombosis, and varicose veins. It also helps to identify vascular damage in the retina, brain, and extremities (limbs, ears, and nose) and in the postoperative period of cardiovascular surgeries to monitor the restoration of blood flow to vessels.

Blood flow measurement determines the amount of blood flowing in a body region per time unit (ml/s, l/min) and whenever possible is desirable to use noninvasive methods. Flow measurements can be made both *in vivo* and *in vitro* and *in vivo* measurements can be made directly and invasively or indirectly and noninvasively. The techniques most commonly used to measure blood flow *in vivo* require the use of special transducers, which must have adequate linearity and accuracy in the working ranges of the vessels of interest. The ideal flowmeter must exhibit compact size and low weight and an important additional feature is that it should be biocompatible, that is, be inert to biological tissues.

The arterial and venous blood flows have values in the range of 250 ml/min to 5 l/min and is usually measured by electromagnetic or ultrasonic flowmeters. Flowmeters are also used to obtain the cardiac output, which is the amount of blood pumped by each heart chamber in a unitary period. The same amount of blood passes through pulmonary and systemic circulations; for an adult at rest is about 5 l/min but it varies from 4 to 25 l/min (Saladin, 2011). Cardiac output is measured by thermodilution, electrical plethysmography, electromagnetic and Doppler flowmeters, among other methods.

It is possible to measure blood flow at different points of the circulatory system. The average velocity of blood is dependent on the vessel diameter and thus, on the vessel cross-sectional area. Equation (7.1) shows the relationship between flow (Q), blood volume and average velocity (*velocity*) and the blood vessel area (*area*) where the flow is measured. Table 7.1 shows typical values of diameter, length, velocity, and pressure for blood vessels.

$$Q = \frac{\text{volume}(\text{m}^3)}{\text{time}(\text{s})} = \text{area}(\text{m}^2) \times \text{velocity}(m/s) \tag{7.1}$$

The complexities of the physiological flows are limiting factors to their measurement. To explain the blood flow characteristics, it is considered as Poiseuille laminar flow. This means to consider blood to be a viscous fluid flowing through a long circular cross-section vessel, with constant flow rate and a parabolic velocity profile along

Table 7.1 Typical values of diameter, length, velocity, and pressure for blood vessels

Blood vessel	Diameter (mm)	Length (mm)	Average velocity (cm/s)	Pressure (mmHg)
Aorta artery	10.50	400	40	100
Artery	0.60	10	<10	40
Arteriole	0.02	2	0.50	40–25
Capillary	0.008	1	<0.10	25–8
Venule	0.03	2	<0.30	12–8
Vein	1.50	100	1	<8
Vena cava	12.50	400	20	3–2

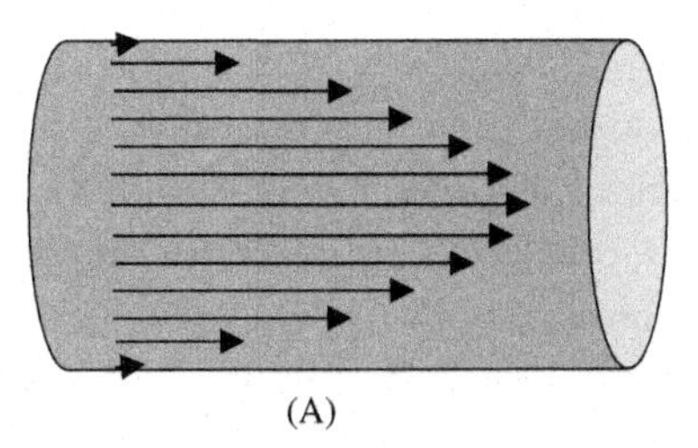

(A)

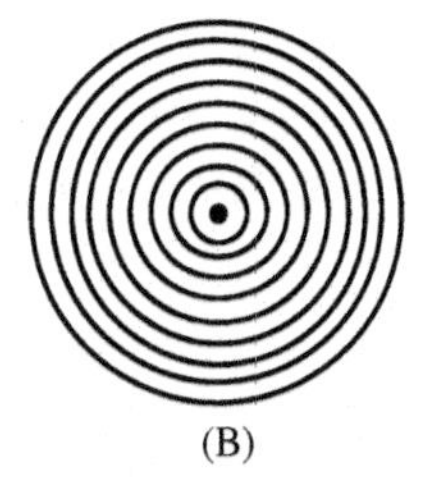

(B)

Figure 7.1 Characteristics of an ideal cylindrical laminar flow. (A) Longitudinal parallel velocity components showing the parabolic profile of the flow in a long and narrow vessel. (B) Cross-sectional view showing concentric fluid layers of increasing velocity from the inner layer to the outer layer, which has zero velocity.

the vessel diameter (zero velocity in the walls and maximum velocity in the center of the vessel), although this concept applies only under conditions of steady laminar flow. The ideal laminar blood flow is organized in concentric layers, which flow parallel to the vessel longitudinal axis, that is, there are only parallel velocity components (Figure 7.1). This can be considered the normal condition of the blood flow in the part of the circulatory system where vessels area long, narrow, uniform, and the blood flows with almost no friction and very low velocity (steady state condition).

The orderly displacement of the layered blood flow through a blood vessel helps minimizing energy losses caused by the interaction of flowing layers of viscous fluid and the blood vessel wall. The flow in the large arteries (e.g., aorta) has nonstationary characteristic and cannot be explained as a Poiseuille flow. The nonuniform geometry and the ramifications of vessels in the vascular system cause the blood flow to present asymmetric velocity profiles, velocity components in different directions than the longitudinal, flow recirculation regions with helical velocity components superimposed to the main velocity axis (longitudinal), in the same vessel. Furthermore, the narrowing of the vessel lumen, for example, due to deposition of fat plaques on the vessel wall, increases the flow velocity, which can cause turbulence. The disruption of the laminar flow into turbulent flow (Figure 7.2) leads to increased energy losses;

turbulent flow has velocity components in all directions, rather than only parallel to the vessel wall. Osborne Reynolds, a mechanical engineer, proposed at the end of nineteenth century, a dimensionless quantity, named the Reynolds number, whose value determines if a flow is laminar or turbulent:

$$\mathrm{Re} = \frac{\rho \cdot \overline{V} \cdot D}{\eta} \tag{7.2}$$

where

ρ is the blood density
$\overline{V}$ is the average velocity of blood flow
D is the vessel diameter
η is the blood viscosity.

At low values, $\mathrm{Re} < 2{,}000$, viscous forces predominate and the flow is laminar; at higher values, $\mathrm{Re} > 3{,}000$, the flow is turbulent (predominance of inertial forces); and for intermediary values, $2{,}000 < \mathrm{Re} < 3{,}000$, the flow is classified as nonuniform laminar.

Volumetric flow equals average flow velocity times vessel cross-sectional area (Eq. (7.1)). Cross-sectional area equals π times squared vessel radius (r^2). Then, velocity is proportional to $1/r^2$ and as the vessel diameter decreases, there is a large increase in mean velocity of blood flow. If stenosis reduces the artery lumen by 50%, flow velocity increases

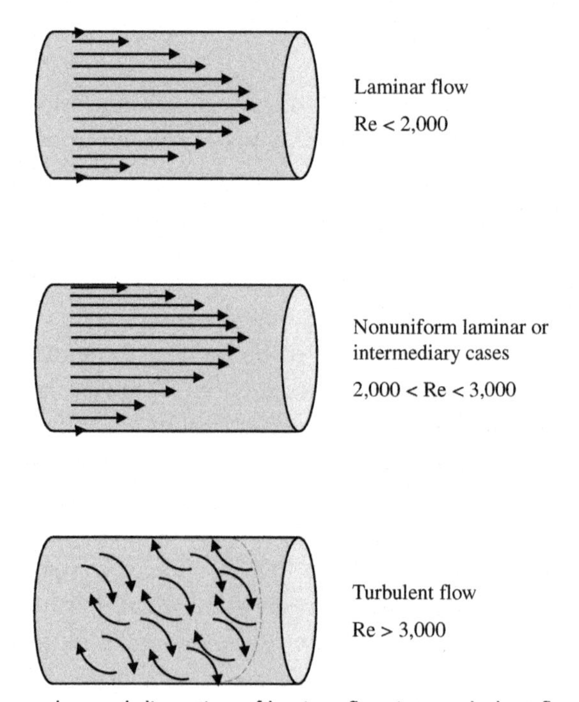

Figure 7.2 Reynolds number and disruption of laminar flow into turbulent flow.

four times, and the Reynolds number also increases four times, bringing Re value closer to turbulence limit. Laminar flow disruption usually occurs distal to narrowed (stenotic) heart valves or arteries, due to the presence of blood clots or atherosclerotic plaques. Turbulent flow also occurs at vessel branch points, and in the ascending aorta, at high cardiac ejection velocities when body blood demand increases (e.g., during exercise).

The pulsatile nature of blood flow, which follows the systole/diastole sequence of heartbeats (cycles of blood ejection and filling of the heart chambers), with the respective changings in the flow velocity, also adds a difficulty in explaining the blood flow as Poiseuille flow.

7.2 FLOW TRANSDUCERS

The classic definition of flow is the fluid volume that crosses a sectional area of the duct in a unitary period of time (Figure 7.3), that is, flow = volume/tempo (m^3/s, SI units). Most flow measuring systems determine the flow rate by measuring the flow velocity of the fluid or the change in kinetic energy thereof. Whereas the cross section is known and constant, and that the flow velocity is maximum at the center and decreases toward the periphery of the cross section (according to a parabolic profile), the flow rate can be calculated from the average velocity, by Eq. (7.3):

$$Q = \int_A V\mathrm{d}A \Rightarrow \overline{Q} = \overline{V} \cdot A \tag{7.3}$$

where

Q is the flow (m^3/s) and $\overline{Q}$ is the average flow (m^3/s)
A is the sectional area of the vessel (m^2)
V is the fluid flow velocity (m/s).

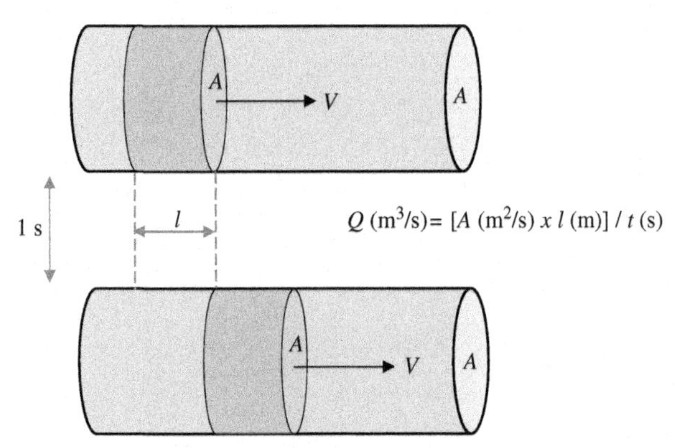

Figure 7.3 Definition of flow: the fluid volume (Q) that crosses a sectional area (A) of the cylindrical vessel in a unitary period of time (1s). l is the distance traveled by the fluid in the unit interval, with velocity V.

In addition to the sectional area of the vessel and the velocity of the fluid, other factors affect flow: viscosity and density of the liquid, the friction of the liquid with the walls of the vessel, and the length of the vessel. Poiseuille's equation describes the relationship between the flow (Q), radius (r), and length (L) of the vessel and perfusion pressure (ΔP) of blood:

$$Q \propto \frac{\Delta P \cdot r^4}{\eta \cdot L} \tag{7.4}$$

As it was mentioned earlier, Poiseuille equation is valid for laminar flow of Newtonian fluid inside long and narrow tubes; in Eq. (7.4) it is evident the radius influence in the flow. Figure 7.4A shows the flow behavior as a function of vessel

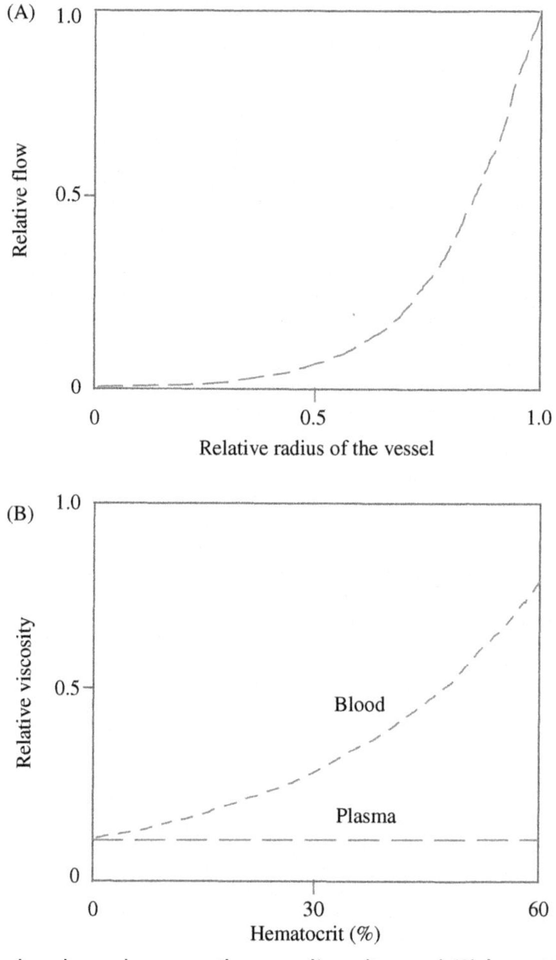

Figure 7.4 (A) Flow value dependence on the vessel's radius and (B) hematocrit influence on the blood viscosity.

radius; as the vessel radius decreases, there is a strong fall in flow due to its dependence with the fourth power of radius. Figure 7.4B shows how hematocrit value influences the blood viscosity, a parameter that is inversely proportional to the blood flow. Viscosity is related to the internal friction of adjacent fluid layers sliding past one another as well as the friction between the fluid and the vessel wall; both friction contributions enlarge the resistance to flow.

Some methods for measuring blood flow will be explained below: differential pressure, variable area, plethysmography, electromagnetic, ultrasonic, laser, and methods for measuring cardiac output. Some methods provide instantaneous flow amount, and others provide an average value. Some methods are invasive, others can be used both invasively and noninvasively (Cobbold, 1974; Dally, Riley & McConnell 1993; Geddes & Baker, 1968; Klabunde, 2011; OMEGA, 2014; Saladin, 2011; Thiriet, 2008; Webster, 2010).

7.2.1 Differential pressure flow transducers

A transducer that measures flow through differential pressure uses an element to restrict the fluid flow, which increases the fluid velocity and reduces its pressure (Figure 7.5). If the fluid flow is turbulent, the pressure drop is proportional to the square of the flow rate. A differential pressure transducer determines the pressure drop resultant of the insertion of the flow restriction element and the flow is calculated from its square root. There are different ways to restrict the fluid flow, but the flow rate always results proportional to the square root of the differential pressure and is determined from Bernoulli's and flow continuity equations.

In 1783, Bernoulli published *Hydrodynamica* and introduced the concept of energy conservation for fluid flows. Bernoulli's equation describes the relation between velocity, density, and pressure for an incompressible fluid flowing through a tube with changing cross-sectional area, which is a common situation for blood vessels. He determined that an increase in the flow velocity causes kinetic energy to increase and static energy to

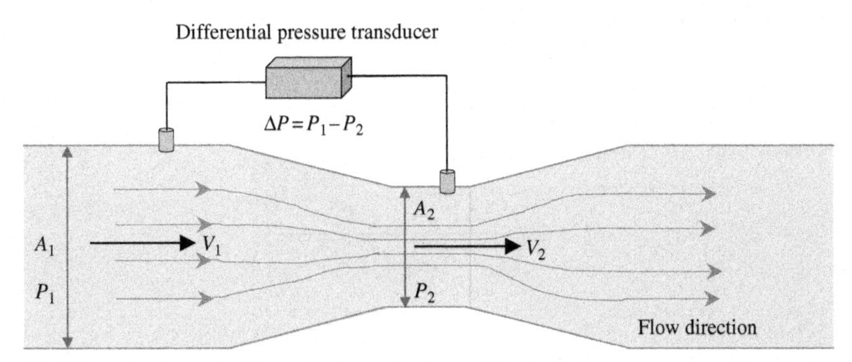

Figure 7.5 Effects in the velocity and pressure due to Venturi's tube type insertion in the vessel's lumen to restrict the fluid flow.

decrease (Bernoulli, 1738; Darrigol, 2009). Bernoulli's equation states that the sum of the static energy (pressure), kinetic energy (speed), and potential energy (elevation) remains constant to an incompressible fluid flowing in steady state through an obstruction:

$$\underbrace{\frac{P_1}{\rho}+\frac{V_1^2}{2g}+z_1}_{\text{energy per unit volume before restriction}} = \underbrace{\frac{P_2}{\rho}+\frac{V_2^2}{2g}+z_2}_{\text{energy per unit volume after restriction}} \tag{7.5}$$

where

P_1 and P_2 are the pressure values in the vessel before and right after the obstruction element

V_1 and V_2 are the velocities of the fluid flow before and after the restriction

z_1 and z_2 are the heights of the fluid before and after the restriction

ρ is the fluid density

g is the gravity acceleration.

Along a streamline in the center of the vessel the height change is negligible and Eq. (7.5) becomes:

$$\frac{P_1}{\rho}+\frac{V_1^2}{2g}=\frac{P_2}{\rho}+\frac{V_2^2}{2g} \tag{7.6}$$

The equation of continuity states that the flow along a vessel with rigid wall must remain constant regardless of its diameter:

$$Q = A_1 \cdot V_1 = A_2 \cdot V_2 \tag{7.7}$$

where

A_1 is the vessel area before the restriction

A_2 is the restriction area.

The example shown in Figure 7.5 is a restriction of the type Venturi's tube. Equation (7.6) can be written as

$$\Delta P = P_1 - P_2 = \frac{1}{2}\rho V_2^2 - \frac{1}{2}\rho V_1^2 \tag{7.8}$$

Combining Eqs. (7.7) and (7.8) results in

$$Q = C\sqrt{\frac{2\Delta P}{\rho}}\frac{A_v}{\sqrt{(A_v/A_r)^2-1}} \tag{7.9}$$

where

C is a constant that depends on the Reynolds number

ΔP is the differential pressure.

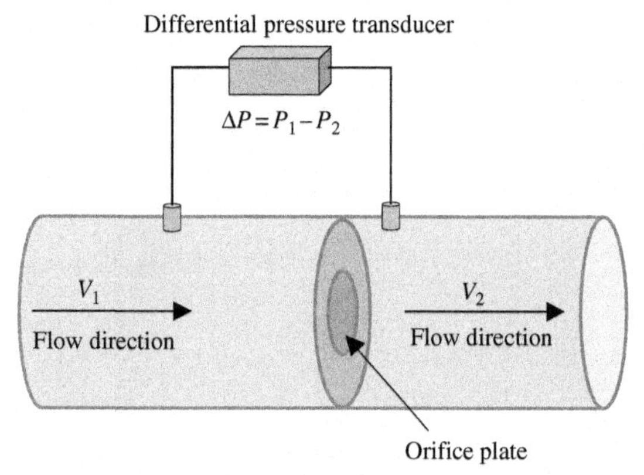

Figure 7.6 Effects in the flow velocity and pressure when a restriction element, orifice plate type, is inserted in the lumen of the tube to restrict the fluid flow.

Figure 7.6 shows another way to apply a restriction to determine the fluid flow, the orifice plate. The flow can be described, after some manipulation of Eqs. (7.7) and (7.8) as

$$Q = \frac{C_1}{\sqrt{1-\beta^4}} C_2 \frac{\pi}{4} D_o^{\,2} \sqrt{\frac{2\Delta P}{\rho}} \tag{7.10}$$

where

C_1 and C_2 are correction factors that depend on the Reynolds number

$\beta = D_o/D_v$ is the ratio between orifice (D_o) diameter and vessel diameter (D_v).

The orifice plate restriction usually causes larger differential pressure losses than Venturi's tube (of the order 40% for orifice plate and 10% for Venturi's tube, when $\beta = D_o/D_v = 0.7$), which implies in lower accuracy.

Differential pressure flowmeters are found in many types of biomedical equipment, as for example, spirometers, ventilators, oxygen analyzers, apnea monitors, nebulizers, and autoclaves.

7.2.2 Variable area flow transducers (flowmeters or rotameters)

Variable area flowmeters are gravity operated devices that provide a roughly linear flow indication of liquid, gas, and steam. They are constructed with several design variations and the most common one, the rotameter, consists of a transparent tapered tube with a calibrated and graduated scale on its wall and a float inside (Figure 7.7A). The flowmeter is used in the vertical position and the flow gets into the tube through the bottom end and goes out through the top of the tube. The cross-sectional area of the tube progressively increases with height and the fluid flow velocity decreases with height (Cole-Parmer).

Floats can have different shapes, but spheres and spherical ellipses are the most commonly used. The float is shaped so that it moves freely inside the tube, rotating

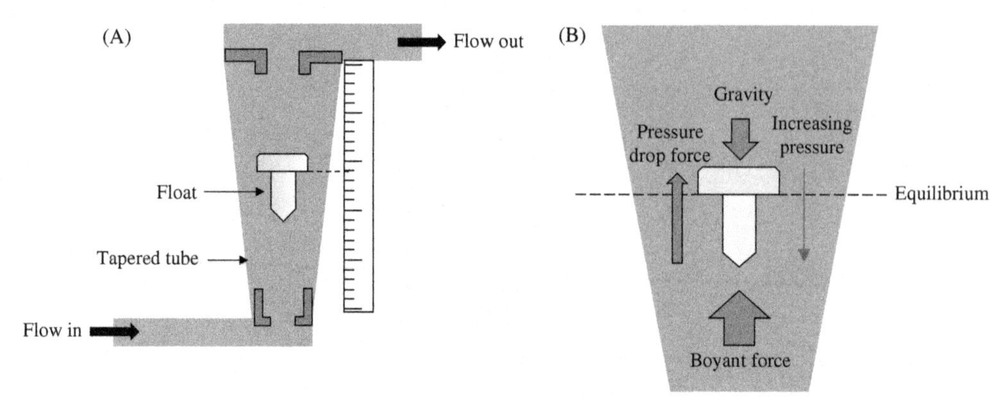

Figure 7.7 Schematic representation of the functioning of variable area flow transducer. (A) Rotameter consists of a transparent tapered tube with a calibrated and graduated scale on its wall and a float inside. (B) Flow value indication depends on the fluid net force in the float: pressure drop across the float and buoyant force against gravity force.

axially as the fluid passes and forces it upwards through the tube. The flow indication is obtained from the balance of the fluid forces underneath the float, pressure drop across the float and buoyant force, with the gravity force (Figure 7.7B). The pressure drop depends on the velocity of fluid flow, which varies with height along the tube. At the position of equilibrium, there is an annular area between the float and the tube wall, which is enough to allow the fluid flows without moving the float. As flow increases, the float is pushed higher in the tube with a corresponding increase in the annular area around it. The float height at equilibrium is proportional to the flow rate and its value is read against the calibrated and graduated scale in the wall tube.

Float is typically made from PVC, glass, and stain steel to be resistant to corrosion and flow tube is made from borosilicate glass, usually with a plastic shield around it, because it is susceptible to breaking if subjected to thermal or pressure shocks.

Rotameter is also used to control the flow of a particular fluid, instead of just measuring its flow. In this case, a needle valve is added between the inlet port and the flow tube, allowing fine adjustments of small flows. Rotameter accuracy is dependent on the accuracy of the pressure, temperature, and flow control during calibration and operation. Typical accuracy error is about $\pm 5\%$ FS, but can be as little as $\pm 2.0\%$ of reading or $\pm$ one scale division with highly accurate and precise calibration procedures. Rotameter operation is independent of factors influencing electronic meters as quality of energy supply, electronic noise, and electromagnetic interference. It is commonly used in anesthesia systems (rotameters and vaporizers) and hospital gas lines.

7.2.3 Ultrasound flow transducers

The ultrasonic flow transducer generates mechanical waves with frequencies that are imperceptible to the human ear (frequency >20 kHz); these waves propagate in the biological tissue and interact with the moving particles of the blood. Parameters

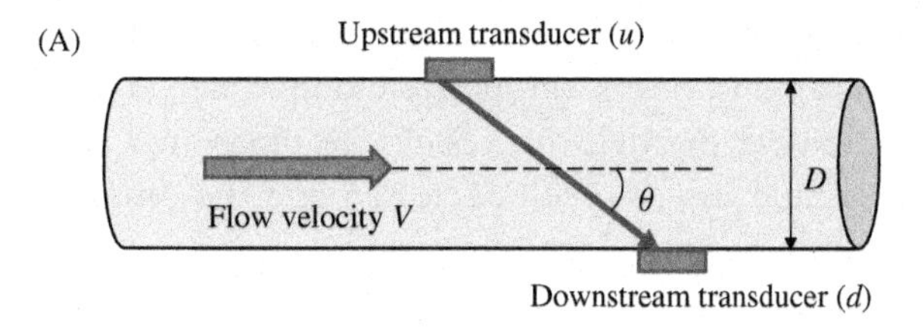

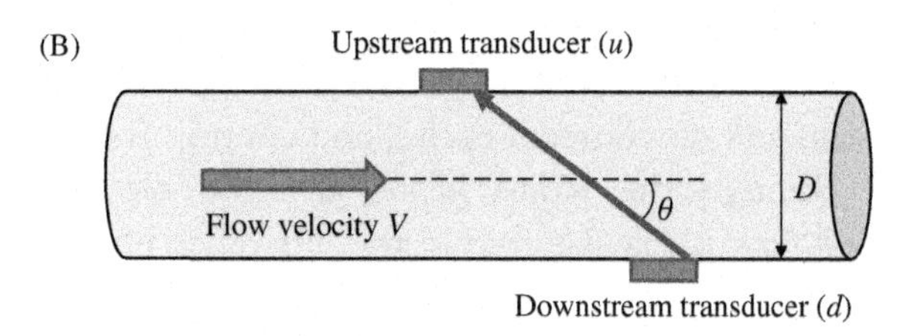

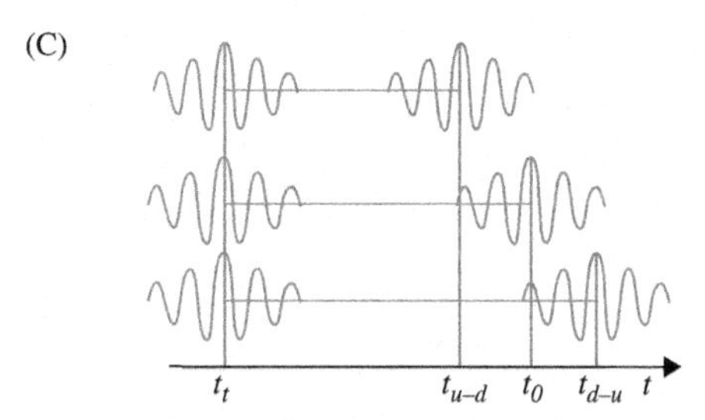

Figure 7.8 Schematic representation of transit-time ultrasonic flowmeters functioning: (A) upstream cycle (B) downstream cycle and (C) t_t is the instant of the ultrasound pulse emission; t_0 is the instant of the ultrasound wave reception without blood movement; t_u is the instant of the ultrasound wave reception in the upstream cycle; t_d is the instant of the ultrasound wave reception in the downstream cycle; and Δt is the time difference between upstream and downstream cycles.

extracted from the acoustic energy that is transmitted or reflected by the flow allow flow computing. Two ultrasound methods are commonly used to do flow measurement: transit time, an invasive (perivascular) method, and Doppler shift (continuous wave Doppler—CW Doppler and pulsed wave Doppler—PW Doppler), a noninvasive (transcutaneous) method, whose functioning are explained below.

7.2.3.1 Transit-time ultrasound flow transducer

A transit-time flowmeter is a perivascular clamp-on probe and measures blood flow invasively. The fundamental measurement principle of transit-time ultrasonic flowmeters can be explained with the schematic representation shown in Figure 7.8. To explain how the transit-time flow transducer works, one considers that the propagation velocity of the ultrasonic wave through a moving fluid is equal to the velocity that the wave would have if the fluid was stopped, plus the fluid velocity. The propagation time of an ultrasound beam, through a blood vessel, is affected by the movement of the blood flowing through the vessel: the ultrasound that propagates in the same direction as the fluid has its speed decreased and the ultrasound that propagates in the opposite direction, has its velocity increased.

During the upstream cycle, the received sound wave travels in the same direction of flow and the total propagation time is reduced by an amount, which depends on the flow velocity value. In the downstream cycle, the received sound wave travels in the opposite direction of flow and the total propagation time is increased by an amount, which depends on the flow velocity value. An electronic circuit alternatively drives the transducers in upstream and downstream cycles, and controls the reception of acoustic energy transmitted through the blood vessel and the biological tissues nearby. The volumetric blood flow is calculated from the difference between the durations of downstream and upstream cycles.

An ultrasound beam propagating at velocity c, in the same direction as the bloodstream (Figure 7.8A from the upstream transducer u to the downstream transducer d), takes a time t_{u-d}:

$$t_{u-d} = \frac{D/\sin\theta}{(c + V\cos\theta)} \tag{7.11}$$

where

D is the diameter of the vessel

c is the ultrasound propagation velocity in blood

V is the blood flow velocity

θ is the angle between blood flow velocity and the direction of ultrasound propagation

$V\cos\theta$ is the component of the blood flow velocity in the direction of ultrasound propagation.

The same ultrasound beam propagating against the bloodstream direction (Figure 7.8B from downstream transducer d to upstream transducer u) takes a time t_{d-u}:

$$t_{d-u} = \frac{D/\sin\theta}{(c - V\cos\theta)} \tag{7.12}$$

The difference between the propagating times of the paths $(t_{d-u} - t_{u-d})$ allows calculating the flow velocity:

$$\Delta T = t_{d-u} - t_{u-d} = V\frac{t_{d-u} \cdot t_{u-d} \cdot \sin 2\theta}{D} \tag{7.13}$$

$$V = \frac{D}{\sin 2\theta} \cdot \frac{t_{d-u} - t_{u-d}}{t_{d-u} \cdot t_{u-d}} \tag{7.14}$$

Then, the volumetric blood flow is calculated from flow velocity:

$$Q = V \cdot A = V \cdot \pi\left(\frac{D^2}{4}\right) \tag{7.15}$$

$$Q = \frac{\pi D^3}{4\sin 2\theta} \cdot \frac{t_{d-u} - t_{u-d}}{t_{d-u} \cdot t_{u-d}} \tag{7.16}$$

Transit-time flow transducers are constructed in a variety of sizes to adjust to different vessel diameters. The transducer is placed around the blood vessel and should not compress it during the systole and diastole phases of the cardiac cycle; the angle θ is constant.

The most common transit-time flowmeter configuration has two ultrasonic transducers positioned on one side of the vessel, and an acoustic reflector positioned between the two transducers, on diametrically opposite side of the blood vessel (Figure 7.9). Both transducers are alternatively activated in upstream and downstream cycles. Figure 7.9 represents the upstream cycle when transducer Tr_1 is excited and transducer Tr_2 acts as receptor, collecting the beams that crossed the vessel and were reflected back by the reflector. In the next cycle, downstream, Tr_2, which beam travels against the blood flow, acts as transmitter and Tr_1 is the receptor.

The transducers in the transit-time flowmeter produce wide ultrasound beams that cut the entire cross section of the vessel and the beam propagation time becomes a function of the flow volume intersected by the beam, independent of the diameter size of the vessel. Thus, transit-time flowmeter provides volumetric flow and sensing acoustic window coincides to the area of the reflector. Ultrasound beams that propagate outside the blood flow, and interact with the surrounding tissues, do not

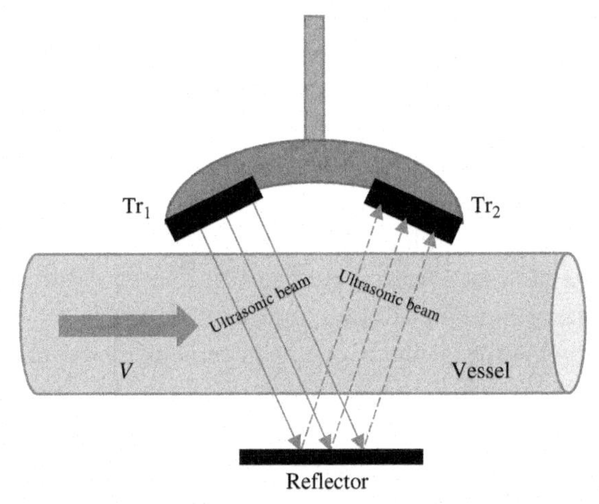

Figure 7.9 Transit-time flowmeter with two ultrasound transducers and a reflector diametrically positioned on both sides of the vessel.

contribute to the flow computing because the blood flow velocity does not modify their travel time; in other words, they arrive in the receptor out of phase, compared to the reflected beams that crossed the blood vessel. Moreover, the propagation time measured results from sampled beams at all points of vessel diameter and then, volume flow measurement is independent of the velocity profile of the flow.

The volumetric flow measurement made with transit-time technique allows to detect bidirectional flow pulsatile waveform as well as the average flow value. It is used during cardiovascular surgeries, to measure and monitor blood flow in arteries and veins, and in extracorporeal blood circulation circuits. Transit-time clamp-on flowmeter detects bidirectional blood flow and in inline version is used to measure water and saline solution flows. Commercial equipment has typically $\pm 1\%$ accuracy, $\pm 0.5\%$ repeatability, working range from a few ml/min to a few tens of l/min and resolution of 10^{-3} fs.

7.2.3.2 Doppler shift (continuous and pulsed) flow transducer

The Doppler principle is based on the fact that if a moving object reflects an incoming ultrasound wave, the frequency of the wave changes. An object moving towards the ultrasonic beam compresses the wave, thereby increasing the signal's frequency, whereas an object moving away from the beam reduces the signal's frequency. The change in frequency, which is also termed the Doppler shift, provides information about the object's speed and direction of motion.

Doppler shift flow transducer measures blood flow in a noninvasively transcutaneous way. The transducer is positioned over the skin, near the vessel whose flow is to be measured. An acoustic coupling gel, applied between the transducer and the skin, reduces their acoustic impedance difference and enhances the transmission efficiency of the ultrasound waves.

Doppler shift method allowed the use of ultrasound into the evaluation of normal and abnormal flow states in blood vessels of the circulatory system, as cerebral and carotid arteries, and within the heart. It provides quantitative data, which are important to disease diagnosis and clinical decision-making procedures. First studies of Doppler flowmetry analyzed the umbilical and uterine arteries with continuous Doppler waves (FitzGerald & Drumm, 1977). Doppler echocardiography is a method for detecting the direction and velocity of moving blood within the heart. This technique is used for detection of cardiac insufficiency due to valves malfunctioning and stenosis, as well as a large number of other abnormal flows.

Doppler echocardiography depends on measurement of the relative change in the reflected ultrasound frequency when compared to the transmitted frequency. Depending on the relative changes of the returning frequencies, Doppler echocardiographic system identifies flow characteristics as direction, velocity, and the presence of turbulence, helping to differentiate between normal and abnormal flow patterns. The quantification of flow characteristics is helpful to classify the severity of abnormal states of intravascular blood flow or within the heart chambers.

Doppler flowmetry is also used for extracorporeal flow measurements, as in blood flow determination in vascular shunts (e.g., carotid shunt) and in cardiopulmonary bypass procedures.

The Doppler shift flowmeter has a transmitter transducer, which generates ultrasound beams that travel through the moving fluid (blood), and a receptor transducer, which collects the ultrasound reflected by the blood particles. Figure 7.10 shows the schematic representation of the Doppler flow transducer operation.

Red blood cells are the main ultrasound reflectors in the circulatory system. When transmitted beams reach blood cells that are moving away from transmitter (Figure 7.10A), ultrasound beams reflected back to the receptor transducer having lower frequency than the transmitted. The resultant Doppler shift, in this case, positive, brings information about flow direction and is proportional to the flow velocity. When the flow approaches the transducer (Figure 7.10B), the frequency of the reflected ultrasound beam is bigger than the transmitted frequency (negative Doppler shift).

The Doppler shift can be obtained with continuous wave (CW Doppler) and pulsed wave (PW Doppler) ultrasound. CW Doppler needs two transducers: one continuously transmits the ultrasound beam, while the other continuously receives the

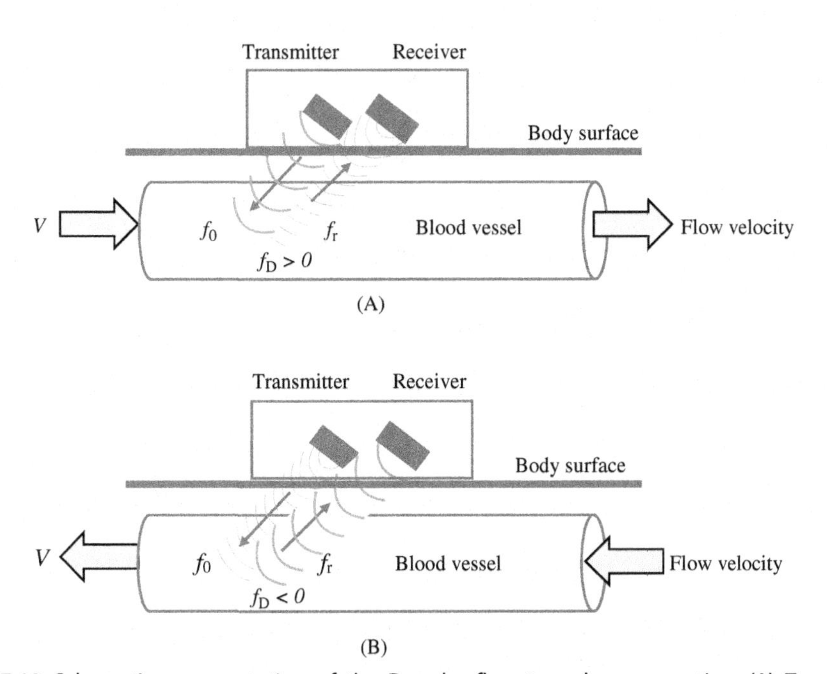

Figure 7.10 Schematic representation of the Doppler flow transducer operation. (A) Transmitted beams reach blood cells that are moving toward transmitter and ultrasound beams reflected back to the receptor transducer having higher frequency than the transmitted one. (B) Transmitted beams reach blood cells that are moving away from transmitter and ultrasound beams reflected back to the receptor transducer having lower frequency than the transmitted one.

reflected beams. PW Doppler can use only one transducer, which alternately emits and receives ultrasound beams to Doppler shift achievement (Figure 7.11A).

The pulse repetition frequency (PRF) in PW Doppler should be carefully chosen, since the transducer must be pulsed only after the previous reflected beam (eco) is

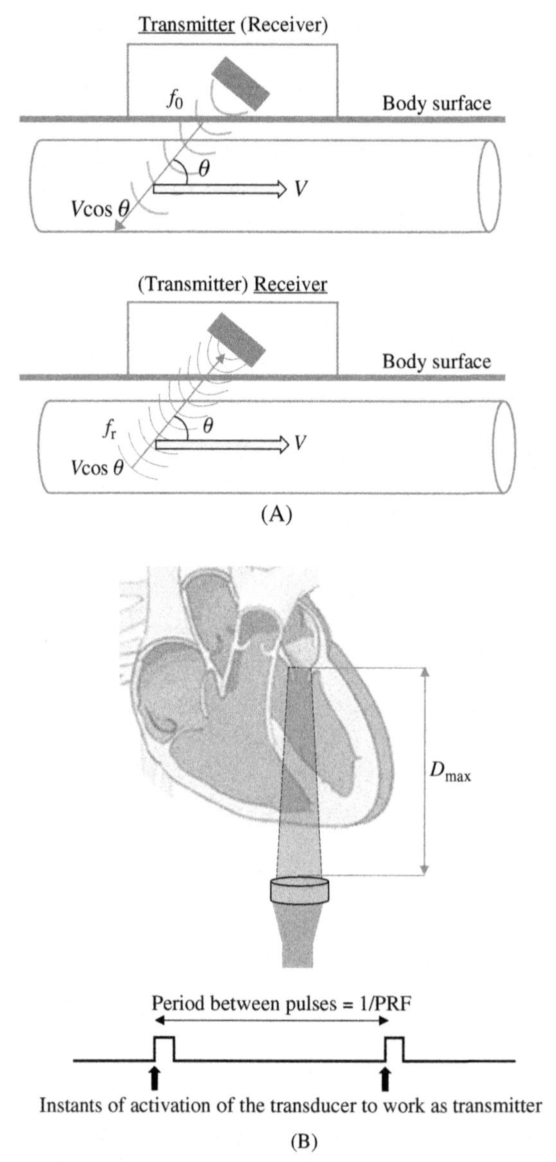

Figure 7.11 (A) PW Doppler can use only one transducer, which alternately emits and receives ultrasound beams to Doppler shift achievement. (B) PRF depends on the frequency of the transducer and the distance D_{max} between transducer and reflectors (blood cells) in the sample volume (heart valve); each echo must be completely received before sending the next pulse.

completely received by the transducer. Each emitted pulse has a corresponding reflected beam and is possible to determine where the reflection has occurred and calculate reflector distances. It is also possible to predefine a sample volume to analyze reflected signals from specific regions of interest in the heart or vessel by choosing an adequate PRF value. PRF depends on the frequency of the transducer and the distance between transducer and reflectors (blood cells) in the sample volume (Figure 7.11B). There is a maximum PRF from which to a certain flow velocity, known as Nyquist limit velocity, Doppler shift is no longer measurable:

$$\mathrm{PRF} > 2f_D \tag{7.17}$$

and

$$\mathrm{PRF} < \frac{c}{2D_{max}} \tag{7.18}$$

where

D_{max} is the maximum distance between transducer and sample volume

c is the velocity of ultrasound transmission in the blood

f_D is the Doppler *shift.*

The higher the velocity of blood flow and thus, the Doppler shift, the higher the required PRF and the lower the distance between the transducer and the region of interest allowed to be examined. There is a maximum limit to the PRF value, or pulse repetition frequency. From this value, the echoes from the region of interest do not have enough time to return to the transducer before transmitting the next pulse, and the Doppler shift is no longer properly detected. The maximum flow velocity, which can be detected with PW Doppler, decreases as the sample volume is positioned farther away from the transducer.

Equation (7.19) shows the relation between Doppler and blood flow velocity:

$$f_D = \frac{2f_0}{c} V \cos\theta \tag{7.19}$$

Blood flow velocity is calculated by

$$V = \frac{c}{2f_0 \cos\theta} f_D \tag{7.20}$$

where

f_0 is the emitted ultrasound frequency

c is the velocity of ultrasound transmission in the blood

f_D is the Doppler shift

θ is the angle between blood flow and ultrasound beam directions (beam inclination).

Volumetric flow estimation requires previous knowledge of the beam-to-flow angle and the blood vessel cross-sectional area; then velocity is integrated across the vessel area. 2D Doppler flowmetry calculates the volumetric flow in an integration plane, which is perpendicular to the beam (Cobbold, 2007; Hoskins, 2002; Jensen, 1996; Richards, Kripfgans, Rubin, Hall, & Fowlkes, 2009).

7.2.3.3 Laser Doppler (shift) flow transducer (LDF)

Laser Doppler flowmetry (LDF) is a continuous and noninvasive method for tissue blood flow monitoring. The Doppler shift of low power laser light ($\approx$1 mW) that has been scattered by moving red blood cells carries information about tissue perfusion. Flow is the amount of blood flowing through an organ, tissue, or vessel at a given time, while perfusion implies the amount of flow per given volume or mass of tissue.

LDF does not give an absolute measure of blood perfusion, but its measurements are expressed as Perfusion Units (PU), which are arbitrary units. LDF is said to measure microcirculation due to the small volumes of tissue this technique works with, where only microscopic blood vessels exist.

Main applications of LDF are pharmacological trials, allergy patch testing, wound healing, physiological assessments, and skin disease research. Some areas of major interest for LDF studies are cochlear, retinal blood, peripheral nerves and central nervous system, kidney, liver, gastrointestinal, skeletal muscle, bone and skin blood flows.

The perfusion in the skin relates the blood flow microcirculation, that is, the blood circulation through capillaries, arterioles, venules, and shunting vessels, localized in the dermis layer of the skin. The perfusion through capillaries (typically about 0.3 mm long and 10 μm in diameter and covering an area of approximately 30 m^2) takes nutrients flow to the junction between the dermis and epidermis, where cells regeneration takes place, while microcirculation through other vessels refers to the regulation flow of body temperature, feed and drain of the capillary network. Average skin perfusion is 10–20 ml/min/100 g, but it may vary from 1 to 200 ml/min/100 g, indicating a remarkable plasticity of regulatory control in dermis vascular bed and making cutaneous tissue of great importance for the investigation of microcirculatory events.

Diseases can disturb skin perfusion, which can cause ulcerations as well as skin necrosis. LDF technique allows monitoring skin blood perfusion in real time, continuously and noninvasively, which is of great importance in medical applications, such as visualization of skin tumors, diagnosis and monitoring of diabetes complications, obstructive and occlusive diseases, ischemia and others.

The first experimental studies using LDF were developed in the 1970s (Riva, Ross, & Benedek, 1972; Stern, 1975) and its functioning principle is represented in Figure 7.12. A monochromatic (single frequency) laser beam transmits photons into the tissue, which are scattered and reflected. Every photon that meets a moving blood particle undergoes a shift in frequency, called Doppler frequency shift, which is a frequency broadening of the incoming monochromatic light. The size of this shift (ω_D) is determined by the scattering angle (α), the velocity (V), the wavelength of the light in the tissue (λ_t) and the angle (θ) between the direction of the velocity and the scattering vector (Eq. (7.21)).

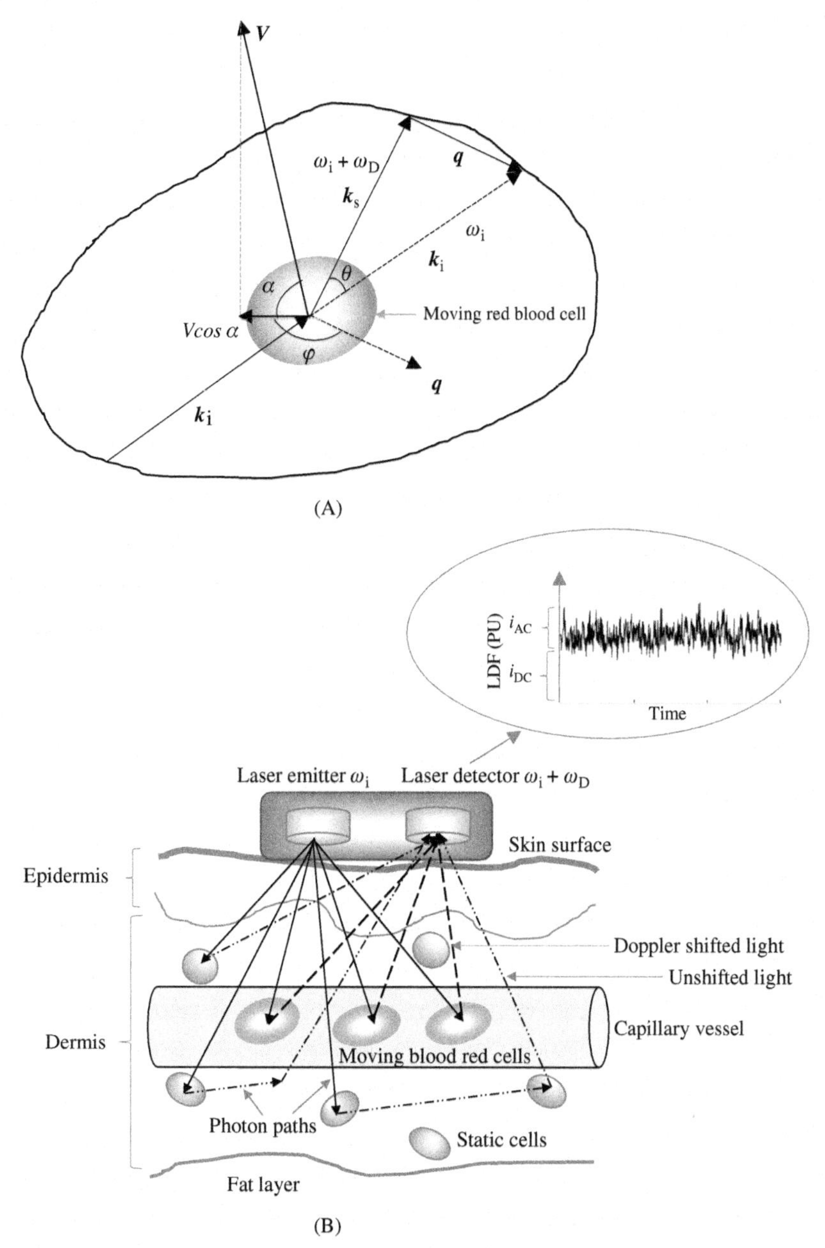

Figure 7.12 Schematic representation of LDF functioning. (A) Incoming photon ($\boldsymbol{k}_i$, ω_i) is scattered by a moving blood cell with velocity $\boldsymbol{V}$ and starts to propagate according to the new vector $\boldsymbol{k}_s$ and angular velocity $\omega_i + \omega_D$. (B) The incoming light from the laser emitter illuminates a small size area of tissue and interacts with static cells and blood flow. α is the angle between the velocity of red blood cell and the plane of scattering; φ is the angle between scattering vector $\boldsymbol{q}$ and blood cell velocity in the plane of scattering; and θ is the scattering angle of photon trajectory. The backscattered photons leaving the tissue are collected by a laser detector, which converts them into a DC output current (i_{DC}), due to the nonshifted photons, superimposed to an AC (i_{AC}) component, due to the Doppler shifted photons, which interacted with the moving blood cells. The frequency spectrum of i_{AC} brings information about blood velocity.

The scattering vector ($\boldsymbol{q}$) is defined as the difference between the incident light vector ($\boldsymbol{k}_i$) and the scattering light vector ($\boldsymbol{k}_s$). The incoming light, usually from a semiconductor laser diode, is delivered by a fiber-optic probe with one multimode fiber and illuminates a small size area of tissue. Another multimode fiber transmits the backscattered photons leaving the tissue light to a semiconductor laser photodiode (PD), which converts them into current. This output current (Figure 7.12B) has a DC component (i_{DC}) due to the nonshifted photons and an AC superimposed component (i_{AC}) due to the Doppler shifted photons. Frequency-weighted signal processing algorithms were developed to compute the frequency spectrum of the AC photocurrent, to extract information about the Doppler shift and thus, about the blood perfusion of the tissue (Briers, 2001; Fredriksson, Fors, & Johansson, 2007; Rajan, Varghese, van Leeuwen, & Steenbergen, 2009; Shepherd & Öberg, 1990).

LDF technique is used in laser Doppler perfusion monitoring (LDPM) and laser Doppler perfusion imaging (LDPI) (Nilsson, Salerud, Strömberg & Wårdell, 2003). LDF instrument output often gives flux, velocity, and concentration of the moving blood cells.

$$\omega_D = -V \cdot \boldsymbol{q} = (\boldsymbol{k}_i - \boldsymbol{k}_s) = -\frac{4\pi}{\lambda_i} \sin\frac{\theta}{2} V \cos\alpha \, V \cos\varphi \tag{7.21}$$

where

$\boldsymbol{k}_i$ is the incoming light
$\boldsymbol{k}_s$ is the scattered light
θ is the scattering angle of photon trajectory
$\boldsymbol{q}$ is the scattering vector
$\boldsymbol{V}$ is the blood velocity
α is the angle between the velocity of red blood cell and the plane of scattering
φ is the angle between scattering vector $\boldsymbol{q}$ and blood cell velocity in the plane of scattering
λ_i is the wavelength of the incoming light $\boldsymbol{k}_i$ with angular frequency ω_i, and

$$\lambda_i = \frac{2\pi}{|\boldsymbol{k}_i|} = \frac{2\pi c}{\omega_i} \tag{7.22}$$

where c is the velocity of light in the tissue.

The wavelength and the fiber-to-fiber distance are chosen according to the blood flow measurement depth and sampling volume. Light with wavelength in the 600–1,600 nm spectral range has good penetration in the human skin. The most often used wavelengths by commercial systems are 630, 780, and 830 nm, with typical standard fiber separation of 0.25, 0.5, and 0.78 mm. LDF transducer with 0.25 mm fiber separation and 780 nm wavelength is adequate to blood flow measurement in 0.5–1 mm depth range and sample volume of approximately 1 mm^3. The moving red blood cells cause Doppler frequency shift from 30 Hz to 12 kHz.

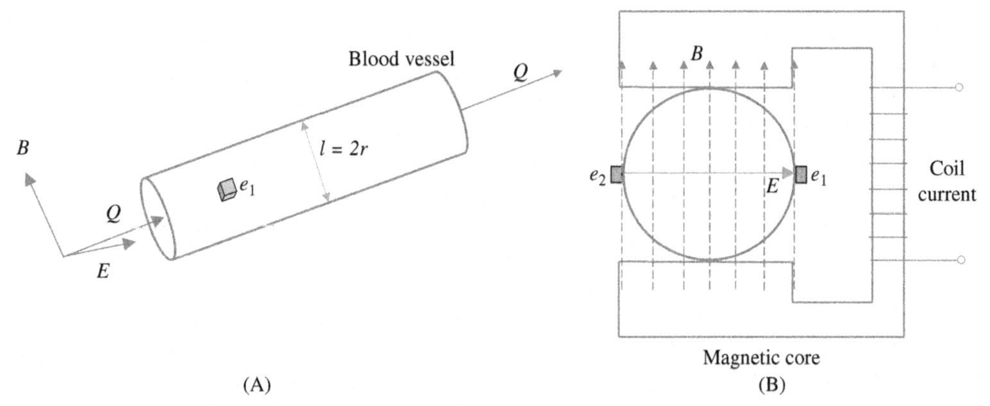

Figure 7.13 Schematic representation of the Faraday's law of induction. (A) Blood flowing through a magnetic field (normal component ***B***) generates an EMF ***E***, detected by electrodes positioned on the outside of the blood vessel. (B) Front view of the blood vessel showing the magnetic core and the electrodes e_1 and e_2.

LDF offers many advantages when compared with other methods relatively to blood flow measurement in microcirculation. Various studies show that this is a method with high sensitivity to local blood perfusion, it is a versatile and easy method for continuous measurements, and it is a noninvasive method, so it does not disturb the normal microcirculation of the patient.

7.2.4 Electromagnetic flow transducers

Electromagnetic flowmeters detect conductive fluid flow and their functioning is based on the laws of electromagnetic induction developed in the nineteenth century. They measure the instantaneous pulsatile blood flow in the circulatory system, blood vessels, and prostheses, by invasive means, during surgical cardiovascular procedures and they are the flow transducers that provide the best accuracy for *in vivo* flow measurements. First electromagnetic flowmeters required 1–5 μS/cm minimum conductivity, while nowadays equipments have sensibility for conductivities as low as 0.05–0.1 μS/cm.

The flow of a conductive fluid, such as blood, across an electromagnetic field (B), induces an electromotive force (EMF), which is measured by diametrically opposed electrodes placed on the outside of the blood vessel. Figure 7.13 shows a representation of the Faraday's law of induction.

Electromagnetic flowmeter functioning is based on the fact that the EMF is proportional to the conductive fluid velocity. According to the Faraday's law of induction:

$$E = \int_0^{l_1} VB\mathrm{d}l \tag{7.23}$$

where

$\boldsymbol{E}$ is the induced EMF

V is the blood velocity

$\boldsymbol{B}$ is the normal component of the magnetic field

l is the distance between electrodes e_1 and e_2, considered equal to the vessel diameter.

In the ideal case, $\boldsymbol{B}$ and V are time invariant, the magnetic field is uniform and the velocities profile is uniform along the vessel diameter; thus, Eq. (7.23) can be written as

$$\boldsymbol{E} = \boldsymbol{BV}l \tag{7.24}$$

From Eq. (7.24), it is observed that the induced EMF is proportional to the magnetic field. Usually the distance between the electrodes (vessel diameter) and the magnetic flow density are known. So, EMF measurement allows to determine the flow velocity value:

$$V = \frac{\boldsymbol{E}}{\boldsymbol{B}2r} \tag{7.25}$$

where $r = l/2$ is the vessel radius.

If the blood flow velocity is nonuniform in different transversal sections of the vessel, like in the laminar flow, which has parabolic profile, but is symmetric in relation to vessel longitudinal axis, Eq. (7.25) can be written as

$$V_{\mathrm{m}} = \frac{\boldsymbol{E}}{\boldsymbol{B}2r} \tag{7.26}$$

where V_{m} is the average blood velocity.

Volumetric blood flow Q is the volume of blood that passes through the cross-sectional area of a given vessel per unit time, which is also equal to the average blood velocity times cross-sectional area:

$$Q = V_{\mathrm{m}}A \tag{7.27}$$

or

$$Q = \frac{\boldsymbol{E}}{2\boldsymbol{B}r}\boldsymbol{A} = \boldsymbol{E}\frac{50\pi r}{\boldsymbol{B}} \tag{7.28}$$

where $A = \pi r^2$ is the section area of the blood vessel, with r in cm, $\boldsymbol{V}$ in cm/s, $\boldsymbol{E}$ in μV, and $\boldsymbol{B}$ in Gauss (weber/cm^2).

Typical flow velocities result in very low EMF values, of the order of units to tens of μV, and often the measured values are lower than the expected values. To quantify this difference, there is the electromagnetic flowmeter sensibility:

$$S = \frac{E_{\mathrm{meas}}}{E_{\mathrm{exp}}} = 50\frac{E_{\mathrm{meas}}}{rBV_{\mathrm{m}}} \tag{7.29}$$

$S = 1$ for an ideal flowmeter and practical flowmeters have $S < 1$. If there is a biological fluid layer between the blood vessel and the flow transducers, its sensibility decreases, as well as if the conductivity of the blood vessel wall is higher than the blood conductivity. The electromagnetic flow transducer, also called perivascular probe, must adjust well to the blood vessel wall during all the cardiac cycle, without leaving space between the electrodes and the blood vessel wall during diastole, when the vessel diameter diminishes or compressing the vessel during systole, when the vessel diameter increases about 7%. Usually the probe diameter is chosen according to vessel diameter during diastole and several sizes are commercially available from 1 to 24 mm diameter to fit the different needs of diameter values of blood arteries and veins.

Figure 7.14 shows some examples of perivascular probe designs, including one without ferromagnetic core (Figure 7.14C) in order to be lighter and smaller, but at the cost of loss of sensitivity.

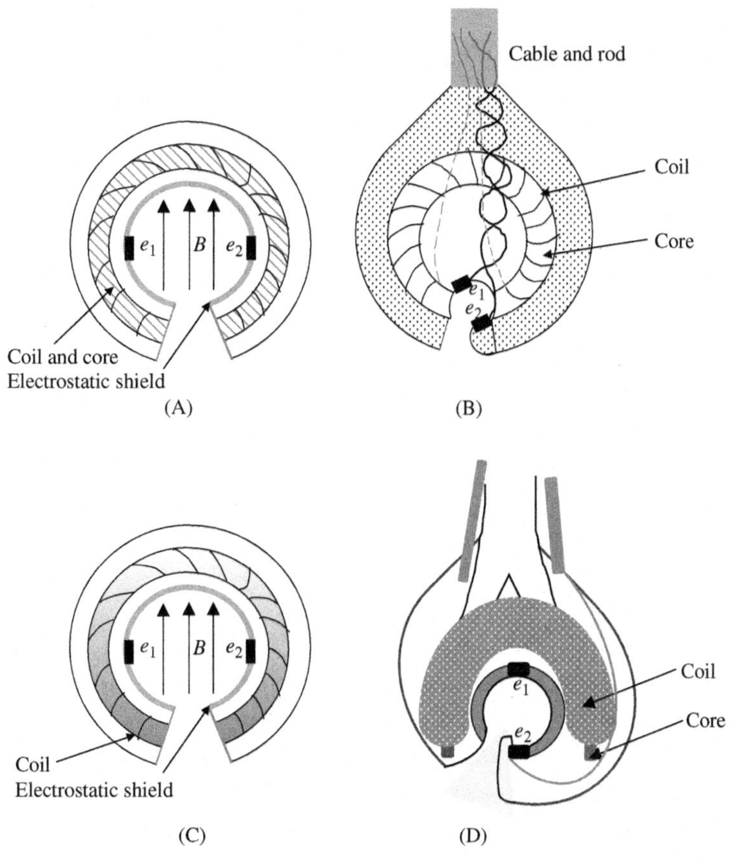

Figure 7.14 Examples of perivascular probe designs: (A) toroidal core; (B) C core; (C) coreless probe; and (D) U core.

Magnetic coil current excitation: DC (Direct Current) and AC (Alternate Current)

Coil excitation current (Figure 7.13B) can be DC or AC. With DC current, magnetic field and magnetic flow density (B) are time invariant. AC current replaced DC excitation used in the first electromagnetic flowmeters due to series offset voltage of the electrode/vessel wall interface, which cannot be easily separated from the blood flow signal. Biopotentials such as ECG and EEG, and electrical noise (proportional to $1/f$), which have spectral components in the same band as the flow signal (0–30 Hz), also cannot be extracted from the main signal.

200 Hz to 1 kHz current is usually used to produce magnetic field:

$$i = I\sin(\omega t) \tag{7.30}$$

where I is the peak-to-peak amplitude of the sinusoidal current and the ideal induced EMF is:

$$E = E_f sin(\omega t) \tag{7.31}$$

where E_f is the peak-to-peak amplitude of the sinusoidal voltage output.

Equation (7.31) is true if the plane defined by electrodes e_1 and e_2 and their lead cables are perfectly parallel to the magnetic field density. In any other case, there will be a perpendicular component of the magnetic density, which will induce a proportional EMF between the electrodes, called transformer voltage, which is added to the desired output. The transformer voltage, E_T, is out of phase compared to the flow signal and its amplitude, E_t, is proportional to frequency:

$$E_T = k_1 \frac{d\Phi_B}{dt} = k_2 \frac{di}{dt} = \underbrace{k_3\omega}_{E_t} \cos(\omega t) \tag{7.32}$$

where

$d\Phi_B$ is the magnetic field density

$E_t = k_3\omega$ is the peak-to-peak amplitude of the transformer voltage

k_1, k_2, k_3 are constants

ω is the angular frequency.

And the output voltage of the electromagnetic flow transducer is

$$E = E_f \sin(\omega t) + E_t \cos(\omega t) \tag{7.33}$$

When the excitation voltage of the magnetic field is sinusoidal, transformer voltage is also sinusoidal, but 90° out of phase with the input. Usually E_T amplitude, which is proportional to the frequency, is large and must be electronically suppressed from output EMF, for example, with a discriminator circuit of quadrature signal, in order to get to know the flow value from E_F. Other types of time-variable waveforms of magnet current can be used. Square wave is one of the magnetic excitation options, but its derivative waveform presents impulses with high amplitude in the transitions, which cause the circuit output amplifiers to saturate. A better choice is trapezoidal waveform, which generates E_T with the format of low amplitude pulses only in the transitions, rise and fall of the waveform, with no transformer components during the plateaus of the trapezoidal current. As E_F has the same format as excitation, E_F can be sampled during its positive plateaus, when E_T is null (Figure 7.15) (Cobbold, 1974; Doebelin, 2004; Webster, 2010; Wyatt, 1982; Yanof, 1960).

In addition to the perivascular electromagnetic flowmeters, intravascular flowmeters can be constructed in very small sizes to be coupled to a catheter tip and introduced into the vessels. Intravascular electromagnetic flowmeters are not as accurate as perivascular ones and can show errors as great as 20%; due to difficulty to determine

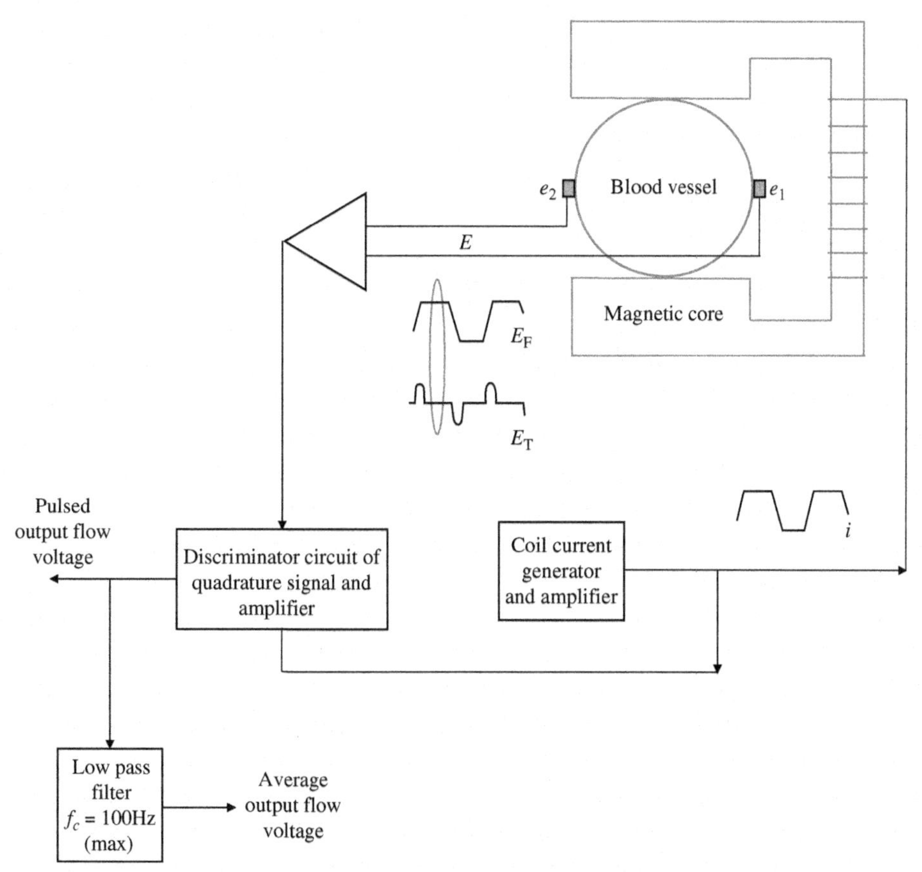

Figure 7.15 Schematic diagram of an electromagnetic flowmeter with trapezoidal magnet excitation current and a discriminator circuit to suppress the transformer voltage in quadrature. Pulsed output flow voltage is obtained sampling EMF during the plateau of the excitation current, in which transformer voltage is null.

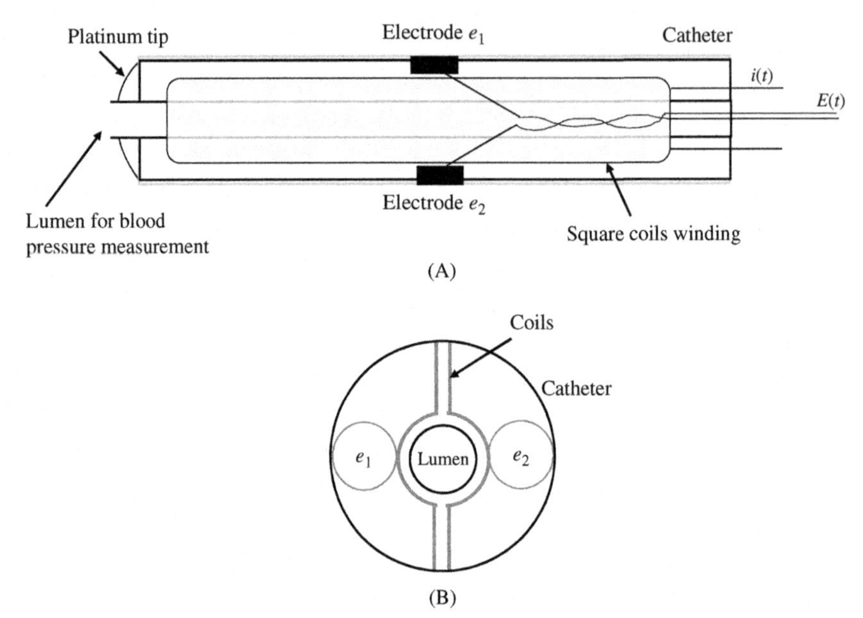

Figure 7.16 Representation of an intravascular electromagnetic flowmeter. (A) Lateral view ($i(t)$ is the excitation current and the EMF, $E(t)$ is the flow signal). (B) Frontal view (cut through electrodes).

if the probe is at the center of a vessel or close to its wall, the blood velocity is determined considering the blood to have an uniform velocity profile along the cardiac cycle. Being sensible to the direction of the blood flow, an intravascular electromagnetic flowmeters is useful, for example, to identify reverse flow and to determine the percentage of regurgitation of a leaking aortic valve.

Some intravascular pressure transducers incorporate an electromagnetic flowmeter and their functioning is similar to the first intravascular flowmeter successfully used, the intravascular probe of Mills (Mills, 1966; Mills and Shilingford, 1967). Figure 7.16 shows a schematic diagram of this type of probe. The magnetic field is produced by the rectangular coil inside the catheter and its flux lines cross the blood flow around the transducer tip. The blood flowing through the magnetic field induces an EMF measured as a voltage difference between the electrodes. Mill's probe had 3 mm external diameter and the frequency of the magnet current was 935 Hz. X-ray determined the artery diameter and its sensibility was 13 μV/100 cm/s with flat response from DC to 35 Hz (Cobbold, 1974).

Macalpin, Kolin, and Stein (1976) modified Kolin's electromagnetic flowmeter (Kolin, 1970) and developed a flow transducer constructed with a fine, insulated wire loop, which had a small electrode on each side of the loop. This loop probe had reduced dimensions, 0.5 mm diameter, and was inserted like a guidewire in the blood vessel through standard cardiac catheter. When emerged from the catheter tip, the loop automatically adjusted to the vessel diameter and the electrodes were in contact

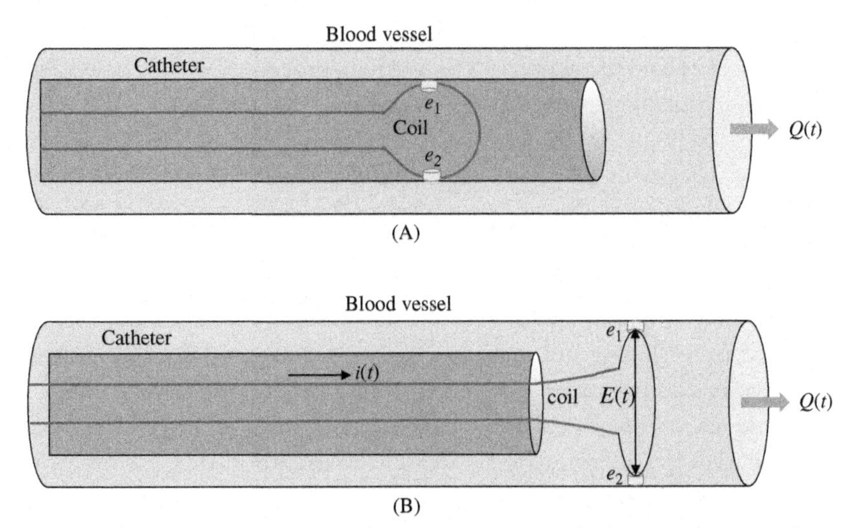

Figure 7.17 Representation of an intravascular flowmeter with extracorporeal magnetic field. The coil winding has only one loop, which is inserted in the vessel as a guided wire through a catheter (A). Once the tip of the loop is released, it expands and the electrodes touch the blood vessel inner wall (B).

to diametrically opposite sides of the inner wall of the vessel. This flow sensor miniaturization was achieved generating the magnetic field from a coil located outside the body. The blood flows through the vessel across the magnetic field, inducing an EMF, measured between the electrodes, proportional to the blood flow velocity. The loop probe allowed simultaneous measurement of the arterial diameter (Figure 7.17).

Electromagnetic blood flowmeters have low-level output voltage, in the range $1-100\ \mu V$. They operate in corrosive environment and the electrodes used must be made of resistant and inert material, usually platinum. Brilliant platinum is used in flowmeters in which the electrodes touch the vessel wall. Its high impedance minimizes current circulation between the vessel wall and the electrodes, but is more susceptible to noise. Black platinum (platinized platinum) has lower impedance than brilliant, and is indicated if the electrodes are placed in recessed cavities, which minimizes noise and current flow in the interface between the vessel wall and the electrode.

7.2.5 Plethysmography

Plethysmography is a technique used to quantify volume changes in parts of the body, such as arms, legs, and digits, or organs like lungs. Measuring the time that takes to a volume change to occur, the fluid flow (blood, air) is obtained in different parts of the body. Plethysmography, also known as pulse volume recording, is a useful technique to help identify blood clot presence in arms and legs, through the measurement of the time of venous return of the limb, or to measure the total amount of air that lungs can hold. Volume plethysmography combined with the venous occlusion procedure has become the standard method for estimating peripheral blood flow in humans since the first decades of twentieth century. The current procedure is still based essentially on the method originally developed by Schäfer and Moore (1896) and adapted to human limb measurements by Hewlett and van Zwaluwenburg (1909). This method seals the limb or a segment of it in a rigid jacket, so the venous blood return stops and any volume changes of the enclosed part will be due to arterial blood inflow, causing a corresponding volume displacement of the sealed space, filled with water or air, which is connected to a volume recorder (Whitney, 1953).

Lung or pulmonary plethysmography is a test used to measure how much air the patient can hold in his lungs, and pressure-corrected integrated flow plethysmographs provide sensitive recordings of pressure and volume events over a wide range of volume displacements. They permit accurate recording of maximal expiratory flow—volume curves in addition to measurement of intrathoracic gas volume and specific airway resistance. Lung plethysmography is usually performed in a whole-body plethysmograph, which measures changes in lung volume over a range of volumes, from the scale of milliliters to liters, and helps identifying lung diseases often associated with a decrease in total lung capacity (Coates, Peslin, Rodenstein, & Stocks, 1997; Goldman, Smith & Ulmer, 2005; Mead, 1960).

Physicians usually perform limb plethysmography on the legs to help diagnose leg artery disease, and it is also be used in patients with suspected arm artery disease, thoracic outlet syndrome, or spasms of the digits (fingers and toes), arteries (Raynaud's disease). Forearm venous occlusion plethysmography with local brachial artery infusion of hormones and vasoactive drugs has been used extensively to study human vascular function (Wilkinson & Webb, 2001). If plethysmography suggests that a patient has a blockage in one or more arteries, a physician may order additional tests, such as an arteriogram, computerized tomographic angiography (CTA), and magnetic resonance angiography (MRA) to confirm a diagnosis of peripheral arterial disease. The diagnosis of vascular disease is done with several types of plethysmography, each one with its own advantages and indications. The functioning of the techniques of air chamber, strain gage, photoelectric and electrical plethysmography is presented below.

7.2.5.1 Chamber plethysmography

Chamber plethysmography, also called venous occlusion, air chamber, and pneumoplethysmography, is a noninvasive technique that allows the measurement of the blood flow from the monitoring of blood volume changes in body extremities. Figure 7.18 shows schematic representations of the chamber plethysmography. It requires venous flow occlusion, which is obtained with a cuff, applied in the proximal region of the limb being examined, with pressure adjusted to 50 mmHg. After venous flow occlusion, the arterial inflow continues, because of the higher arterial pressure, and changes the volume of the limb (arm, leg, finger, or a segment of a member) inserted in the

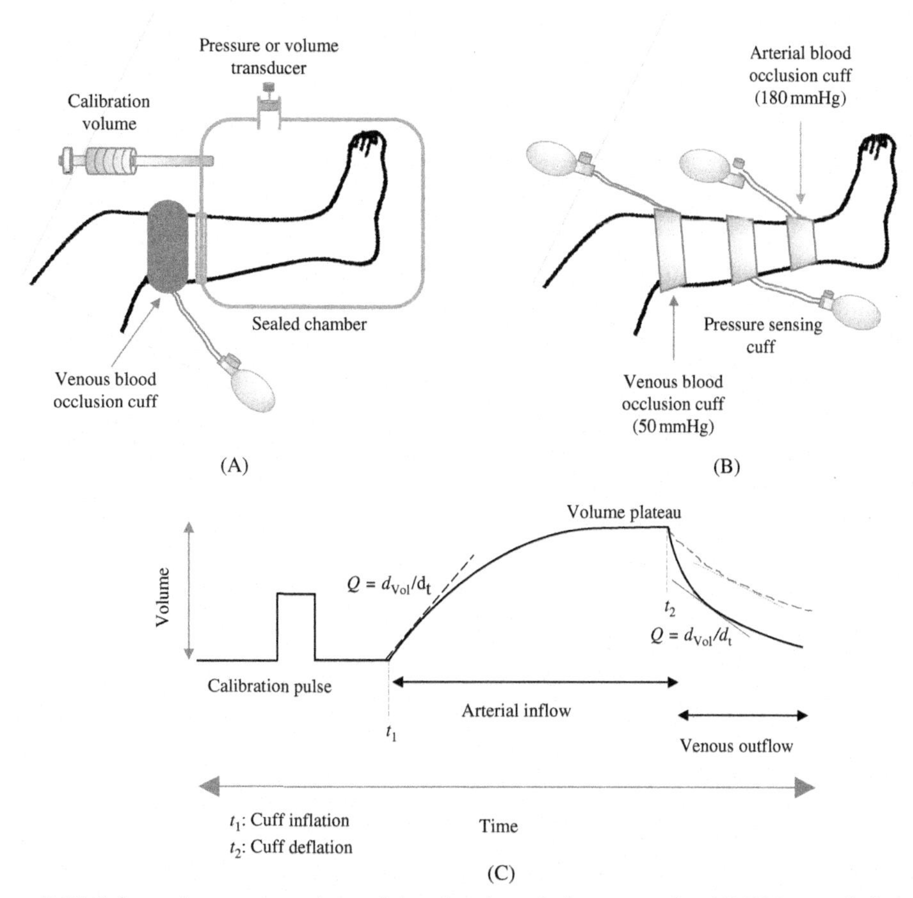

Figure 7.18 Schematic representations of the chamber plethysmography. (A) With a sealed chamber with rigid walls where the limb is placed and (B) with a sensing cuff to measure blood flow in a leg segment. (C) Typical output waveform of chamber plethysmography test. Decreased flow velocity during venous outflow may indicate blood clot presence (dashed line).

sealed chamber; the volume change is detected by a volume or pressure transducer installed in the sealed chamber (Figure 7.18A). The pressure in the chamber increases with the arterial blood inflow. Blood flow (Q) is computed as the derivative of volume with time ($Q = \mathrm{dVol}/\mathrm{d}t$). The veins are filled with blood and when the venous pressure, due to blood accumulation in the limb, reaches 50 mmHg, venous return is reestablished and the volume, and thus, the pressure in the chamber becomes constant (Figure 7.18C). The venous occlusion cuff is then quickly released, the excess blood accumulated in the leg is readily removed, and the limb volume back to normal. Time and shape of the decay of blood volume is evaluated by physicians to identify the presence of vascular diseases. For example, the speed of outflowing blood is significantly reduced in case of an outflow obstruction like a thrombosis.

The venous occlusion plethysmography is generally used for evaluating maximum venous outflow, waveform shapes, and relative amplitude changes. It can be calibrated by adding or subtracting a known volume of air to the system and observing the corresponding output changes. Chamber plethysmography is the noninvasive method that has the best accuracy for volume change measurement (Webster, 2010).

Air plethysmographic measurements are based on Boyle's law, a principle that describes the relationship between the pressure and volume of a gas: the volume of a gas at constant temperature varies inversely with the pressure exerted on it. With venous outflow occluded, the arterial inflow makes the volume of the leg increase, which in turn, increases the pressure with ΔP_{cham} within the chamber, since it is a closed system and the volume of the limb, measured with transducer, has increased by $\Delta V_{\text{leg}} = -\Delta V_{\text{cham}}$, provided that temperature is constant. Since the initial pressure P_{cham} and volume V_{cham} (transducer measurements) are also known, ΔV_{leg} can be computed as

$$\Delta \text{Vol}_{\text{leg}} = -\frac{\text{Vol}_{\text{cham}}}{P_{\text{cham}}} \Delta P_{\text{cham}} \tag{7.34}$$

And blood flow is computed by

$$Q = \frac{\text{dVol}_{\text{leg}}}{\text{d}t} = -\frac{\text{Vol}_{\text{cham}}}{P_{\text{cham}}} \frac{\text{d}P_{\text{cham}}}{\text{d}t} \approx -\frac{\text{Vol}_{\text{cham}}}{P_{\text{cham}}} \frac{\Delta P_{\text{cham}}}{\Delta t} \tag{7.35}$$

A similar procedure is used to develop the flow equation of whole-body or pulmonar plethysmography. It is possible to measure blood flow in a limb without the use of sealed chamber. Figure 7.18B shows a measurement configuration in which the changes in the volume of leg are detected from the pressure changes in a sensing cuff, wrapped around the leg segment. In addition to the cuff of venous occlusion, an artery occlusion cuff (180 mmHg) is placed in the distal region, isolating the leg segment from the foot, so only the leg volume change is sensed. The sensing cuff is placed around the calf, inflated to a low pressure (acts like calibration volume). Any limb change in volume, due to arterial blood inflow, is reflected by a pressure change within the cuff, which is shown on a display or chart recorder.

7.2.5.2 Strain gage plethysmography

The plethysmography technique originally developed by Schäfer and Moore (1896), adapted to human limb measurements by Hewlett and van Zwaluwenburg (1909), was perfected to a simple and practical implementation by Whitney in 1953, who used a strain gage made of silastic tubing filled with mercury as volume change sensor. The strain gage was part of a bridge circuit, whose output voltage was amplified and the relationship between gage resistance and limb circumference was determined by calibration at the start of each study (Gamble, Gartside, & Christ, 1993).

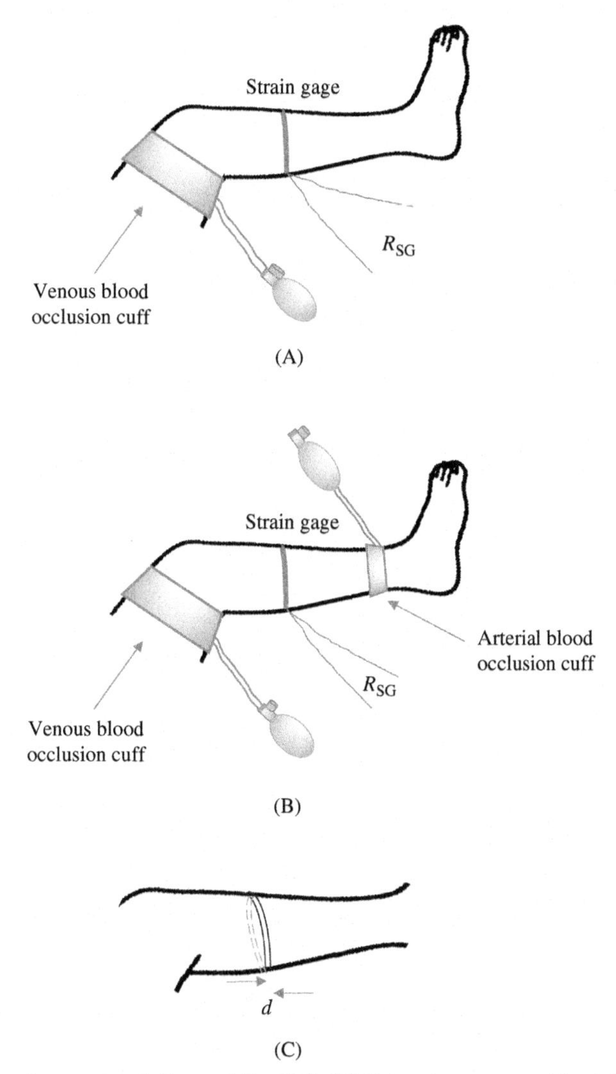

Figure 7.19 Schematic representations of the SGP. (A) Setup to measure blood flow in the leg and (B) with an arterial blood cuff to measure blood flow in a leg segment. (C) A small segment of the limb with circumference *l* and width *d*.

The classical equation to get flow from strain gage plethysmography (SGP) is deduced considering a small limb segment with length *l* and width *d* (Figure 7.19C). The segment volume is computed by

$$\mathrm{Vol} = \frac{l^2 \mathrm{d}}{4\pi} \tag{7.36}$$

If the limb volume increases, the limb segment volume also increases (Vol + ΔVol), its circumference changes to $(l + \Delta l)$ and width remains the same:

$$(V+\Delta V)=\frac{(l+\Delta l)^2 \mathrm{d}}{4\pi} \tag{7.37}$$

As $\Delta l << l$:

$$\Delta \mathrm{Vol}=\frac{2l\,\Delta l\,\mathrm{d}}{4\pi} \tag{7.38}$$

and

$$\frac{\Delta \mathrm{Vol}}{\mathrm{Vol}}=\frac{2\Delta l}{l} \tag{7.39}$$

Considering that the limb circumference and the strain gage length are the same, and that strain gage resistance R can be approximate by $R = k\,l$, where k is a constant, for a particular gage length l_L, comes that:

$$\frac{\Delta \mathrm{Vol}}{\mathrm{Vol}}=\frac{2\Delta R}{k\,l_L} \tag{7.40}$$

From Eq. (7.40), flows are computed as volume variation along a time Δt:

$$Q=\frac{\Delta \mathrm{Vol}}{\mathrm{Vol}\Delta t}=\frac{2\Delta R}{k\,l_L\Delta t} \tag{7.41}$$

Equation (7.41) is dependent on the strain gage sensitivity, and thus, dependent on the gage calibration. Hokanson, Summer, and Strandness (1975) and Taylor, Coghlan, Beasley, and King (1978) contributed to modify Eq. (7.41) into a flow equation independent of gage calibration, allowing measurement automation:

$$Q=\frac{\Delta \mathrm{Vol}}{\mathrm{Vol}\Delta t}=\frac{\Delta R}{R\Delta t} \tag{7.42}$$

From Eq. (7.42), the flow into a limb under venous occlusion is computed from the resistance measurement of the strain gage at all times along Δt (Taylor et al., 1978).

Actual devices are in the loop form of a very thin distensile silicon rubber tube, filled with mercury or indium-gallium most often. The loop is adjusted around the limb or digit under test. The active portion of the elastic strain gage has a slightly smaller length than the limb or digit circumference to stay under tension. Volume changes of the limb or digit, within the period of each heartbeat, modify the electrical resistance of the strain gage, which value is processed and displayed as a waveform.

Same way as in the chamber plethysmography, a proximal cuff (50 mmHg) is used to prevent venous blood return allowing arterial blood inflow (Figure 7.19A). If the volume change is to be measured in only a segment of the limb, for example, the forearm or thigh, it is necessary to use an additional distal arterial occlusion cuff (180 mmHg) (Figure 7.19B).

Common applications of the strain gage include measuring arterial blood flow into the limbs and digits, and venous capacitance, and maximum venous outflow to detect deep venous thrombosis in the legs and also to study physiological functions (Alomari et al., 2004). SGP is the standard mode for testing endothelial dysfunction and reactive hyperemia.

7.2.5.3 Photoelectric plethysmography

Photoelectric plethysmography (PPG) is an optical measurement technique that uses an invisible infrared light sent into the tissue and the amount of the backscattered light corresponds to the variation in the volume of blood in vessels on microvascular beds. Hertzman was the first to find a relationship between the intensity of backscattered light and blood volume in 1938 (Hertzman, 1938).

Microvascular blood flow in the human skin presents a pulsed rhythm that reflects heartbeat, respiration frequency, intrinsic myogenic activity, neurogenic factors, and endothelial activity. LDF and PPG are noninvasive methods that allow blood flow evaluation from cutaneous microcirculation (Allen, 2007; Jones, 1987; Nitzan, Turivnenko, Milston, Babchenko, & Mahler, 1996). PPG is a noninvasive technique for detection of blood volume changes at tissues capillary bed. It provides a qualitative measurement of the increase of blood volume in the capillary bed during systole and decrease during diastole, by light attenuation through the tissue as a function of time. The PPG output signal reflects the blood movement in the circulatory system, which goes from the heart to the fingertips and toes through the blood vessels in a wave-like motion, which is proportional to changes in the volume of red blood cells in the peripheral microvascular beds.

PPG technique detects and processes optical radiation after interaction with tissue microvascular bed, mainly red blood cells, at different body locations, such as fingertip, toe, earlobe, foot, forehead, and forearm. When tissue is illuminated by visible or near-infrared radiation, the amount of light that is absorbed depends mainly on the optical properties of the capillary bed (arterioles and venules). These properties are different according to blood volume changes in vessels during heartbeat period. Optical input signal is generated by light emitting diode (LED) and optical output levels are detected by PD of PPG transducers. Usually PD output is associated with an optical filter to pass light wavelengths of interest. The PPG output signals are originated by absorption of input optical radiation by the pulsed blood volume; therefore, they contain valuable cardiovascular information on the blood pumping and nutrients transport (Elgendi, 2012; Kamal, Harness, Irving, & Mearns, 1989).

Figure 7.20A shows a representation of the radiation transmission through skin, light interaction with capillary bed and backscattering to the surface. Figure 7.20B shows disposition of LED and PD in transmission PPG and Figure 7.20C in reflection PPG.

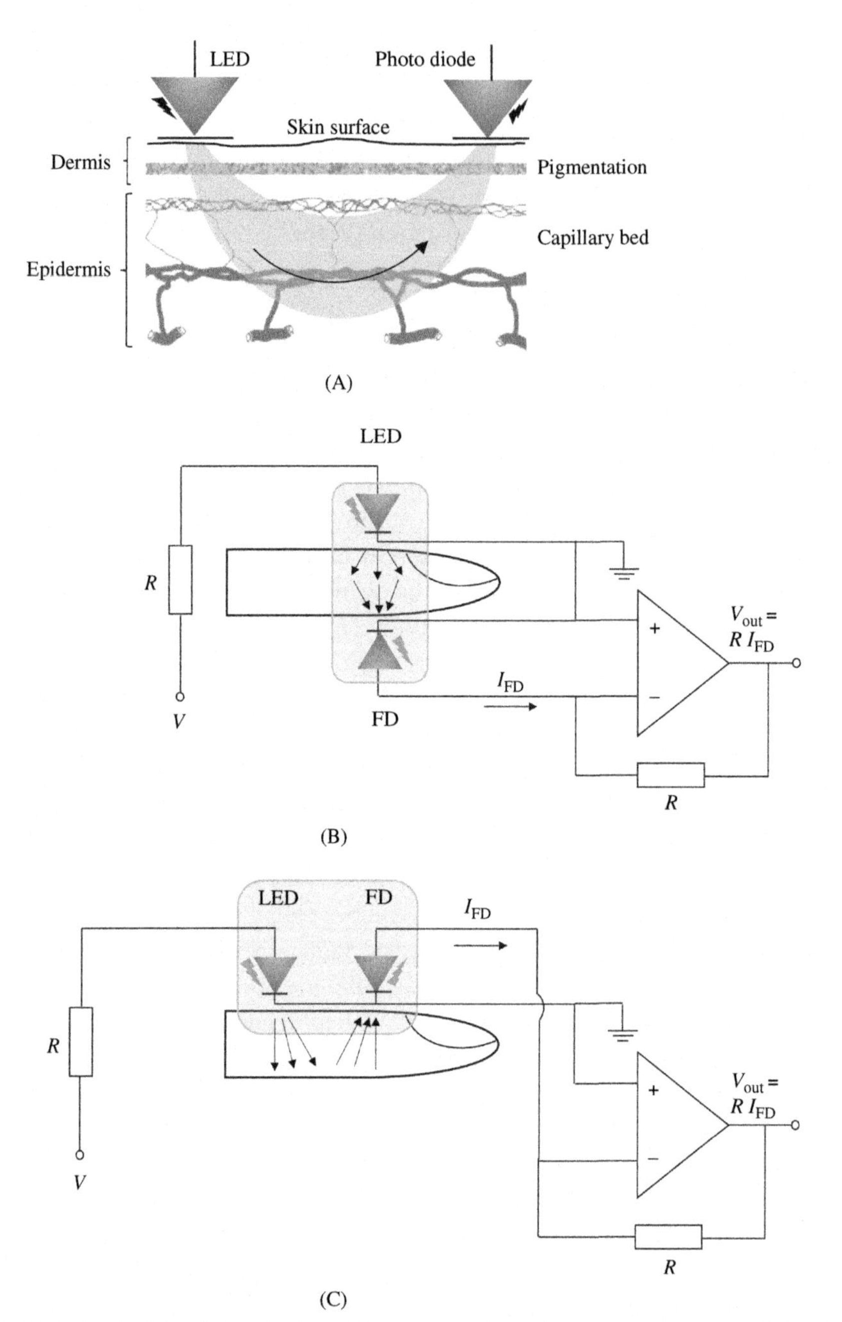

Figure 7.20 PPG principle of functioning: (A) representation of the radiation transmission through skin, interaction of the light with capillary bed, and backscattering to the surface; (B) disposition of LED and PD in transmission PPG and transimpedance amplifier; and (C) disposition of LED and PD in reflection PPG.

In transmission PPG, LED and PD are placed in opposite sides of the finger (in this example). The radiation emitted by the LED is scattered, absorbed, and reflected in the different tissues (skin, muscle, nerve, blood, and bone), and part of the radiation is transmitted and detected by the photodetector. The changes in blood volume can be quantified from the amount of reflected light and the optical properties of blood and tissues. The PD must have spectral characteristics matched with LED characteristics; its output (reverse current) is amplified ($\times 300-500$) by a transimpedance amplifier, conditioned in analog circuits or digitalized and processed in microcontrolled systems and displayed.

LED wavelength is chosen in the red or near-infrared region, 650 nm to 1 μm (e.g., GaAs with $\lambda \sim 940$ nm), due to preferable absorption of this length by blood cells. This way, the larger the amount of blood in the vessel, the larger is the amount of absorbed light and smaller is the amount of light detected by PD.

In reflection PPG, both optical devices, LED and PD are placed side by side on the same side of the finger. Part of the radiation that is not transmitted or absorbed in the tissues reflects back and gets to the PD.

Output signal of both types of PPG devices (Figure 7.21A) occurs at the same frequency as heartbeat and has a pulsatile or AC component superimposed to an almost DC baseline. Baseline is due to constant constituents of the path (average blood volume, nerve, muscle, tendon, bone) and its low frequency components are related to respiration, thermoregulation, and sympathetic nervous system activity. AC component is due to additional blood volume, which is added and removed at each heartbeat, during systole and diastole, respectively.

Pulsatile component of the PPG signal is easily separated from DC component by a high-pass filter and is synchronized with heartbeat (frequency around 1 Hz). Figure 7.21B shows AC component of a typical PPG signal waveform. Hertzman and Spealman (1937) described two main characteristics of the PPG pulsatile waveform morphology: the rising and falling phases of the pulse, called anacrotic and catacrotic, respectively. Anacrotic phase is due primarily to systole and reflects heart conditions. Catacrotic phase is due to diastole and is determined by the elasticity of components of the vascular system; healthy arteries commonly exhibit a dicrotic notch in the catacrotic phase.

Transmission-type finger and earlobe PPG devices are routinely used for monitoring of heartbeat rate and tissue blood supply. Transmission PPG can also be used in newborn foot due to its delicate, thin, and almost transparent tissues. In addition to ear and fingers, reflection PPG is used in forehead and forearm, regions that have thin layer of tissues over a bone. Transmission PPG signals travel a path twice as long the transmission path, are less intense and therefore noisier, than the transmitted ones.

PPG is a simple, low cost, fast response technique used, among other applications, to detect peripheral flow pulse waveform, through blood volume variation along cardiac cycle. Its output is synchronized with heartbeat and qualitatively related to blood

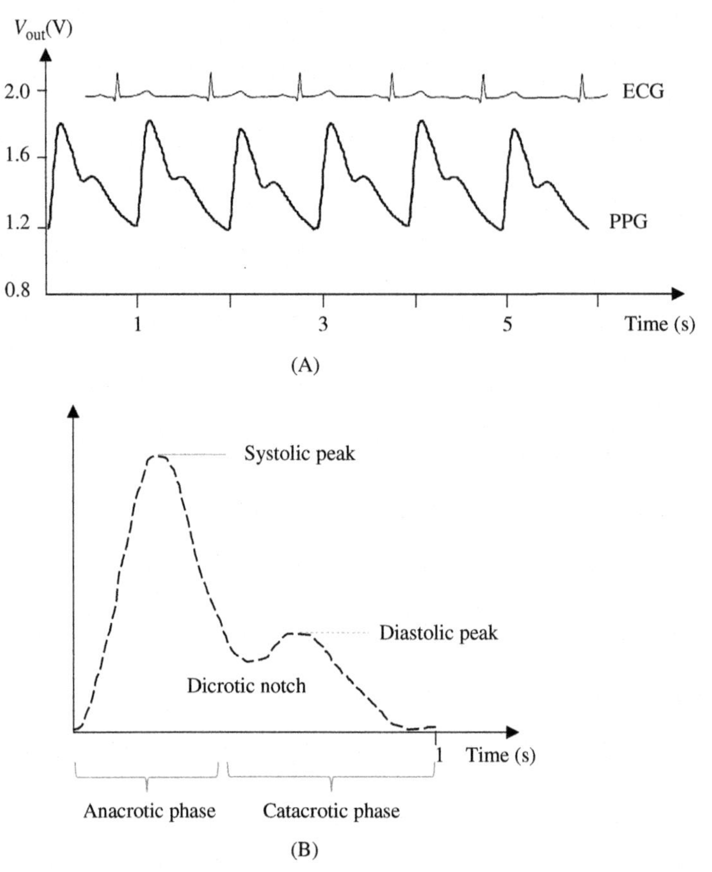

Figure 7.21 (A) Output signal of PPG devices occurs at the same frequency as heartbeat and has a pulsatile or AC component superimposed to an almost DC baseline. (B) AC component of a typical PPG signal waveform showing its parameters.

flow, not quantitatively. Skin color, nail polish, perfusion restriction, ambient illumination, anemia, and polytrauma are limitation factors of PPG application. PPG measurements are quite sensitive to patient movement and probe–tissue movement artifacts and the method of application preclude volume calibration.

7.2.5.4 Impedance plethysmography

Impedance plethysmography (IPG) technique was developed in 1932 through Atzler and Lehman's observation that a capacitor formed by metallic parallel plates applied across the human chest exhibited a variable capacitance and that it varied in synchronism with heartbeat frequency (Atzler & Lehman, 1932). Few years later, in 1940, Nyboer et al. introduced a technique that allowed measuring the impedance of a body segment, as a function of time, by injecting constant current between surface

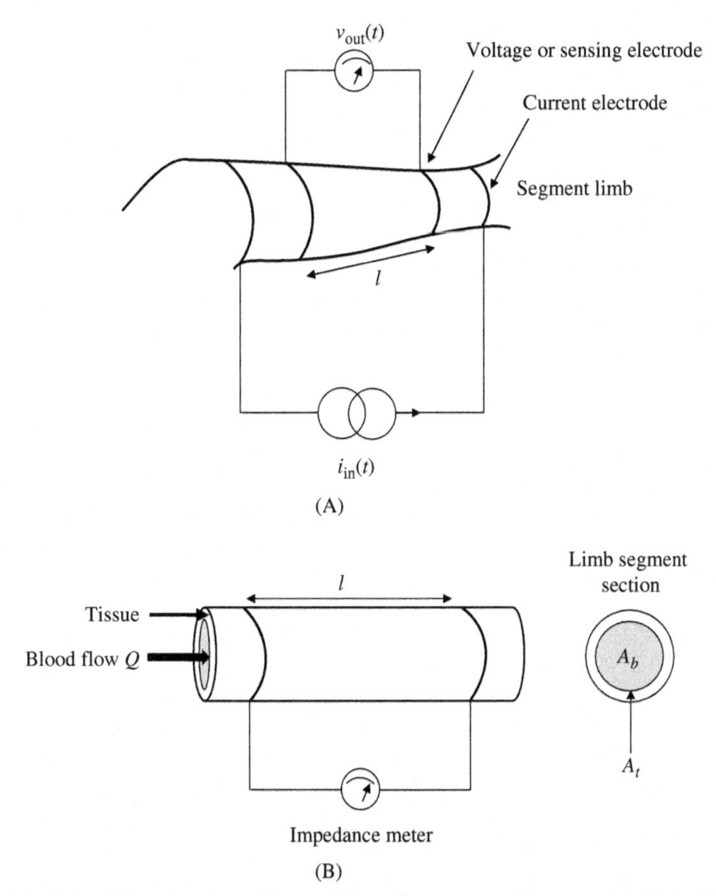

Figure 7.22 Principle of functioning of impedance flowmeter: (A) setup for blood flow measurement in a segment limb and (B) model to determine impedance and blood volume change.

electrodes placed in the limbs (Nyboer, Bango, Barnett, & Halsey, 1940). The measurement of electric impedance at the body surface is the basis of IPG, a noninvasive technique that quantifies body fluid volumes and estimates tissue blood flow.

The wide range of values of electrical resistivity of biological tissues, from 30 Ω cm (urine) to 16.6 kΩ cm, is useful for acquiring parameters that help to understand the operation of various types of tissues and cells. The electrical resistivity of blood is 150 Ω cm, a much higher value than the electrical resistivity of good electricity conductors as copper, for example, which resistivity is 1.724 mΩ cm. Thus, pulsatile blood volume along cardiac cycle modifies the impedance of a body segment. The impedance decreases proportionally to the blood volume increase during systole and increases again during diastole, when the blood volume decreases.

Figure 7.22 shows the principle of functioning of IPG for measurement of the blood flow in a limb segment. The segment receives four metal electrodes. RF current ($i(t)$) injected between the outer and inner electrodes is used to measure output voltage $v_{out}(t)$ in the limb region where electric current lines are approximately parallel to vessels and current density is more uniform (Figure 7.22A).

According to two compartment model, a constant resistivity blood volume, with cylindrical format of length l and area A_b, surrounded by tissue of length l and area A_t, acts like the limb segment and blood vessels (Figure 7.22B) (Schwan & Kay, 1956). Blood and surrounding tissue cylinder has area A. Blood (Vol_b) and surrounding tissue (Vol_t) volumes are computed as

$$Vol_b = lA_b \tag{7.43}$$

$$Vol_t = lA_t = l(A - A_b) \tag{7.44}$$

Changes in the volume of a limb, due to blood flow, cause variations of the electrical impedance associated. Impedances of blood and tissue in the limb segment are:

$$Z_t = \rho_t \frac{l}{A - A_b} \tag{7.45}$$

$$Z_b = \rho_b \frac{l}{A_b} \tag{7.46}$$

where

ρ_b is the resistivity of blood in ohm-cm
ρ_t is the resistivity of blood in ohm-cm
l is the length between sensing electrodes
Z_t is the electrical impedance of tissue in the body segment
Z_b is the electrical impedance of blood in the body segment.

The impedance Z of the limb segment is the parallel association of Z_t and Z_b:

$$\frac{1}{Z} = \frac{1}{Z_t} + \frac{1}{Z_b} \tag{7.47}$$

and

$$Z = \frac{\rho_t \rho_b l^2}{\rho_b l(A - A_b) + \rho_t l A_b} \tag{7.48}$$

$$Z = \frac{\rho_t \rho_b l^2}{\rho_b Vol_t + \rho_t Vol_b} \tag{7.49}$$

During systole, limb segment area increases ΔA uniformly along length l, due to arterial blood inflow, which corresponds to a ΔVol increase, but tissue volume remains the same. The impedance variation due to blood volume variation is computed as the derivative equation (7.49) in function of blood volume variation:

$$\frac{dZ}{d\mathrm{Vol_b}} = -\frac{\rho_b\, \rho_t{}^2 l^2}{(\rho_b \mathrm{Vol_t} + \rho_t \mathrm{Vol_b})^2} \tag{7.50}$$

and

$$d\mathrm{Vol_b} = -\frac{(\rho_b \mathrm{Vol_t} + \rho_t \mathrm{Vol_b})^2}{\rho_b\, \rho_t{}^2 l^2} dZ \tag{7.51}$$

Replacing the numerator of Eq. (7.51) by $(\rho_t \rho_b (l^2/Z))^2$ results:

$$d\mathrm{Vol_b} = -\frac{l^2 \rho_b}{Z^2} dZ \tag{7.52}$$

Equation (7.52) is equal to Nyboer et al. (1940) and Nyboer (1960) solution derived from parallel conductor theory, and allows estimating the blood volume inflow into the limb segment. The impedance variation is obtained by injecting alternate current between current electrodes and measuring the voltage between sensing electrodes in the setup shown in Figure 7.22A. The variation of blood flow during the cardiac pulse is computed from the volume change of the limb segment with time. Blood volume variation and flow are directly proportional to impedance variation and thus, to the output voltage.

Adequate signal to noise ratio depends on using sinusoidal current intensities larger than 1 mA. The frequency of the alternate current must be chosen between 20 and 100 kHz, to avoid the discomfort of shock sensation, which occurs at low frequencies, and to avoid high frequencies stray capacitance effect. In addition, the impedance of the electrode–skin interface decreases with increasing frequency (Webster, 2010).

7.2.6 Methods for obtaining cardiac output

Adequate hemodynamic evaluation is crucial in the management of critically ill patients. Although noninvasive diagnostic tools have reduced the need for invasive procedures, cardiac catheterization is still mandatory for absolute quantification of pressures, flows, and vascular resistances. Cardiac output is one of hemodynamic variables evaluated.

Cardiac output (*CO*) is the blood volume ejected by the ventricle in 1 min. It is equal to the stroke volume (systolic volume, $\mathrm{Vol_{sys}}$) multiplied by the number of heart beats per minute (cardiac frequency, *CF*). Venous return is the blood volume that returns to any of the atriums. In normal conditions, blood volumes inflow and outflow of any of the heart chambers are the same.

$$\mathrm{CO} = \mathrm{CF} \times \mathrm{Vol_{sys}} \tag{7.53}$$

Typical values of the cardiac output are 6 l/min in men and 5 l/min in woman. These values decrease with aging and depend on the body surface (mass), gender, and metabolic demand. Cardiac output is the most important hemodynamic parameter for tissue perfusion, being responsible for the supply of oxygen and nutrients. *CO* helps clinicians to quantify the severity of cardiac diseases and their response to treatment. In addition, *CO* participates in the calculus of other hemodynamic variables and oxygenation, such as systemic vascular resistance, pulmonary vascular resistance, and oxygen delivery. It is used also in many areas of research, like for instance, in the evaluation of the cardiac adaptation to physical training.

The measurement of cardiac output should be made preferably by a noninvasive technique that does not require anesthesia or surgical procedures that is simple and of fast implementation and that provides reliable and reproducible results. Stroke volume can be measured separately by Doppler ultrasound flowmeter, electromagnetic flowmeter, echocardiography, impedance cardiography, or other methods of flow measurement, and then multiplied by the cardiac frequency to obtain the cardiac output. There are techniques that allow measuring cardiac output as a single entity. In the following, the principle of functioning of Fick's, dye indicator and thermodilution techniques are explained.

7.2.6.1 Method of Fick

This method is based on the Principle of Fick, dated from 1870, when Fick announced that blood flow through an individual organ might be calculated by measuring the arteriovenous concentration gradient of an indicator, a known mass of which having previously been added to the arterial circulation (Jhanji, Dawson, & Pearse, 2008). According to the Principle of Fick, when applied to pulmonary flow, the rate of O_2 uptake in the pulmonary capillaries at the lungs, from the inspired air (ml O_2/min), is equal to the arteriovenous difference in O_2 concentration in the blood (ml O_2/min), multiplied by the pulmonary blood flow (l/min) (Levick, 2009). Figure 7.23A shows a representation of the pulmonary oxygen transport to explain Fick's principle of blood flow measurement.

Oxygen uptake from pulmonary blood is:

$$V_{O_2} = Q \times (\mathrm{ConcO}_{2\mathrm{art}} - \mathrm{ConcO}_{2\mathrm{ven}}) \tag{7.54}$$

where

Q is the pulmonary blood flow
V_{O_2} is the oxygen uptake
$\mathrm{ConcO}_{2\mathrm{art}}$ is the oxygen concentration in the arterial blood
$\mathrm{ConcO}_{2\mathrm{ven}}$ is the oxygen concentration in the venous blood.

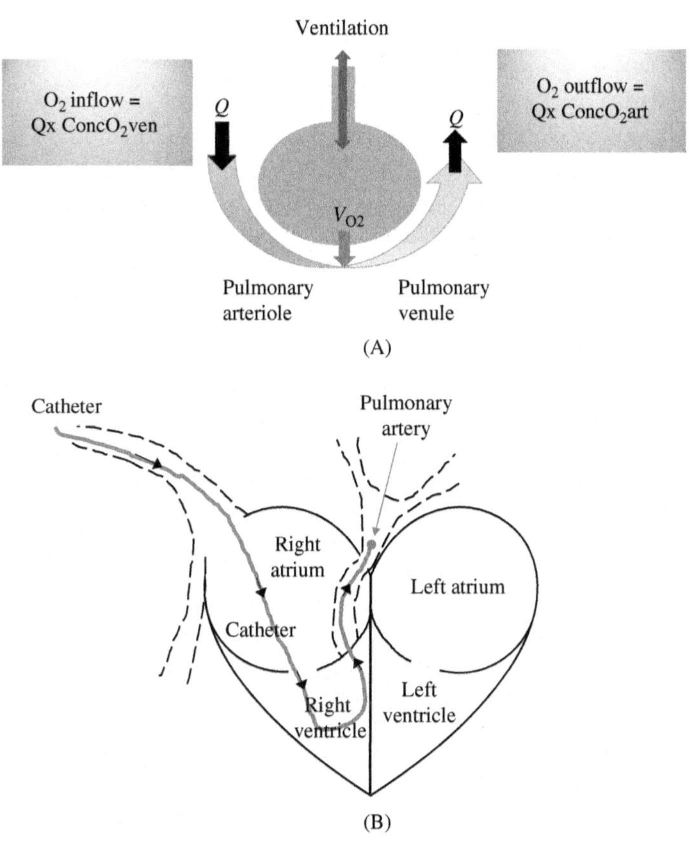

Figure 7.23 Fick method for cardiac output measurement. (A) Principle of Fick and pulmonary oxygen transportation. (B) Oxygen uptake is obtained by spirometry and blood samples are collected from pulmonary blood vein and from an artery in the periphery circulation.

Pulmonary blood flow is equal to the right ventricular output. Thus, cardiac output can be calculated from measurements of O_2 uptake:

$$\mathrm{CO(l/min)} = \frac{V_{O_2}(\mathrm{ml/min})}{\mathrm{ConcO}_{2\mathrm{art}}(\mathrm{ml}/l) - \mathrm{ConcO}_{2\mathrm{ven}}(\mathrm{ml}/l)} \tag{7.55}$$

For cardiac output calculus by Fick's equation (Eq. 7.53), it is necessary to obtain oxygen uptake, as well as the oxygen concentration in arterial and venous blood. Figure 7.23B shows where the measurements are made.

Oxygen consumption is determined by spirometry, from a resting subject, for 5–10 min. The determination of oxygen consumption represented a limitation for the use of the Fick method, in the first years of this technique application. When tables of presumed oxygen consumption for gender, age, and body surface area are used, the error associated with this method can increase up to 10%, compared to the direct measurement of O_2 consumption by spirometry, for example. Nowadays modern methods of obtaining oxygen uptake, as indirect calorimetry and mass spectroscopy respiratory, contributed to increase the accuracy of the technique (Levick, 2009; Martins et al., 2003; Visscher & Johnson, 1953).

The concentration of arterial oxygen can be determined from a blood sample taken in any artery, usually an artery of an arm (brachial, radial) or leg (femoral). The venous oxygen concentration is determined from a mixed venous blood sample taken in the output of the right ventricle, at the pulmonary artery, that has the average O_2 concentration entering the lungs. This requires the introduction of a catheter into a vein, usually a Swan–Ganz catheter, in order to get access to the right heart. This requirement results from the fact that the concentration of oxygen in venous blood varies depending on the vascular site it is taken. Oxygen concentration in venous blood from the upper part of the body (neck, head, and in particular cerebral circulation) is different from the concentration of oxygen in venous blood from the lower body (blood outflow from kidneys, torso and legs muscles, etc.). For example, O_2 concentration in renal venous blood is 170 ml/l, while in coronary venous blood is 70 ml/l. The different streams of venous blood, which come into the right atrium from superior and inferior cava veins, only become fully mixed in the right ventricle (Barrat-Boyes & Wood, 1957; Edwards & Mayall, 1998; Levick, 2009; Mahutte & Jaffe, 1995; Martins et al., 2003).

The Fick method is an invasive method that requires relatively steady state physiological conditions, but it takes several minutes to be executed and, therefore, does not provide cardiac output immediately. It does not allow beat-to-beat stroke volume observation. Its fundamental assumption is based on the fact that the volume of oxygen received by pulmonary ventilation is equal to the volume of oxygen uptake by the tissues and the largest errors in its implementation occur in situations of rapid changes in circulatory and pulmonary ventilation conditions.

7.2.6.2 Dye dilution method

At the end of nineteenth century, Stewart developed the indicator dilution concept that was described more than a hundred years before, by Haller (Stewart, 1897). He detected electrical conductance changes in circulating blood using hypertonic saline solution as indicator. Based on Stewart's work, Hamilton developed an indicator dilution technique to measure cardiac output using phenolphthalein (Hamilton, Moore, Kinsman, & Spurling, 1948). He plotted the oxygen concentration in arterial blood versus time, showing that cardiac output is inversely proportional to the area under the curve, described as Stewart–Hamilton equation (Jhanji et al., 2008).

In dilution method, a known bolus of an indicator substance (I) is injected in the pulmonary trunk and the time the blood flow takes to dilute the substance, introduced into the circulatory system, is measured. The indicator becomes diluted in the venous bloodstream, then carried through the lungs and left heart chambers and ejected into the systemic arteries. At the same time, dye concentration in blood is sampled and measured, downstream in a point of the arterial system, usually in radial or femoral artery. By definition, concentration C is the amount of injected bolus I (mg) distributed by a volume of blood plasma, Vol (ml), that is:

$$C = \frac{I(t)}{\mathrm{Vol}} \tag{7.56}$$

Concentration C is not constant and varies with time. In addition, if dilution volume Vol takes Δt seconds to reach the sampling point, this means that the left ventricle must be ejecting plasma (blood) at the rate $\mathrm{Vol}/\Delta t$, which is the cardiac arterial blood output:

$$\mathrm{CO} = \frac{\mathrm{Vol}}{\Delta t} = \frac{I(t)\Delta t}{C(t)\Delta t} \tag{7.57}$$

$C(t)$ represents the variation of the indicator concentration versus time, called dilution curve and $I(t)$ is the amount of indicator passing through the sampling point. Cardiac output is inversely proportional to the dye concentration in the blood sample collected in the arterial site, and is computed by

$$\mathrm{CO} = \frac{I}{\int_0^t C(t)\mathrm{d}t} \tag{7.58}$$

where I is the total amount of indicator bolus injected integration limit and t is the time that I takes to be eliminated from arterial blood flow.

Figure 7.24A shows the points in the circulatory system where dye bolus is injected and arterial blood sample is taken. Figure 7.24B shows a typical curve of the dilution method output, dye concentration versus time.

The dilution curve presented in Figure 7.24B shows that the dye concentration reaches a maximum value, a few seconds after bolus injection, and then decays in an approximate exponential way, but instead of reaching null concentration, the curve exhibits a recirculation effect, that is, blood with diluted dye passes again at the sampling point, which causes the concentration to increase. This happens because only about two-third of ventricle volume is ejected at each systole, and in the next cycle, residual blood with diluted dye mixes with fresh venous blood and reaches the sampling point. To allow computing cardiac output, the recirculation effect is overwhelmed by extrapolating to zero the descending branch, exponentially (dashed line), to get the primary curve that would be obtained if there was no recirculation. If $C(t)$ is plotted on a logarithmic scale, the descending branch of the curve is linear and the extrapolation portion is a straight line, which makes computing easier. Thus, cardiac

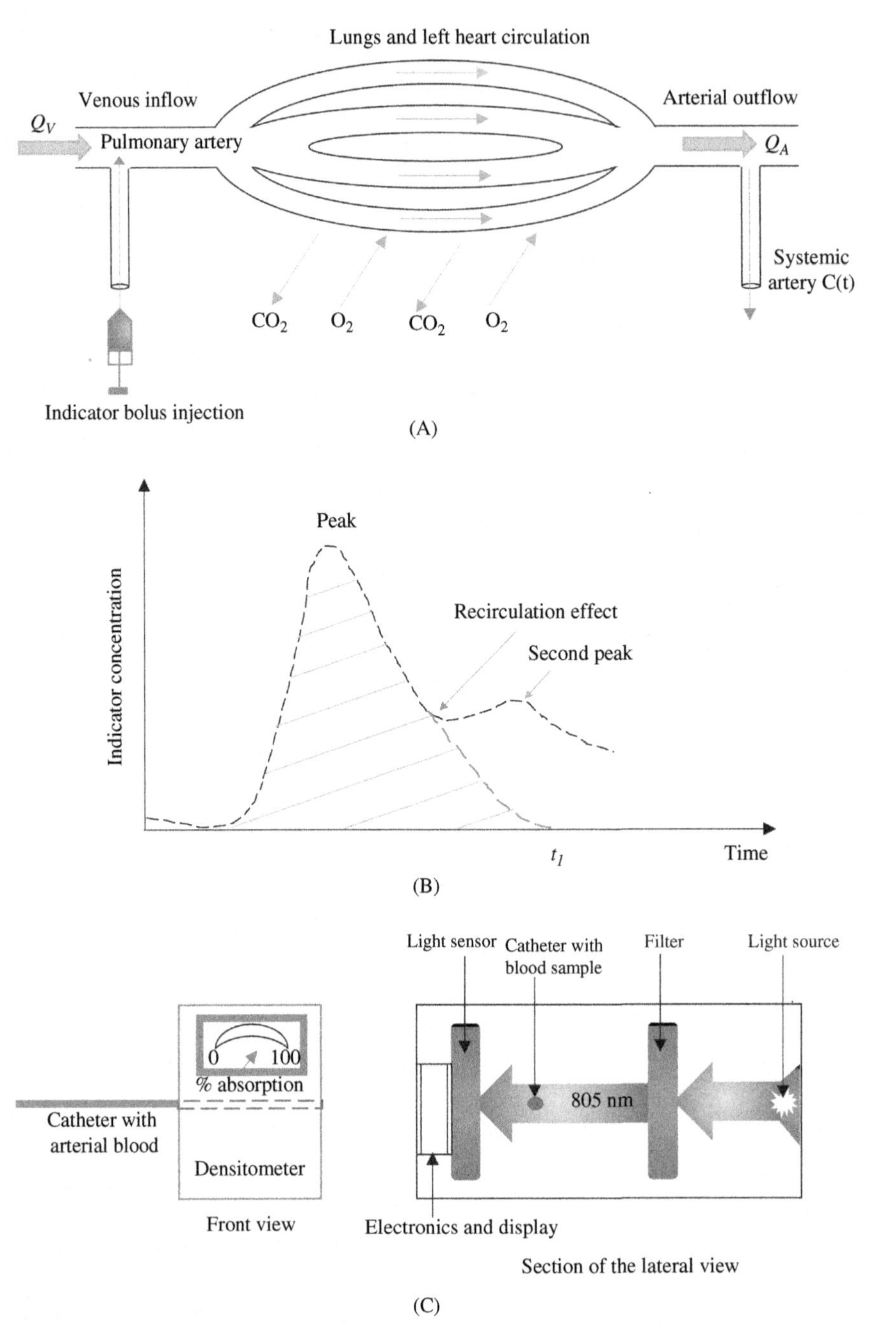

Figure 7.24 Dye dilution method for cardiac output measurement. (A) The dye bolus is injected in pulmonary artery and blood sample is taken in the arterial stream. (B) Dilution curve. Dashed line is the extrapolation of dilution curve to zero to eliminate recirculation effect. (C) Setup for measurement of the absorption coefficient of diluted indicator.

output is calculated dividing the indicator bolus volume by the area under the dilution curve as if there was no recirculation.

In the performance of dye dilution curves, a known amount of dye is usually injected as a single bolus as rapidly as possible via a cardiac catheter. When the indicator is injected into venous stream, it modifies blood optical properties. The Indocyanine Green (ICG) is a standard indicator to measure cardiac output by dye dilution technique. ICG is hydrophilic and binds to plasma protein, which yields it to stay confined to the intravascular site. The usual dose of the indicator used in the bolus is typically 5 mg for an adult patient and is injected in a 1 ml volume (ICG powder is dissolved in sterile water). A typical diagnostic cardiac catheterization exam requires an average of five dilution curves and the total dose of dye injected should be kept below 2 mg/kg (BioPortfolio, 2014). The indicator ICG is inert, harmless, and is cleared rapidly from the blood, through the liver (at a rate of 18–24% per minute, in a healthy person), and can be given every 5 min to reassess blood volume and cardiac output (Fox & Wood, 1960; Reekers et al., 2009). Optical absorption peak of ICG occurs at 805 nm, the same spectrum wavelength at which blood absorption coefficient is independent of oxygen saturation.

The concentration sampling points of $C(t)$ are obtained measuring the absorption coefficients of blood samples. Early methodology required the analysis of blood samples withdrawn at short intervals from a system artery. Later, the use of a direct arterial sampling cuvette simplified the technique, yielding continuous recording with a dichromatic densitometer, of the indicator concentration in the blood, withdrawn through a catheter from the arterial flow. Figure 7.24C shows a schematic representation of the densitometer functioning. This transmission densitometer has a light source (805 nm) and a light sensor, that is, a photoelectric cell. It measures the optical density of the blood sample in the catheter, placed between the light source and the photoelectric cell, from the decrease of the amount of light that gets to the light sensor, in relation to the light sent by the source. The color filter allows only part of the spectrum (805 nm) to pass. According to Beer's law, concentration is proportional to optical density. Thus, the smaller the amount of light that gets to the sensor, the larger is the ICG concentration in the blood.

In addition to the established standard dye dilution method, that requires continuous withdrawal of blood from an arterial site for indicator assay in the cuvette densitometer, alternative techniques have been developed in an effort to obtain a less invasive method of measuring. Estimation of cardiac output by indirect (transcutaneous) earpiece densitometry (monochromatic and dichromatic) has been reported since 1950 (Gabe & Shillingford, 1961; Nicholson, Burchell & Wood 1951), but its use was not widely accepted due to the difficulty of device calibration and lack of reliability of the use of the ear as a recording site (Reed & Wood, 1964).

Pulsed dye dilution (PPD) has been used for cardiac output and blood volume determination, among other applications since the late 1990s; it uses the indicator dilution technique and requires only intravenous access to deliver the ICG bolus. It detects indicator concentration in blood using noninvasive spectrophotometric methods with a finger photosensor or nose probe. Its reliability and clinical applicability to *CO* determination have not yet been validated, but available results recommend transcutaneous densitometry use for total blood volume calculation and for quantitative circulatory studies in specific cases, as in infants and adults with congenital heart diseases (Baulig, Bernhard, Bettex, Schmidlin, & Schmid, 2005; Imai, Takahashi, Goto, & Morishita, 1998; Iijima et al., 1997; Reekers et al., 2009; Sakka, Reinhart, Wegscheider, & Meier-Hellmann, 2002).

Lithium indicator dilution for cardiac output determination was first described by Linton, Band, and Haire (1993). A computerized version of the indicator dilution method is based on intravenous lithium ion injection. A small dose of lithium chloride is injected as an intravenous bolus via a central venous catheter and the concentration of Li^+ ion in arterial plasma is detected by a Li^+ ion-selective electrode attached to the arterial line. Cardiac output is derived from the lithium dilution curve using a modified Stewart–Hamilton equation. Because lithium is only distributed in plasma, the stroke volume calculation needs a correction for hematocrit to transform plasma flow into blood flow. Lithium is an appropriate indicator because its plasma concentration is normally negligible, and it does not bind to plasma or tissues protein. Results obtained with lithium dilution technique suggest good correlation with other cardiac output measurement techniques (Garcia-Rodriguez et al., 2002; Jonas & Tanser, 2002; Linton, Band, O'Brien, Jonas, & Leach, 1997).

7.2.6.3 Thermodilution method

The main problems of the indicator dilution techniques are indicator stability, accumulation or loss of the indicator in the blood, and inaccurate measurement of the indicator concentration. Fegler introduced thermal indicators in 1954 to measure cardiac output, based on the same concept as indicator–dilution methods. A cold saline solution in injected in venous blood and temperature is detected downstream (Fegler, 1954). Fegler development resulted in significant indicator loss during blood transit. The incorporation of a temperature measuring thermistor in the tip of a pulmonary artery catheter by Branthwaite and Bradley in 1968 contributed to minimize indicator loss. The cold bolus was injected in the right atrium and temperature was detected in the pulmonary artery, reducing the indicator transit path (Branthwaite & Bradley, 1968).

In 1970, Swan et al. developed a "flow-directed balloon-tipped" multiple lumen catheter, the Swan–Ganz catheter (Swan et al., 1970). It was introduced into the bloodstream via a vein to reach the right side of the heart and then the pulmonary artery. One lumen is connected to a small balloon situated at the catheter tip, which can be inflated during positioning; other lumen has an orifice, used to deliver the cold bolus at the right atrium and a thermistor to monitor the injectate temperature; another lumen is used to put a thermistor at the pulmonary artery (Figure 7.25A) and measure blood temperature. A fourth lumen can be used as a port to couple a pressure transducer to help catheter positioning.

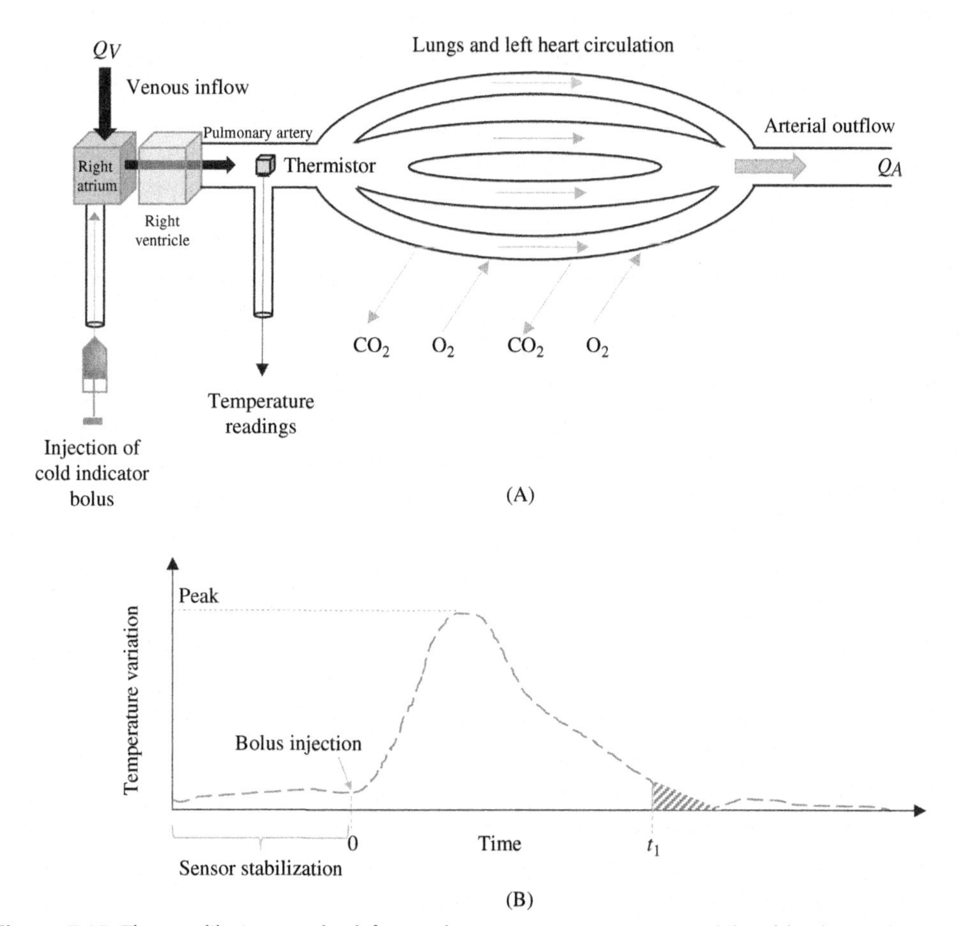

Figure 7.25 Thermodilution method for cardiac output measurement: (A) cold saline solution is injected at the right atrium and temperature is measured at the pulmonary atrium and (B) thermodilution curve.

When a thermal indicator is used to measure cardiac output, a modified Stewart–Hamilton equation is used to calculate cardiac output:

$$CO = \frac{\mathrm{Vol_I}\cdot(T_B - T_I)\cdot K}{\int_0^{t_1}\Delta T_B(t)\mathrm{d}t} \quad (7.59)$$

where

CO is the cardiac output
$\mathrm{Vol_I}$ is the injected bolus volume
T_B is the blood temperature measured at the pulmonary artery
T_I is the temperature of the saline solution injected at the right atrium
K is the correction constant

$\Delta T_B(t)$ is the integral of temperature change over time

t_1, the integral limit, is the time.

The correction constant K must be fed into the computer program that calculates CO and depends on the physical characteristics of the catheter (i.e., size and composition) and the indicator used (i.e., specific heat, specific gravity, and volume). The integral of temperature change over time is equal to the area under the thermodilution curve (Figure 7.25B). Any factor that reduces this area will overestimate the true cardiac output. Usually a series of three cardiac output measurements performed in rapid succession are averaged to provide a more reliable result.

Additional technical issues must be considered to interpret thermodilution measurements properly. The thermodilution technique measures right ventricular output and pulmonary artery blood flow. In the presence of some pathologies, the cardiac outputs of right and left sides of the heart are not the same, as are the cases of patients that have large left-to-right or right-to-left shunt, or severe tricuspid regurgitation. Other errors in the measurement of thermodilution cardiac output occur when pulmonary artery blood temperature changes because of rapid fluid infusion through a peripheral intravenous site.

An indicator bolus at room temperature volume of 10 ml is typically used in adults, and a smaller volume, 3–5 ml, in children. Iced indicator is more time-consuming and expensive to prepare and the use of injectate at room temperature results in equivalent accuracy in the cardiac output determinations. After decades of its development, thermodilution method is still considered the clinical gold standard technique for cardiac output monitoring measurement, due to its unique characteristics. It can be performed quickly and repeatedly and it employs a nontoxic, nonaccumulating, and nonrecirculating indicator.

7.3 REVIEW THE LEARNING

1. Choose one of the different types of differential pressure flow transducer, show its schematic diagram and explain its functioning. Discuss advantages and disadvantages of its use.
2. Show a schematic diagram of a variable area flow transducer. Can it be used to measure blood flow? Justify your answer.
3. How does a transit-time ultrasound flowmeter works? Show drawings and equations to complement your answer.
4. Show the schematic diagrams of Doppler ultrasound and Laser Doppler blood flowmeters. Explain their functioning and discuss the differences in their medical applications.
5. Explain how the electromagnetic induction principle is applied in an electromagnetic flowmeter. Show the schematic diagram of an invasive extravascular

electromagnetic flowmeter and explain its functioning. Show the construction solution to obtain an intravascular electromagnetic flowmeter. Discuss advantages and disadvantages of the use of intra- and extravascular flowmeters.

6. The "transformer voltage," which is generated when sinusoidal voltage excitation is applied in the core of the electromagnetic flowmeter, is an undesired output that saturates the flowmeter amplifiers in the conditioning circuitry. Show a solution to suppress voltage transformer and explain its operation.
7. What is plethysmography? Explain the working principle of chamber (or venous occlusion or limb) plethysmography technique and how it is used to measure blood flow. Complement your answer with a drawing showing how this technique is used to measure blood flow in a limb, arm, or leg. Show and explain the resulting curve. Discuss the advantages and disadvantages of this technique application for blood flow measurement.
8. Explain the working principle of PPG technique and how it is used to measure blood flow. What are the differences between transmission and reflection PPG? Complement your answer with drawings showing how this technique is used to measure blood flow in a limb, arm, or leg. Show and explain the resulting curve. Discuss the advantages and disadvantages of this technique application for blood flow measurement.
9. Explain the working principle of the SGP technique and how it is used to measure blood flow. Show and explain the resulting curve. Discuss the advantages and disadvantages of this technique.
10. Explain the working principle of IPG technique and how it is used to measure blood flow. Show and explain the resulting curve. Discuss the advantages and disadvantages of this technique application for blood flow measurement.
11. What is and how is the Fick method used for measurement of cardiac output? Complement your explanation with drawings showing the locations where substances are inserted/removed from the circulatory system to enable the calculus of the cardiac output. Discuss about advantages, disadvantages, and sources of errors of this method.
12. What is and how is the dye dilution technique used for measurement of cardiac output? Complement your explanation with drawings showing the locations where substances are inserted/removed from the circulatory system to enable the calculus of the cardiac output. Discuss about advantages, disadvantages, and sources of errors of this method, comparing it with Fick's technique.
13. What is and how is the thermodilution technique used for measurement of cardiac output? Complement your explanation with drawings showing the locations where substances are inserted/removed from the circulatory system to enable the calculus of the cardiac output. Discuss about advantages, disadvantages, and sources of errors of this method, comparing it with Fick's and dye dilution techniques.

REFERENCES

Allen, J. (2007). Photoplethysmography and its application in clinical physiological measurement. *Physiological Measurement, 28*, R1–R39.

Alomari, M. A., Solomito, A., Reyes, R., Khalil, S. M., Wood, R. H., & Welsch, M. A. (2004). Measurements of vascular function using strain-gauge plethysmography: technical considerations, standardization, and physiological findings. *American Journal of Physiology—Heart and Circulatory Physiology, 286*, H99–H107.

Atzler, E., & Lehman, G. (1932). Über ein neus verfahren zur darstellung de herztätigkit (dielektrogua-phie). *Arbeitsphysiologie, 5*, 636–680.

Barrat-Boyes, B. G., & Wood, E. H. (1957). The oxygen saturation of blood in the vena cavae, right heart chambers and pulmonary vessels of heathy subjects. *Journal of Clinical Medicine, 50*, 93–106.

Baulig, W., Bernhard, E. O., Bettex, D., Schmidlin, D., & Schmid, E. R. (2005). Cardiac output measurement by pulse dye densitometry in cardiac surgery. *Anaesthesia, 60*, 968–973.

Bernoulli, D. (1738). Hydrodynamica sive de viribus et motibus fluidorum commentarii. Argentorati, Johann Reinhold Dulsecker, <http://books.google.com.br/books?id = 3yRVAAAAcAAJ&pg = PP7 &hl = pt-BR&source = gbs_selected_pages&cad = 2#v = onepage&q&f = false> Accessed 10.06.14.

BioPortfolio. (2014). Biotech, Healthcare and Medical Resource. Indocyanine Green for Injection USP—Indocyanine Green. <http://www.bioportfolio.com/resources/drug/18311/Indocyanine-Green.html> Accessed 19.07.14.

Branthwaite, M. A., & Bradley, R. D. (1968). Measurement of cardiac output by thermal dilution in man. *Journal of Applied Physiology, 24*, 434–438.

Briers, J. D. (2001). Laser Doppler, speckle and related techniques for blood perfusion mapping and imaging. *Physiological Measurement, 22*, R35–R66.

Coates, A., Peslin, R., Rodenstein, D., & Stocks, J. (1997). Measurement of lung volumes by plethysmography. *European Respiratory Journal, 10*, 1415–1427.

Cobbold, R. S. C. (1974). *Transducers for biomedical measurements: Principles and applications.* New York: John Wiley & Sons.

Cobbold, R. S. C. (2007). *Foundations of biomedical ultrasound.* New York: Oxford University Press.

Cole-Parmer. Rotameters. Variable Area Flowmeters Tech Info. <http://www.coleparmer.com/TechLibraryArticle/813> Accessed 20.06.14.

Dally, J. W., Riley, W. F., & McConnell, K. G. (1993). *Instrumentation for engineering measurements* (2nd ed.). New York, Chichester: John Wiley & Sons.

Darrigol, O. (2009). *Worlds of flow: A history of hydrodynamics from Bernoulli to Prandtl.* Oxford: Oxford University Press.

Doebelin, E. O. (2004). *Measurements systems—Application and design* (5th ed.). New York: McGraw Hill.

Edwards, J. D., & Mayall, R. M. (1998). Importance of the sampling site for measurement of mixed venous oxygen saturation in shock. *Critical Care Medicine, 26*, 1356–1360.

Elgendi, M. (2012). On the analysis of fingertip photoplethysmogram signals. *Current Cardiology Reviews, 8*(1), 14–25.

Fegler, G. (1954). Measurement of cardiac output in anaesthetized animals by a thermodilution method. *Quarterly Journal of Experimental Physiology and Cognate Medical Sciences, 39*, 153–164.

FitzGerald, D. E., & Drumm, J. E. (1977). Non-invasive measurement of human fetal circulation using ultrasound: a new method. *British Medical Journal, 2*, 1450–1451.

Fox, I. J., & Wood, E. H. (1960). Indocyanine green: physical and physiologic properties. *Staff Meetings Mayo Clinic, 35*, 732–744.

Fredriksson, I., Fors, C., & Johansson, J. (2007). *Laser Doppler flowmetry—A theoretical framework.* Department of Biomedical Engineering, Linköping University <www.imt.liu.se/bit/ldf/ldfmain.html> Accessed 21.06.14.

Gabe, I. T., & Shillingford, J. P. (1961). The photoelectric earpiece techniques for recording dye dilution curves. *British Heart Journal, XXIII*, 271–280.

Garcia-Rodriguez, C., Pittman, J., Cassell, C. H., Sum-Ping, J., El-Moalem, H., Young, C., et al. (2002). Lithium dilution cardiac output measurement: A clinical assessment of central venous and peripheral venous indicator injection. *Critical Care Medicine, 30*(10), 2199–2204.

Gamble, J., Gartside, I. B., & Christ, F. (1993). A reassessment of mercury in silastic strain gauge plethysmography for microvascular permeability assessment in man. *Journal of Physiology, 464*, 407–422.

Geddes, L. A., & Baker, L. E. (1968). *Principles of applied biomedical instrumentation*. New York, NY: John Wiley & Sons.

Goldman, M. D., Smith, H. J., & Ulmer, W. T. (2005). Whole-body plethysmography. *European Respiratory Monograph, 31*, 15–43.

Hamilton, W., Moore, J., Kinsman, J., & Spurling, R. (1928). Simultaneous determination of the greater and lesser circulation time, of the cardiac output and an approximation of the amount of blood actively circulating in the heart and lungs. *American Journal of Physiology, 85*, 377–378.

Hamilton, W., Riley, R. L., Attyah, A. M., Cournand, A., Fowell, D. M., Hommelstein, A., et al. (1948). Comparison of the Fick and dye injection methods of measuring the cardiac output in man. *American Journal of Physiology, 153*, 309–321.

Hewlett, A. W., & van Zwaluwenburg, J. G. (1909). The rate of blood flow in the arm. *Heart, 1*, 87–97.

Hertzman, A. B. (1938). The blood supply of various skin areas as estimated by the photoelectric plethysmography. *American ournal of Physiology, 124*, 329–340.

Hertzman, A. B., & Spealman, C. R. (1937). Photoelectric plethysmography of the fingers and toes in man. *Proceedings of the Society for Experimental Biology and Medicine, 37*, 529–534.

Hokanson, D. E., Summer, D. S., & Strandness, D. E., Jr (1975). An electrically calibrated plethysmograph for direct measurement of limb blood flow. *IEEE Transactions on Bio-Medical Engineering, 22*(1), 25–29.

Hoskins, P. R. (2002). Ultrasound techniques for measurement of blood flow and tissue motion. *Biorheology, 39*(3-4), 451–459.

Iijima, T., Aoyagi, T., Iwao, Y., Masuda, J., Fuse, M., Kobayashi, N., et al. (1997). Cardiac output and circulating blood volume analysis by pulse dye densitometry. *Journal of Clinical Monitoring, 13*, 81–89.

Imai, T., Takahashi, K., Goto, F., & Morishita, Y. (1998). Measurement of blood concentration of indocyanine green by pulse dye densitometry: comparison with the conventional spectrophotometric method. *Journal of Clinical Monitoring and Computing, 14*, 477–484.

Jensen, J. A. (1996). *Estimation of blood velocities using ultrasound, a signal processing approach*. New York: Cambridge University Press.

Jhanji, S., Dawson, J., & Pearse, R. M. (2008). Cardiac output monitoring: basic science and clinical application. Review article. *Anaesthesia, 63*, 172–181.

Jonas, M. M., & Tanser, S. J. (2002). Lithium dilution measurement of cardiac output and arterial pulse waveform analysis: an indicator dilution calibrated beat-by-beat system for continuous estimation of cardiac output. *Current Opinion on Critical Care, 8*, 257–261.

Jones, D. P. (1987). Medical electro-optics: measurements in the human microcirculation. *Physics in Technology, 18*, 79–85.

Kamal, A. A. R., Harness, J. B., Irving, G., & Mearns, A. J. (1989). Skin photoplethysmography—A review. *Computer Methods and Programs in Biomedicine, 28*(4), 257–269.

Levick, J. R. (2009). *An introduction to cardiovascular physiology* (5th ed.). CRC Press.

Linton, R., Band, D., & Haire, K. M. (1993). A new method of measuring cardiac output in man using lithium dilution. *British Journal of Anaesthesia, 71*, 262–266.

Linton, R., Band, D., O'Brien, T., Jonas, M., & Leach, R. (1997). Lithium dilution cardiac output measurement: a comparison with thermodilution. *Critical Care Medicine, 25*, 1796–1800.

Klabunde, R. E. (2011). *Cardiovascular physiology concepts* (2nd ed., <http://www.cvphysiology.com/Hemodynamics/H007.htm> Accessed 16.06.14). Lippincott Williams & Wilkins <http://www.cvphysiology.com/Hemodynamics/H007.htm> Accessed 16.06.14.

Kolin, A. (1970). An electromagnetic catheter blood flow meter of minimal lateral dimensions. *Proceedings of the National Academy of Sciences of the United States of America, 66*(1), 53–56.

Macalpin, R. N., Kolin, A., & Stein, J. J. (1976). The external field intravascular electromagnetic flowmeter system as applied to standard arteriographic catheters and conscious humans. *Catheterization and Cardiovascular Diagnosis, 2*(1), 23–37.

Mahutte, C. K., & Jaffe, M. B. (1995). Effect of measurement errors on cardiac output calculated with O_2 and modified CO_2 fick methods. *Journal of Clinical Monitoring, 11*, 99–108.

Martins, M. A., Campos Filho, W. O., Viana, J. M., Nicolini, E. A., Campos, A. D., & Basile-Filho, A. (2003). Comparative analysis of cardiac output (CO) calculated by Fick's method and measured by indirect calorimetry in septic patients. *Revista Brasileira de Terapia Intensiva*, *1*(1), 5–14.

Mead, J. (1960). Volume displacement body plethysmograph for respiratory measurements in human subjects. *Journal of Applied Physiology*, *15*, 736–740.

Mills, C. J. A. (1966). A Catheter tip electromagnetic velocity probe. *Physics in Medicine and Biology*, *11*, 323–324.

Mills, C. J., & Shillingford, J. P. A. (1967). Catheter tip electromagnetic velocity probe and its evaluation. *Cardiovascular Research*, *1*(3), 263–273.

Nyboer, J., Bango, S., Barnett, A., & Halsey, R. H. (1940). Radiocardiograms: electrical impedance changes of the heart in relation to electrocardiograms and heart sounds. *Journal of Clinical Investigation*, *19* 773 (Abstract).

Nicholson, J. W., Burchell, H. B., & Wood, E. H. (1951). A method for the continuous recording of Evan's Blue dye curves in arterial blood and its application to the diagnosis of cardiovascular abnormalities. *Journal of Laboratory and Clinical Medicine*, *37*, 353–364.

Nilsson, G. E., Salerud, E. G., Strömberg, N. O. T., & Wårdell, K. (2003). Laser Doppler perfusion monitoring and imaging. In T. Vo-Dinh (Ed.), *Biomedical photonics handbook* (15, pp. 1–24). CRC Press.

Nitzan, M., Turivnenko, S., Milston, A., Babchenko, A., & Mahler, Y. (1996). Low-frequency variability in the blood volume and in the blood volume pulse measured by photoplethysmography. *Journal of Biomedical Optics*, *1*(2), 223–229.

Nyboer, J. (1960). Plethysmograph: impedance. In O. Gasser (Ed.), *Medical Physics* (vol. 3). Chicago: Yearbook Publishers. 459–471.

OMEGA (2014). *Transactions on measurement and control. Vol. 4 Flow and level measurement.* <http://www.omega.com/literature/transactions/Transactions_Vol_IV.pdf> Accessed 10.06.14.

Riva, C., Ross, B., & Benedek, G. B. (1972). Laser Doppler measurements of blood flow in capillary tubes and retinal arteries. *Investigative Ophthalmology*, *11*(11), 936–944.

Rajan, V., Varghese, B., van Leeuwen, T. G., & Steenbergen, W. (2009). Review of methodological developments in laser Doppler flowmetry. *Lasers in Medical Science*, *24*, 269–283.

Reed, J. H., & Wood, E. H. (1964). Use of dichromatic earpiece densitometry for determination of cardiac output. *Final report.* The Mayo Clinic and Mayo Graduate School of Medicine. <http://contrails.iit.edu/DigitalCollection/1964/AMRLTR64-134.pdf> Accessed 30.06.14.

Reekers, M., Simon, M. J. G., Boer, F., Mooren, R. A. G., van Kleef, J. W., Dahan, A., et al. (2009). Cardiovascular monitoring by pulse dye densitometry or arterial indocyanine green dilution. *Anesthesia & Analgesia*, *109*, 441–446.

Richards, M., Kripfgans, O., Rubin, J., Hall, A., & Fowlkes, J. (2009). Mean volume flow estimation in pulsatile flow conditions. *Ultrasound in Medicine & Biology*, *35*, 1880–1891.

Sakka, S. G., Reinhart, K., Wegscheider, K., & Meier-Hellmann, A. (2002). Comparison of cardiac output and circulatory blood volumes by transpulmonary thermo-dye dilution and transcutaneous indocyanine green measurement in critically ill patients. *Chest*, *121*, 559–565.

Saladin, K. S. (2011). *Anatomy and physiology* (6th ed.). Boston: McGraw-Hill.

Schäfer, E. A., & Moore, B. (1896). On the contractility and innervation of the spleen. *Journal of Physiology*, *20*, 1–51.

Schwan, H. P., & Kay, C. F. (1956). Specific resistance of body tissues. *Circulation Research*, *4*(6), 664–670.

Shepherd, A. P., & Öberg, P. Å. (1990). *Laser-Doppler blood flowmetry.* Boston: Kluwer Academic Publishers.

Stern, M. D. (1975). *In vivo* evaluation of microcirculation by coherent light scattering. *Nature*, *254* (5495), 56–58.

Stewart, G. N. (1897). Researches on the circulation time and on the influences which affect it. IV. The output of the heart. *Journal of Physiology*, *22*(3), 159–183.

Swan, H. J., Ganz, W., Forrester, J., Marcus, H., Diamond, G., & Chonette, D. (1970). Catheterization of the heart in man with use of a flow-directed balloon-tipped catheter. *New England Journal of Medicine*, *283*, 447–451.

Taylor, M. G., Coghlan, B. A., Beasley, M. G., & King, D. H. (1978). Automated strain-gauge plethysmograph. *Medical and Biological Engineering and Computing*, *16*(5), 554–558.

Thiriet, M. (2008). *Biology and mechanics of blood flows. Part 1: Biology. Part II: Mechanics and medical aspects. Series: CRM Series in Mathematical Physics.* Springer.

Visscher, M. B., & Johnson, J. A. (1953). The Fick principle: analysis of potential errors in its conventional application. *Journal of Applied Physiology, 5*, 635–645.

Webster, J. (Ed.), (2010). *Medical instrumentation. Application and design* (4th ed.). Hoboken, NJ: John Wiley & Sons.

Whitney, J. R. (1953). The measurement of volume changes in human limbs. *Journal of Physiology, 121*, 1–27.

Wilkinson, I. B., & Webb, D. J. (2001). Venous occlusion plethysmography in cardiovascular research: methodology and clinical applications. *British Journal of Clinical Pharmacology, 52*(6), 631–646.

Wyatt, D. G. (1982). Blood flow and blood velocity measurement *in vivo* by electromagnetic induction. *Transactions of the Institute of Measurement and Control, 4*, 61–78.

Yanof, H. M. (1960). A new trapezoidal-wave electromagnetic blood flowmeter and its application to the study of blood flow in the dog. PhD Thesis. University of California. Lawrence Radiation Laboratory, Berkeley, CA.

CHAPTER 8

Optical Transducers for Oximetry and Capnography

Contents

8.1 INTRODUCTION

Respiration provides oxygen (O_2) to tissues and removes carbon dioxide (CO_2) from tissues. The physiological function of respiration results from ventilation, which consists of mechanical actions to promote the cyclic exchange of alveolar gas with atmospheric air; diffusion of oxygen (O_2) and carbon dioxide (CO_2) between the alveoli and the blood; and transportation, through the blood, of O_2 and CO_2 between the lungs and other body tissues. Information about the adequacy of ventilation, the efficiency of gas exchange in the lungs, the transport of gases in blood and tissue oxygenation are essential in patients monitoring, especially if they are subjected to artificial ventilation or under anesthesia (adult, infant, and neonatal). The need for such information has led to the development of equipment for measuring the concentration of O_2 and CO_2 from blood samples, collected from vessels, and analyzed and tested *in vitro* in the laboratory (invasive methods), and also *in vivo*, by noninvasive methods, such as pulse oximetry and capnography.

Gas analyzers determine oxygen partial pressure (pO_2) using a specific electrode. Hemoximeters use spectrophotometric principle to measure directly the blood

Principles of Measurement and Transduction of Biomedical Variables.
DOI: http://dx.doi.org/10.1016/B978-0-12-800774-7.00008-8

oxyhemoglobin to hemoglobin ratio or hemoglobin saturation (SaO_2). The analysis of arterial blood performed with these devices, although accurate, requires the collection of a blood sample and laboratory analysis is invasive, slow, and oxygenation of the patient could change before lab results get ready.

Pulse oximetry is a noninvasive technique that monitors in arterial blood the percentage of available hemoglobin that is saturated with oxygen (SaO_2). This technique is based on the color changings of blood according to different levels of oxygen saturation, which are detected through optical transducers placed on the surface of the body, usually in the extremities, such as fingertip and ear lobe. Pulse oximetry is often used to monitor the blood oxygenation level in ICU, surgical room, during any procedure executed under anesthesia, as well as in burned units, ambulance transportation, sleep study, physical effort study, etc.

Capnography is also a noninvasive technique and it is used to determine CO_2 partial pressure in inhaled and exhaled air of the lungs of a patient during ventilation cycles. It helps to evaluate the cell metabolism through the amount of CO_2 removed from blood circulation, the adequacy of pulmonary perfusion and alveolar ventilation, the integrity of the artificial ventilation system connected to the airways of a patient who is receiving respiratory support or artificial ventilation. Capnography is also useful in the diagnosis of circulatory problems and malignant hyperthermia in patients under general anesthesia. An optical transducer coupled to the ventilation tube of the patient analyzes the concentration of CO_2 in the inhaled and exhaled breaths. The concentration of CO_2 in the exhaled air from the lungs, in the artificial ventilator, reflects indirectly the elimination of CO_2 by tissues and its transportation to the lungs, through circulatory system. Capnography is the golden pattern to detect intubation error, if the tube went to esophagus instead of the patient airways during the procedure, when little or none CO_2 is detected.

The principle of functioning of optical transducers is usually explained through the changes of intensity or phase of the light transmitted in or reflected by the measurand. The pulse oximeter functioning is based on a modification of Beer–Lambert's law, which relates the absorption of light by a solute to its concentration, and to its optical properties at a given light wavelength.

Using the premise that arterial blood is the only pulsatile absorbance between the light source and the photodetector, oximeter operation uses the absorbance characteristics of hemoglobin in the red and infrared range. The oxygen saturated hemoglobin, oxyhemoglobin, absorbs less light than the hemoglobin, deoxyhemoglobin, in the red region; in the infrared region, the inverse is true. Pulse oximeter utilizes two wavelengths of light, red and infrared, to measure the pulsatile changes in light transmission through living tissues, which are due to alteration of the arterial blood volume in the tissue along cardiac cycle. Measuring the pulsatile component eliminates the variable absorption of light by bone, nerve, tendon, fat, skin, pigment, venous blood, and steady volume of arterial blood.

In infrared spectroscopy, the samples under test should be in liquid or gaseous state, and this is one of the techniques used to determine the concentration of CO_2 in exhaled air, in the capnography examination. Capnography readings give information about the respiratory process and are obtained irradiating the inhaled or exhaled air with infrared light, with a wavelength at which occurs an absorption peak of CO_2 (4.26 μm). The amount of infrared radiation absorbed is proportional to the number of molecules of CO_2 (partial pressure of CO_2) present in the air sample, according to the Beer–Lambert law, and allows the calculation of the pressure of CO_2. The following text will show the basic optical techniques used in pulse oximetry and capnography devices.

8.2 PULSE OXIMETRY

In the blood, oxygen is transported dissolved in the plasma and covalently linked to hemoglobin, forming oxyhemoglobin. Under normal conditions, 97% of the oxygen is carried combined with hemoglobin, while only 3% is transported dissolved in the plasma. Oxyhemoglobin, or oxygenated hemoglobin, is bright red, which causes the skin and mucous membranes to have a pink appearance. Hemoglobin, or deoxyhemoglobin, is dark blue and thus, blood color varies according to its oxygenation level, from dark blue to bright red.

The first device used to determine blood oxygen saturation was invented in the 1930s, but it took decades before oxygen saturation measuring method began to be clinically used. Development of oximetry was driven during the 1940s due to lack of pressurization in aircrafts used in the World War II, which obliged pilots to use oxygen mask. Glenn Millikan developed under request of the British Army, a lightweight ear oxygen meter (i.e., the origin of the oximeter term). This device included a large and heavy galvanometer, which did not allow its use in aviation (Millikan, 1942). The oximetry technology was developed in the 1970s and had, since then, progressed into a relatively reliable noninvasive measurement of the blood oxygen saturation. The functioning of the pulse oximeter is based on the optical plethysmography and blood oximetry, to compute the oxygen saturation through the amount of colored light transmitted or reflected in the blood vessels, synchronized with cardiac pulse, which is the origin of the given name, pulse oximetry, to this technique.

Optical plethysmography technique allows to reproduce pulsatile blood waveform through the varying amount of light that is absorbed by blood. Spectrophotometry is a quantitative technique that irradiates a substance with one or more wavelengths (λ) and measures the different amounts of light that are absorbed and transmitted by the substance. The rates of absorption and transmission in a given λ are unique to each substance, and thus analyzing the light absorption in a different λ, the substance can be determined (Beer–Lambert Law). Pulse oximetry technique uses different wavelengths and measures blood oxygen saturation considering that the amount of light absorption by blood is distinct in each wavelengths used, and depends on the blood oxygenation level. In addition, the light transmitted through tissues has a pulsatile component due to the blood volume variation that occurs at each heartbeat, which can be separated from the nonpulsatile component that results from the light absorption by tissues and veins (Aoyagi, 2003; Carlson & Jahr, 1993; Chan, 2008; Geddes & Baker, 1968; Payne & Severinghaus, 1987; Severinghaus & Aoyagi, 2007; Severinghaus & Honda, 1987a, 1987b; Webster, 2010).

Hemoglobin absorbs different amounts of light according to wavelength and to oxygenation level. Oxyhemoglobin (oxy-Hb) and hemoglobin (Hb) have significantly different optical spectra in the wavelength range from 600 nm to 1,000 nm. The blue Hb absorbs red light, while the red oxy-Hb transmits red light. Figure 8.1 shows the absorption or extinction coefficient of Hb and oxy-Hb to wavelengths from 600 nm to 1050 nm.

The molar extinction coefficient (also called molar absorptivity) is a parameter that defines the intensity at which a substance absorbs light at a given wavelength per molar concentration. The isosbestic point, 805 nm, is the light wavelength at which the absorption, or extinction, coefficients of Hb and oxy-Hb are the same. Light absorption at this wavelength is independent of the O_2 saturation and it can be used as measurement reference. At wavelengths larger than isosbestic point, Hb absorption is lower than oxy-Hb and at lower wavelengths, Hb absorption is higher than oxy-Hb.

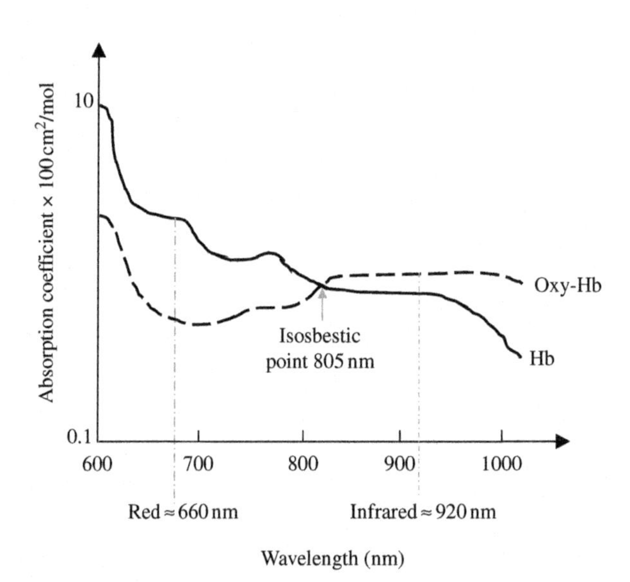

Figure 8.1 Absorption spectra of hemoglobin (Hb) and oxyhemoglobin (oxy-Hb). The isosbestic point is the wavelength at which light absorptions by Hb and oxy-Hb are the same.

8.2.1 Beer–Lambert law

Lambert's law (Johann Lambert, German physicist, 1728–1777) relates the amount of light absorbed and the distance the light travels through an absorbing medium. The intensity of transmitted light exponentially decreases with the increase of the distance:

$$I(\lambda) = I_0(\lambda)e^{-kd} \tag{8.1}$$

where

I is the intensity of the transmitted light

I_0 is the intensity of incident light

k is the absorptivity coefficient (constant) of the absorbing medium or molar extinction coefficient ($cm^2/\mu mol$)

d is the thickness of the absorbing medium or the distance that the light travels (cm).

Beer's law (August Beer, German physicist, 1825–1863) relates light absorption (or optical density) and the concentration of the absorbing substance in a medium. According to Beer's law, the absorptive capacity of a dissolved substance is directly proportional to its concentration. The intensity of the transmitted light in a medium exponentially decreases with the increase of the concentration of the absorbing substance:

$$I(\lambda) = I_0(\lambda)e^{-kc} \tag{8.2}$$

where

I is the intensity of the transmitted light

I_0 is the intensity of incident light

k is the absorptivity coefficient (constant) of the absorbing substance ($cm^2/\mu mol$)

c is the concentration of the absorbing substance in the medium ($\mu mol/cm^3$).

Figure 8.2 represents the Beer–Lambert's law components: the intensity of the transmitted light I decreases with the increase in the concentration c of the absorbing

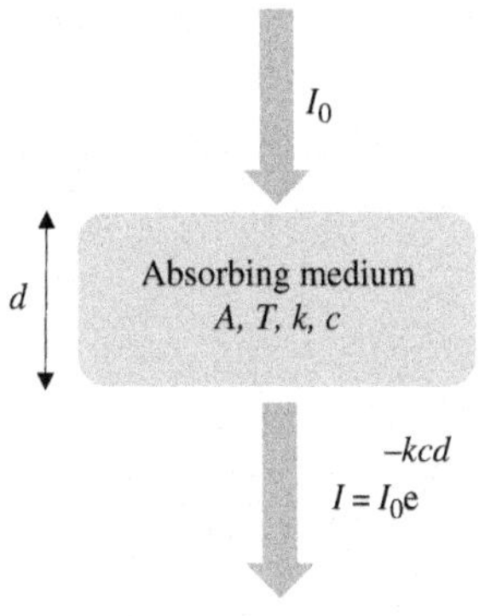

Figure 8.2 Schematic diagram showing the idealized model for validity of Beer–Lambert's law. A collimated, nonscattering monochromatic light source traveling through an absorbing medium with thickness d and absorbance $A = kcd$.

substance and the distance d. This is true for monochromatic light incident in a homogeneous medium. Equation (8.3) describes Beer–Lambert law:

$$I(\lambda) = I_0(\lambda)e^{-kcd} \tag{8.3}$$

where

k is the absorptivity coefficient (constant) of the absorbing substance ($cm^2/\mu mol$)
c is the concentration of the absorbing substance in the medium ($\mu mol/cm^3$)
d is the thickness of the absorbing medium (cm)
$kcd = A$ is the absorbance (also called optical density) of the medium.

The amount of absorbed radiation can be measured in several ways, among them, transmittance and absorbance. Transmittance is defined as

$$T = \frac{I(\lambda)}{I_0(\lambda)} \tag{8.4}$$

The percentage of transmittance is indicated by $\%T = 100T$. The absorbance A is a dimensionless term also called light attenuation. It indicates the order of magnitude of attenuation between the incident light I_0 and the transmitted light I. Absorbance is defined as the logarithmic attenuation of light traveling through an absorbing medium and it was described in the eighteenth century by Lambert and Bouguer. The Lambert–Bouguer law can be written as

$$A = \log\frac{I_0(\lambda)}{I(\lambda)} = kcd \tag{8.5}$$

The absorbance or optical density of a material relates to the tendency of the atoms of a material to maintain the absorbed energy of an electromagnetic wave in the form of vibrating electrons before reemitting it. The higher the absorbance A, the lower is the transmittance T. In terms of percentage of transmittance, absorbance is written as

$$A = \log\frac{1}{T} = \log\frac{100}{\%T} \tag{8.6}$$

$$A = 2 - \log\%T \tag{8.7}$$

In 1949, Wood and Geraci applied Beer–Lambert law to compute blood oxygen saturation, using two wavelengths, the red light wavelength, 605 nm, and the isosbestic point, 805 nm. The resulting equation was

$$SaO_2 = A + B\frac{OpD_{650}}{OpD_{805}} \tag{8.8}$$

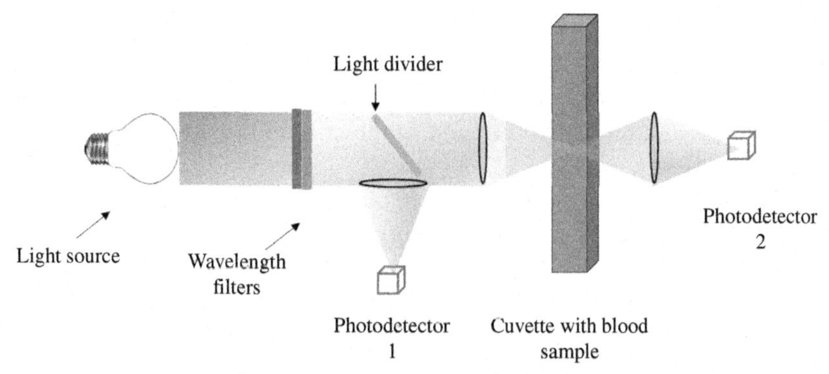

Figure 8.3 Main components of an oximetry instrument for laboratory use.

where

SaO_2 is the oxygen saturation (%)

OpD_{650} is the optical density of blood at 650 nm

OpD_{805} is the optical density of blood at 805 nm

$A = k_{805}/(k_{650\text{Hb}} - k_{650\text{oxy-Hb}})$

$B = k_{650\text{Hb}}/(k_{650\text{Hb}} - k_{650\text{oxy-Hb}})$.

Oximeters used in the laboratory to determine oxygen saturation of blood samples measure the blood absorbance in two wavelengths, which are transmitted through a cuvette where the previously hemolyzed blood is deposited. The blood optical densities at 650 and 805 nm are determined by Beer–Lambert equation (Eq. (8.3)) and then used in Wood and Geraci equation (Eq. (8.8)) to SaO_2 computing. Figure 8.3 shows the main components of a laboratory use oximeter. The wavelength filters are alternately used allowing that light with 650 and 805 nm get to the blood sample. With the help of the light divider, 5% of the emitted light is sent to photodetector 1 (I_0) and 95% to the cuvette and then to photodetector 2 (I). The incident and transmitted light intensities are used to compute OpD_{650}, OpD_{805}, and SaO_2 (Eq. (8.8)).

Equation (8.8) is based on the assumption that the hemolyzed blood sample consists of a two-component homogeneous mixture (Hb and oxy-Hb), that the light absorbance of the mixture of these two components is additive, and that it obeys Beer–Lambert's law, which requires a monochromatic light source and collimated light transmission through the sample, which therefore, does not contain light scattering particles.

8.2.2 Pulse oximetry

Wood and Geraci (1949) solution to obtain a noninvasive oximetry method based on Beer–Lambert's law was an ear oximeter. Ear tissue is far beyond an ideal cuvette and the oxygen saturation measurement had to compensate light scattering and reflection.

A device was used to pressurize ear lobe to a pressure level that would prevent the blood to flow and the light transmission was measured, stablishing a light attenuation baseline. Then the device was released and a second light transmission was performed. Both attenuation measurements, with and without blood, were subtracted to get the blood attenuation.

Further works described the influence of different parameters on the light transmission through intact blood, whose optical density is 7–20 times greater than optical density of solutions with the same hemoglobin concentration. The optical density differences between intact blood and hemoglobin solutions are due to light scattering effect in inhomogeneous medium. In the noninvasive oximetry, light absorption depends on several components. There is a continuous component due to tissue (skin, fat, bone, nerve, and tendon) scattering, reflection and absorption and venous blood absorption; and there is a pulsatile component, due to arterial blood volume added and removed with each heartbeat. In the 1970s, an ear oximeter was developed that measured SaO_2 comparing the intensity of light passing through the ear lobe at eight selected wavelengths in the range 650–1,050 nm. A heater maintained ear lobe temperature controlled at 41°C to increase the local arterial blood flow. A Tungsten lamp was used as a large spectrum light source and the eight wavelengths were obtained from narrow-band interference filters, mounted in a rotating wheel. The eight pulsed light beams were sent to the ear tissue through fiber optic cables, which helped to enlarge the ear probe size, bringing difficulty to neonatal use.

A different optical approach to measure arterial SaO_2 noninvasively was suggested by Aoyagi, Kishi, Yamaguchi, and Watanabe (1974) and Yoshiya, Shimada, and Tanaka (1980). They introduced the concept that the time-varying photoplethysmographic signal, caused by changes in arterial blood volume, associated with cardiac cycle synchronously with each heartbeat, is only due to the arterial blood component and is sensitive to changes in arterial oxygen saturation. Additionally, there is no pulse from the surroundings tissues. Figure 8.4 represents the light transmission through body tissues in a noninvasive SaO_2 measurement. The solution to get the actual noninvasive oximeter was to separate the pulsatile component of the light transmitted through the tissues, by filtering (high-pass filter—HPF) or digital processing, from the nonpulsatile component, resulting from light absorption by tissues, veins, and capillaries.

From Yoshiya et al. (1980) development, pulse oximeters began to use light emitting diodes (LEDs) as light sources. The two wavelengths, one red (~660 nm; 600–700 nm) and one infrared (~930 nm; 800–940 nm), transmitted through the skin, are differently absorbed by hemoglobin and oxygenated hemoglobin. Oxygen saturated blood absorbs less red light than oxygen depleted blood and absorption coefficients are the same at 805 nm. A photodetector is placed on the opposite side of the LEDs and collects the amount of received red and infrared lights. The pulse oximeter processes these signals, separating the time invariant parameters (tissue thickness, skin color, light intensity, and

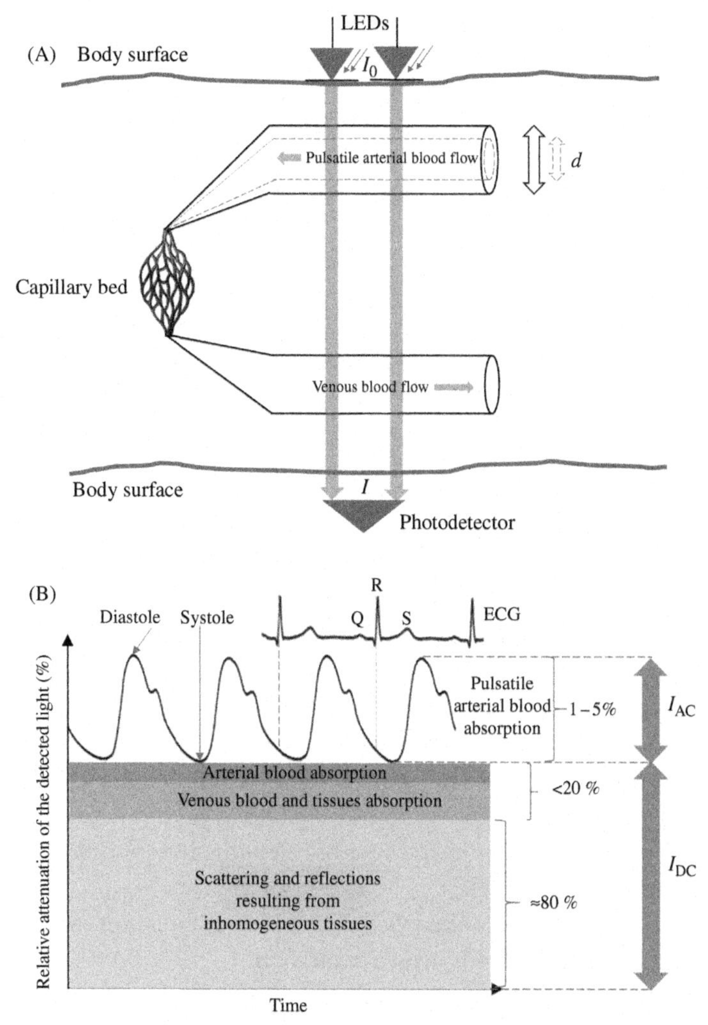

Figure 8.4 Principle of functioning of pulse oximetry. (A) Simplified model showing body tissues, blood vessels, incident and transmitted light. (B) Percentile contribution of the light attenuation components in pulse oximetry output signal. Pulsatile component of the current in the photodetector (1–5%) is commonly called I_{AC} alternate current and constant component is called I_{DC} direct current.

venous blood) from the time variant parameters (arterial volume and SaO_2) and the degree of absorption at each wavelength is used to estimate the Hb to oxy-Hb concentrations ratio, or the level of blood oxygen saturation and to identify the pulse rate. Only one photodetector can be used if the LEDs are alternately activated; usually a microcontroller is used to set the frequency and the sequence of activation of the LEDs. Pulse oximeter determines SaO_2 through the pulsatile component of the light detected by the

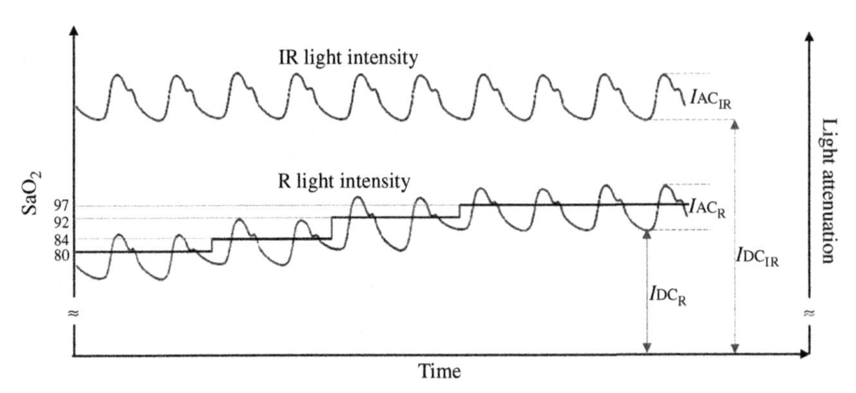

Figure 8.5 Representation of SaO_2 variation along time (straight line) and light attenuation output signals of the red (R) and infrared (IR) LEDs.

photodetector; this component represents <5% of the detected light. The peak amplitude of the pulsatile component (I_{AC}) occurs in the diastole and the minimum intensity corresponds to systole, in each heartbeat. The light attenuation by the nonpulsatile tissues is constant (I_{DC}) during cardiac cycle (Figure 8.4B).

Pulse oximeter usually shows SaO_2 instantaneous value and the curve of oxygen saturation variation along time. Figure 8.5 shows the pulse oximeter output along time while oxygen saturation varies from 82% to 97%. The light intensities at the red and infrared LEDs outputs are also shown. The infrared outputs (IAC_{IR} and IDC_{IR}) do not vary with oxygen saturation and the red light output intensities (IAC_R and IDC_R) variation reflects the blood oxygen saturation (SaO_2). The light absorption of oxyhemoglobin and deoxyhemoglobin in the two wavelengths is very different, which gives good sensitivity to pulse oximetry.

Equation (8.9) shows the modified Wood and Geraci equation used in commercial pulse oximeters to compute blood oxygen saturation:

$$SapO_2 = A + B\frac{\log(IAC_R/IDC_R)}{\log(IAC_{IR}/IDC_{IR})} \tag{8.9}$$

where

A and B are calibration constants, empirically determined and specific for each manufacturer

IAC_R is the current intensity of the pulsatile component at red wavelength

IDC_R is the current intensity of the constant component at red wavelength

IAC_{IR} is the current intensity of the pulsatile component at infrared wavelength

IDC_{IR} is the current intensity of the constant component at infrared wavelength.

Transmission pulse oximetry devices usually have the format of a clip with red and infrared LEDs and the light sensor oppositely located on the inner side of the clip.

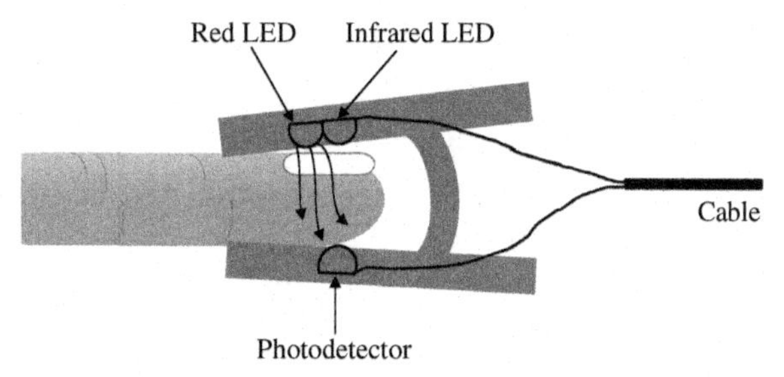

Figure 8.6 Transmission configuration of pulse oximetry.

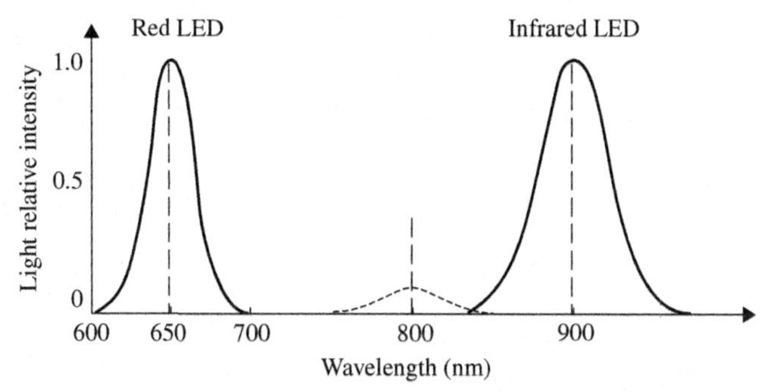

Figure 8.7 Relative light intensity as a function of wavelength of typical red and infrared LEDs used in SaO_2 transducers.

The clip is adjusted to the patient's finger or ear lobe (Figure 8.6). LEDs are fast and sequentially pulsed, while the photodetector synchronously captures the light from each LED as it is transmitted through the blood and tissue. Photodetector output current is sent by a cable, connected to the clip, to a microcontrolled unit. Steady-state absorption components are canceled while blood arterial time-varying component, at each wavelength, is used to calculate the absorption of Hb and oxy-Hb.

Semiconductor LEDs are a good choice as light source for SaO_2 transducers. Red and infrared LEDs are low cost and low power devices that have good light intensity in their outputs with narrow spectral half-bandwidths, but need to be fed with constant and DC current source. Figure 8.7 shows an example of the relative intensity as a function of wavelength of typical red and infrared LEDs used in pulse oximeter. Red LED spectrum is centered at 650 nm and has a half-bandwidth of 20 nm; there is a secondary emission at 800 nm, but its peak intensity is usually $<5\%$ of the peak intensity of the main emission. Infrared LED spectrum is centered at 900 nm and has a half-bandwidth of about 40 nm. They can be found as dual emitter LED, with both red and infrared LEDs mounted in the same package.

8.2.3 IR light sources and detectors

The photodiode has been the best light detector choice for decades, but lately there is a growing interest in using either a light-to-voltage or a light-to-frequency converter. When using a photodiode, considerable effort is made into shielding it from noise and its output is analog. Optical converters as light-to-voltage and light-to-frequency converters eliminate the need for additional shielding, and in addition have digital outputs, and therefore can interface directly with microcontroller units. Light-to-voltage and light-to-frequency converters are currently used in pulse oximeter systems and personal heart rate monitors.

Light-to-voltage optical converters, such as the TSL257 and TSL267 from AMS (AMS TSL257, 2014; AMS TSL267, 2014), detect light with high irradiance sensitivity (1.68 mV/(μW/cm^2) @ $\lambda_p = 645$ nm and 0.45 V/(μW/cm^2) @ $\lambda_p = 940$ nm, respectively) and are a low-noise optical detectors, which combine a photodiode and a trans-impedance amplifier on a single monolithic CMOS integrated circuit. It can make measurements with 16 bits resolution, low power dissipation, responds extremely fast (160 μs output rise time) and its output voltage is directly proportional to the light intensity that comes to the photodiode.

The TSL235R (AMS 235, 2014) light-to-frequency converter combines a silicon photodiode and a current-to-frequency converter on a single monolithic CMOS integrated circuit. It is an attractive choice as photodetector because its output is digital rather than analog and it also can make measurements with 16-bit resolution. The output voltage is a square wave (50% duty cycle), whose frequency is directly proportional to the light intensity that comes to the photodiode. This device is temperature compensated for the ultraviolet-to-visible light range of 320–700 nm and responds over the light range of 320–1,050 nm.

There are medical development kits commercially available that provide development platforms, specially designed to support complete medical applications, such as ECG monitor, stethoscope, and pulse oximeter. The platform usually includes analog front-end board, digital signal processing (DSP) and software for data processing and display. One example is the TMS320C5515 DSP Medical Development Kit da Texas Instrument (Texas Instrument TMS320C5515, 2010).

8.2.4 Transmittance and reflectance pulse oximetry

Transmission pulse oximetry is the most common used configuration. In the transmission or transillumination mode of operation, light source and photodetector are placed on opposite sides of the pulsatile bed. Transmittance oximeter transducer is placed in peripheral regions as fingertip and ear lobe, or even foot (neonates), to minimize light attenuation (Figure 8.6). Sometimes it is not possible to place the transducer in the extremities, due to blood perfusion problems or trauma, and then the reflection

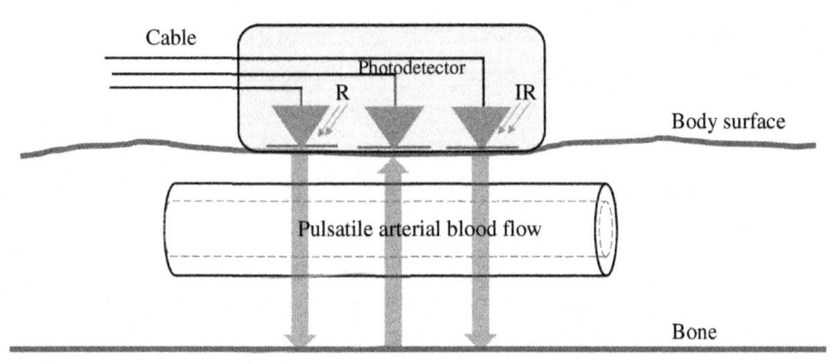

Figure 8.8 Reflectance configuration of pulse oximeter configuration.

configuration is preferred. The reflectance oximeter transducer has red and infrared LEDs and photodetector arranged side by side, facing the skin. In this case, there are fewer restrictions on the body location to place the transducer and light is emitted and collected in the same side of the body. Transducer has to be hold firmly against the skin, usually of the forearm or chest, in order to minimize movement artifact. Light is still reflected by blood and soft tissues, but mainly by the bones (Figure 8.8).

The pulse oximeter output can be connected to a computer, a multiparametric monitor or the measurement result can be displayed on its own screen. In the range of oxygen saturation between 90% and 100%, oximeters have an accuracy of ± 2%; from 70% to 89%, ± 3%; and when the saturation is below 70%, the accuracy greatly decreases (unspecified).

Pulse oximetry monitors continuously and instantaneously blood oxygen saturation and is responsive to little changes; sensibility depends on electronic components used (mainly photodetector) and digital resolution of signal processor. Factors that adversely affect accuracy of pulse oximeter output include transducer movement, peripheral vasoconstriction, low perfusion, edema, a nonpulsating vascular bed, hypotension, anemia, dysfunctional hemoglobin, changes in systemic vascular resistance, hypothermia, presence of intravascular dyes and nail polish, misalignment of LEDs and photodetector and optical interference of other light sources. Optical interference of ambient light is easily resolved, for example, wrapping the transducer with an opaque tape.

8.3 CAPNOGRAPHY

8.3.1 Introduction

Capnography is the monitoring of the concentration or partial pressure of carbon dioxide (CO_2) in the respiratory gases during respiratory cycle. Physiologically, CO_2 produced in the tissues and diffused into the venous blood reaches the right side of the heart and then the lungs, via pulmonary circulation. There, oxygen (O_2) enters the blood and CO_2 is removed and eliminated in the exhaled air by ventilation. Carbon dioxide can be measured in arterial blood gas, by specific electrode, as $PaCO_2$, whose normal range is 35–45 mmHg; it can also be measured in mixed venous blood as $PeCO_2$, which normal range is 46–48 mmHg. CO_2 is quantified by capnography technique, in exhaled air as $EtCO_2$ and its normal range is 35–45 mmHg. $EtCO_2$ (End-tidal CO_2) is the level of carbon dioxide released at the end of an exhaled breath (expiration). Carbon dioxide reflects cardiac output and pulmonary blood flow as the gas is transported by the venous system to the heart and then pumped to the lungs. When carbon dioxide diffuses out of the lungs into the exhaled air, the partial pressure or maximal concentration of the gas at the end of exhalation can be measured. The CO_2 continuous monitoring is obtained through capnography with the device named capnograph or capnometer, and the graphical display of these values along time is the capnogram.

Figure 8.9 shows the four phases of a typical capnogram. Phase I from A to B represents the beginning of expiration, when the exhaled air comes from the dead space from the trachea of the respiratory circuit. It defines the baseline (CO_2 partial pressure = 0 mmHg). Phase II, the fast rise from B to C, represents the initial increase of the CO_2 concentration due to the alveolar gas displacement toward airway where it mixes with the dead space air. The plateau of phase III (from C to D) corresponds to exhalation of the largest part of alveolar gas and CO_2 partial pressure reaches its maximum value (D) at the end of expiration. Phase IV, from D to E, is the inspiration phase when the CO_2 value in the airway becomes null. Then expiration begins again and the cycle is repeated.

Pulse oximetry reflects the status of oxygenation of the patient directly, but it does not help in establishing a differential diagnosis of hypoxia prior irreversible changes take place. Hypoxia is a pathological condition in which body tissues are deprived of oxygen. If hypoxia occurs, irreversible brain damage can be the result.

The capability of measurement of CO_2 in the expired breath of a patient has been an important technological advance in medicine. The measurement of CO_2 in the expired air directly indicates changes in the elimination of CO_2 from the lungs and

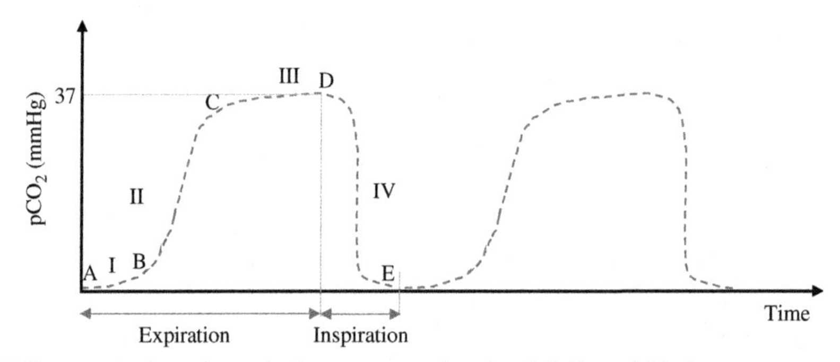

Figure 8.9 Representation of a typical capnogram showing I, II, III, and IV phases.

indirectly indicates changes in the production of CO_2 at the tissue level and in the delivery of CO_2 to the lungs by the circulatory system.

Capnography devices are very sensitive respiratory monitors and they are essential to identify adverse respiratory events in critical state patients, before brain damage occurs. Nonintubated patients undergoing moderate or deep sedation, under postgeneral anesthesia recovery in the immediate postoperative period or under critical care in the ICU, during treatment of respiratory diseases or in resuscitation scenarios, usually are being submitted to oxygen supplementation, which makes it difficult to detect respiratory depression with pulse oximeters, because they are not sensitive respiratory monitors, even more if oxygen is being administered (Downs, 2003; Fu, Downs, Schweiger, Miguel, & Smith, 2004; Hazinski, Samson, & Schexnayder, 2010; Weaver, 2011; Whitaker, 2011). The American Society of Anesthesiologists (ASA) published a guideline in which the use of capnometer is recommended to respiration monitoring (ASA, 2011). The Anesthesia Patient Safety Foundation (APSF) also recommends the capnometer as the most appropriate device for monitoring nonintubated patients in the presence of supplemental oxygen (Weinger & Lee, 2011).

Capnography is the method for determination of the values of the inhaled and exhaled CO_2 pressure over time (capnogram). It constitutes an important noninvasive technique providing data about cellular metabolism, transport of CO_2, alveolar ventilation, pulmonary perfusion, CO_2 production by respiration, respiratory pattern (hipo or hyperventilation), CO_2 elimination from patient circuit in the anesthesia machine, the adequacy of artificial ventilation (ventilator settings and malfunctions, tubing obstructions, disconnections and leaks in the ventilation system), and it helps to diagnose malignant hyperthermia and circulatory problems. It is the gold standard for detecting esophageal intubation, in which very little or no CO_2 is detected; the American Heart Association (AHA) affirmed the importance of using capnography to verify tube placement in their 2005 CPR and ECG Guidelines. Capnography also allows to calculate the amount of CO_2 pressure at the end of expiration phase, which is known as End-tidal CO_2 or $EtCO_2$ or $PetCO_2$ (Farish & Garcia, 2013; Jaffe, 2008; Weaver, 2011; Whitaker, 2011).

Among the various methods that can be used to measure concentrations of gases, the most common is the spectrophotometry, which is divided into four different types: mass, emission, Raman, and infrared. Mass spectrophotometry is the measurement of CO_2 and other gas concentrations based on differing molecular weights. Raman spectrophotometry uses spectral analysis of scattered light energy that results from an argon laser light source exposed to a gas mixture. Atomic emission spectrophotometry is a method of chemical analysis that uses the intensity of light emitted from a flame, plasma, arc, or spark at a particular wavelength to determine the quantity of an element in a sample. Infrared spectrophotometry is the analysis of infrared light interacting with a molecule, measuring absorption, emission, or reflection.

Infrared spectrophotometers are more compact and less expensive than the other methods of measurement and this has been the most popular technique for monitoring CO_2. Then, the capnograph is nothing more than an infrared spectrophotometer for CO_2 gas detection. Different chemical forms, both in gaseous phase and in liquid solutions, absorb radiation in specific bands of the light radiation spectrum. In addition to spectrophotometry, other methods may also be used to measure gas concentrations, including detection of thermal conductivity and detection with paramagnetic sensors (only for O_2).

Wavelengths in the infrared spectrum, from 3 μm to 30 μm, are frequently used to gas characterization. This is because many gases, each with its own chemical composition, absorb infrared radiation in different wavelength ranges in the electromagnetic spectrum, and the morphology of the spectral curve acts as a "fingerprint" of the specific gas. The infrared light is absorbed exclusively by liquid or gaseous state molecules formed by dissimilar atoms, because they have an electric dipole moment with which the electromagnetic wave can interact. CO_2, CO, N_2O (gas), H_2O, and volatile anesthetic agents (vapor) are examples of substances whose molecules are formed by dissimilar atoms.

Figure 8.10 shows absorption of CO_2, CO, N_2O, and water in the 2–8 μm wavelengths spectrum. CO_2 maximum absorption occurs at 4.26 μm and water absorbs a minimum amount of this radiation wavelength. A secondary absorption peak of CO_2 occurs around 2.7 μm and again, water absorbs radiation within the CO_2 spectrum.

O_2 does not absorb infrared radiation, but oxygen interferes with capnography due to the broadening effect on CO_2 absorption peak caused by the collision between O_2 and CO_2 molecules, which leads to a false increase in the CO_2 partial pressure measurement.

Eventually, the presence of N_2O and volatile anesthetic agents in the patient breath can interfere with CO_2 concentration measurement. Nitrous oxide absorption peak (4.5 μm) is near CO_2 maximum absorption, and its presence, in the sample chamber, therefore can

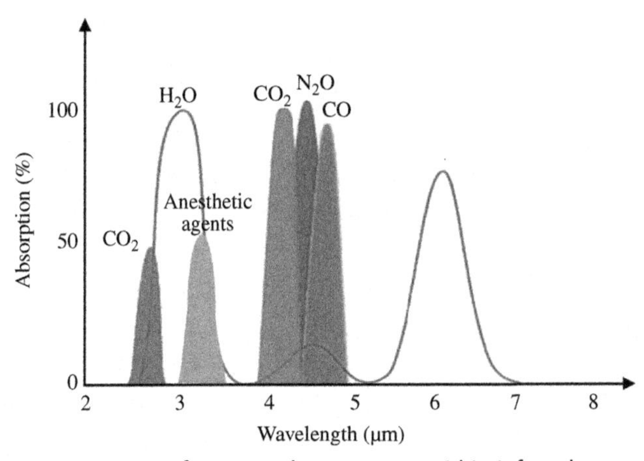

Figure 8.10 Absorption spectrum of water and some gases within infrared range.

result in high CO_2 readings. This N_2O influence can be minimized using a collimated IR light beam and a narrow-band IR filter. Nitrous oxide presence also can cause "collision broadening effect," contributing to an error in the CO_2 reading. The compensation of the other absorptions than CO_2 allows the correct determination of the carbon dioxide concentration value. Most capnographs provide some system of electronic or digital compensation to pressure, O_2, N_2O, and anesthetic agents.

Determining the CO_2 concentration in human breath by measuring its infrared absorptive power was established as a reliable technique by John Tyndall in 1864, though initial devices developed in nineteenth and early twentieth century were not ideal for everyday clinical use due to size and weight (Jaffe, 2008). In 1943, the first infrared carbon dioxide measuring and recording apparatus was developed. It was called URAS or "Ultra Rot Absorption Schreiber" (Infrared Absorption Writer). It was big, heavy, and very impractical to use. In the next decades, capnography technique has evolved and also capnographs with the development of new technologies. The first practical and commercially successful CO_2 mainstream sensor was the HP 4710A Capnometer; it calculated and displayed the end tidal and instantaneous CO_2 values as well as the respiration rate, and had settable alarms for the $EtCO_2$ and respiration rate. In the 1980s, respiratory filters were introduced to prevent infection and contamination and in the 1990s, the use of these filters became patient single use (Ragg, 1994). Until 2003, medical mainstream CO_2 analyzers were limited to capnography, when one Swedish company, PHASEIN, introduced the first fully integrated mainstream anesthesia multigas analyzer (PHASEIN, 2009).

Generally, the infrared capnography gaseous sample of exhaled air, for example, and a gas reference sample with known concentration of CO_2, are irradiated by a light source wavelength equal to 4.26 μm. Carbon dioxide selectively absorbs the specific wavelength 4.26 μm of IR light. A photodetector, usually a photodiode, collects the radiation that passes through the sample at this wavelength, and its output current is directly related to the incident radiation. The amount of infrared radiation absorbed is proportional to the number of molecules of CO_2 (partial pressure of CO_2) in the sample chamber, and according to Beer–Lambert's law (Eq. (8.3)), allows to calculate CO_2 pressure. Figure 8.11 shows a diagram of the basic functioning of capnography by infrared spectrophotometry. Since the amount of light absorbed is proportional to the concentration of the absorbing molecules, the concentration of CO_2 can be determined by comparing the measured absorbance with the absorbance of a known standard.

8.3.2 Electromechanic and solid-state transducers

Capnography technique can be implemented with electromechanic and solid-state transducers. Figure 8.12 shows the schematic diagram of an electromechanic transducer.

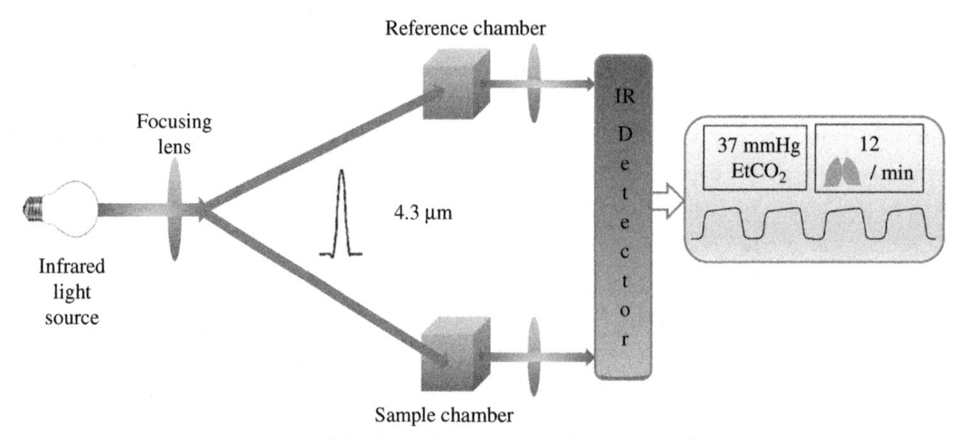

Figure 8.11 Schematic diagram of the basic functioning of a typical infrared capnograph.

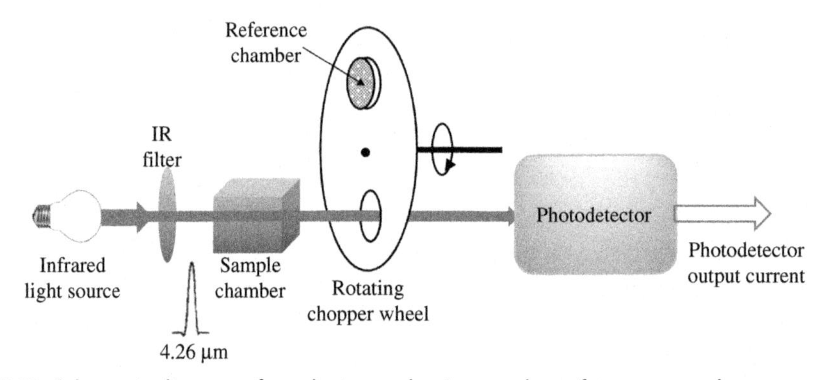

Figure 8.12 Schematic diagram of an electromechanic transducer for capnography.

The electromechanical transducer (Figure 8.12) has an infrared light source that emits broad spectrum radiation (2–16 μm). Infrared radiation sources used in capnography must have high irradiance, uniform emissivity, large radiant area, and spectral uniformity. The radiation from real sources is always less than that from an ideal blackbody, which has maximum emissivity (1.0). The hot filament of quartz tungsten halogen lamps provides strong near-infrared output. There are micromachined IR sources, which are thermal infrared emitters, electrically modulated, that show radiation characteristics similar to the ideal blackbody in the range 2–14 μm, low power consumption, high emissivity (≈ 0.95), and long lifetime. The resistive heating element of MEMS IR source is integrated in a thin and low mass dielectric membrane, which is suspended on a micromachined silicon structure. A Sapphire, CaF_2, BaF_2, or Germanium broadband filter improves the signal to noise ratio, and acts as a spectral low-pass filter (2–6 μm, 2–11 μm, 2–13 μm, and 2–>14 μm, respectively) (Axetris).

In Figure 8.12, the broadband IR light beam passes through an interference filter, which transmits light in the wavelength of the maximum absorption of CO_2, 4.26 μm, with bandwidth equal to 0.07 μm. The light beam is sampled at low frequency (some tens of Hz) by a rotating chopper wheel. As the wheel rotates, there is a position where IR light passes through the sample chamber and the radiation is absorbed by CO_2 molecules present in the exhaled air. In a second position, IR light passes through the sample and the reference chambers. Reference is a sealed chamber with known CO_2 concentration gas. In the remaining positions, no light crosses the rotating wheel or gets to detector. The radiation that passes through the wheel, and was not absorbed by CO_2 molecules, is collected by the photodetector, usually a GeAs photodiode. The pulsed photodiode output current has frequency equal to the sampling and its amplitude is modulated by the amount of transmitted radiation. The intensity of the oscillating signal is processed to determine the carbon dioxide concentration in the patient breath.

Due to mechanical moving parts, electromechanic transducer tends to be fragile. The solid-state transducer is an option. The solid-state transducer (Figure 8.13) uses an electronically pulsed IR light source, eliminating the need of the rotating chopper wheel. The IR source emits a narrow-band radiation centered at 4.26 μm, which passes through the sample chamber and is partially absorbed by CO_2 molecules. The IR emitter can be a hot filament made from Tungsten or special metal alloy. Ideally, it should be very stable, intense, and collimated radiance (4.26 μm) with high emissivity and long lifetime.

A beam splitter divides the IR radiation that was not absorbed; then the IR beams pass through two optical filters before getting to photodetectors (Figure 8.13). The bandwidth of one filter is centered at CO_2 maximum absorption spectrum, and the other, outside this band (<4 μm), to act as reference. Temperature affects narrow-band optical filters causing a shift in the center wavelength, which leads to a loss of sensitivity in the capnometry. This problem is traditionally minimized stabilizing the

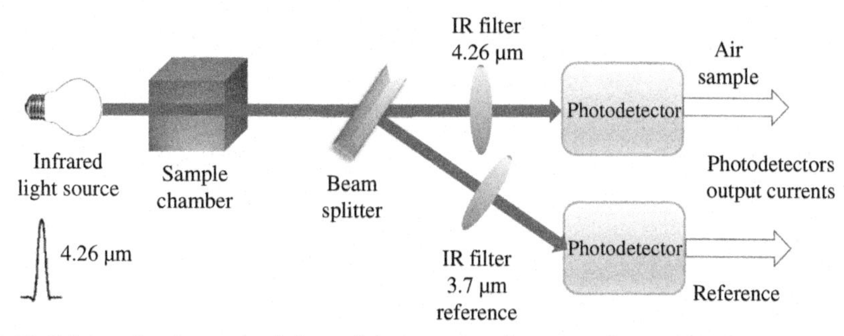

Figure 8.13 Schematic diagram of the solid-state transducer used in infrared spectrophotometry capnography.

device at an elevated temperature, at the cost of higher power consumption and a delay in the startup operation time. Technological solution to minimize this problem arose from a special thin film deposition process that compensates the layer thickness variations due to changes in temperature, and thus, stabilizes the central wavelength of the optical filter (Masimo Sweden AB, 2014; PHASEIN, 2009).

A quantification of the concentration of CO_2 in the gas mixture can be obtained by simultaneously sampling the outputs of the detectors, that is, the intensity of the IR radiation that was not absorbed in the chambers (sample and reference). The ratio of the photodetector output intensities is compared to a lookup table to determine the CO_2 concentration. Typically, photodiodes are used to detect the attenuated infrared beam light. PbSe photoconductive detectors are also used in many mainstream CO_2 analyzers and they respond adequately from 1.5 to 5.2 μm; they present high sensitivity and high-speed response at room temperature, but if cooled, their signal to noise ratio becomes higher.

Pyroelectric detectors are responsive in the spectral range from 4 to 10 μm, have low-noise characteristics at room temperature and are insensitive to temperature variations. Thermopile detectors are used in some multigas analyzers and their response cover the interest spectral range but are slow in response (Masimo Sweden AB, 2014; PHASEIN, 2009). Yang, An, Wang, and Wang (2010) proposed a double-ended sidestream CO_2 monitor with pyroelectric detector, in which air sample is irradiated by 4.0 and 4.3 μm. The nonabsorbed radiations got to reference and sample thermocouple detectors, respectively, that are part of a thermopile. The output EMF is proportional to the difference of detector temperatures, which in turn is due to the difference in radiation absorbed in each detector. Thus, the EMF signal amplitude reflects CO_2 concentration in the exhaled breath. After amplification, filtering, and digitalization, wavelet-based algorithms processing provides CO_2 partial pressure. According to the author, the device can accurately monitor the cardiopulmonary status during anesthesia and mechanical ventilation in real time.

In solid-state transducers, the incoming IR light is electronically pulsed, instead of mechanically sampled. The main advantage of solid-state transducers is the durability of electronic components compared to mechanical moving parts.

Some CO_2 monitors also have multigas monitoring capability. Basically, they have the same IR broadband radiation source, but a larger number of optical filters; specific filter and processing software are selected according to the gas being analyzed.

8.3.3 Sampling systems

There are two basic configurations of capnograph use according to sampling system: mainstream and sidestream. In the mainstream or nonaspirative system, the light absorption chamber is directly attached to the patient-ventilator airway. In the sidestream or aspirative system, a tubing is connected to the patient-ventilator airway and with the help of a pump, the gases mixture is continually aspirated at a rate of 50–400 ml/min to the sample chamber. Sidestream configuration usually affects tidal volume, which is the volume of gas exchanged during each ventilated breath, or the volume of air exhaled per minute. There is a third configuration, which is a side-stream variation, named low flow or microstream system. In this configuration, the sample chamber volume is only 15 μl, the air is aspirated at a low rate (50 ml/min), and the response time is faster than the conventional sidestream. In addition, tidal volume is minimally affected.

8.3.3.1 Mainstream system

Mainstream system is used only with intubated patients under artificial ventilation. Transducer is placed between endotracheal tube and the respiratory circuitry in a flat region of the trachea tube. Coincident windows in this flat region and in the trans-ducer allow the inspired and expired gas to flow directly across the IR light path and the IR radiation to pass through the air that is being breathing in and out the intubated patient, as shown in Figure 8.14A.

The heater and the temperature sensor inside the sample chamber are used to maintain the temperature above the body temperature, preventing water condensation to form and accumulate in the transducer windows, which could block the light pas-sage. In this system, the transducer is connected directly in the patient airway and does not reduce the tidal volume. Due to first models' large size, mainstream CO_2 transducers were considered bulky and difficult to be used directly in endotracheal tube. Modern models are durable, small, and lightweight. Their main advantages are fast response time to CO_2 concentration changes and elimination of water traps needed in the sidestream system. As the transducer casing contains IR source, optical filters, lens and electronics, they should be protected from fallings.

8.3.3.2 Sidestream system

In the sidestream configuration system (Figure 8.14B), the CO_2 transducer is placed outside the patient airway, for example, in the main unit, and requires the air sample to be constantly aspirated from the airway of the breathing circuit, by a pump, and sent to the sample chamber. The patient is not under artificial ventilation, but receiv-ing a ventilation support by means of an oronasal mask or a nasal cannula.

Sidestream system is used in nonintubated patients and transducer is not connected directly in the patient airway, but in the sample chamber, where the air comes through a lateral tubing connected to the airway. Response time to CO_2 concentration changes is not as fast as in the mainstream configuration and the continuous with-drawing of the breath sample can reduce the tidal volume in the patient circuit. Delay in measurement response time depends on the diameter and length of the tubing.

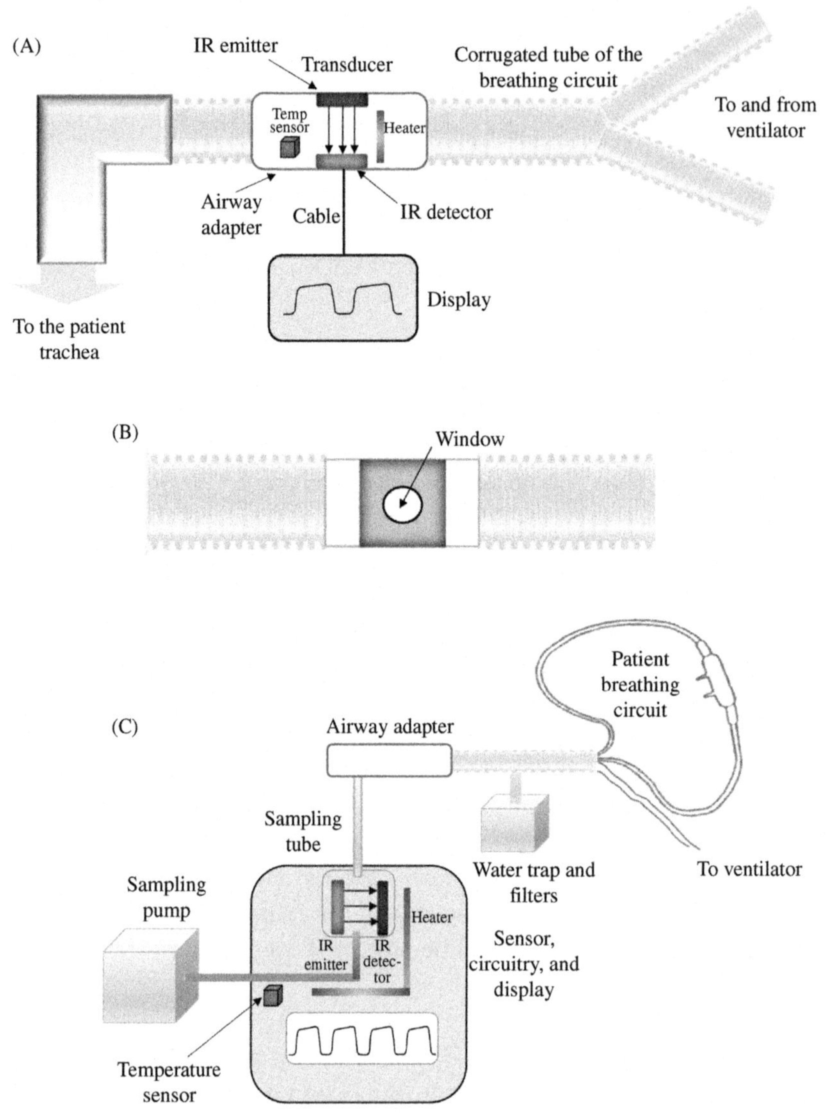

Figure 8.14 Schematic diagram of the positioning of capnography sensors in (A) mainstream and (C) sidestream. (B) The corrugated tube has a flat region where mainstream transducer is connected with a window to allow IR radiation to pass through the air that is being breathing in and out by the intubated patient.

Transducer alone is lightweight and sidestream system allows obtaining accurate capnography values when attached as close as possible to the patient. Maximum recommended air tubing length is 6 ft or 1.8 m, which allows the transducer to be located inside the main unit, with electronic circuitry and display.

The main disadvantage of sidestream system is that condensation of humidified gases and water vapor may cause frequent clogging of the tubing for withdrawing of the air sample. The water trap and filters are used to prevent condensation from reaching the measuring chamber and to prevent machine contamination. A heater is used to increase the chamber temperature to a value a few degrees higher than body temperature, also to prevent water vapor condensation; a temperature sensor (e.g., thermistor) helps to control this temperature.

8.3.3.3 Microstream (low flow) system

In the sidestream system with conventional method of IR spectrophotometry, to CO_2 measurement, the sampling cell uses up to 150 ml of exhaled air and the flow should be between 40 and 200 ml/min, to meet adult and pediatric patients, but may reach 400 ml/min. The microstream system uses molecular correlation spectrography (MCS) that operates at room temperature and emits only CO_2 specific IR radiation, with a high-collimated laser beam focused precisely at 4.26 μm. This CO_2 specificity and sensitivity of the emitter allows the use of an extremely short light path, in other words, the use of very small sample cell (15 μl), which in turn allows the use of low flow rate (50 ml/min), without compromising accuracy and resulting in a fast response time.

Microstream system aspires 50 ml/min of the patient breath, a lower value than the rate typically required by conventional sidestream capnographs. The low flow rate can contribute to reduce the presence of moisture and humidity in the sampling tube and chamber. The moisture and humidity condensation tends to obstruct airflow and optical pathway, which is a common problem with conventional sidestream system. Another advantage of the low flow rate use, without affecting response time, is that the smaller air volume aspired from the patient circuit practically does not affect tidal volume, which is important mainly in infant and neonate patients that have low tidal volumes.

Instead of a black body-like IR source, MCS uses a glass discharge lamp, without an electrode, coupled to an IR transmitting window. The window is made from sapphire, for very high signal to noise ratio, or from high IR transmission glass (nitrogen-based glass), for standard functions. The glass lamp is filled with a balanced mixture of up to seven gases, including Nitrogen (N) and CO_2, at low pressure. Electrons generated by a radio frequency voltage excite N molecules, which in turn, collide with CO_2 molecules. When the excited CO_2 molecules are back to their energy resting state, they emit the CO_2 signature wavelength, which is the radiation emitted by the source. The output of the glass lamp is electronically modulated at a frequency of 40 Hz. The amplitude of each signal that leaves the photodetector every 25 ms is proportional to the radiation absorbed in the sample chamber, which is proportional to the CO_2 concentration in the patient breath. The photodetector output is processed (amplified, digitalized, and compared to stored absorption curves) to provide the partial pressure of CO_2 in the patient breath. The high sensitivity and specificity of MCS absorption characteristic provides high signal to noise characteristics in the final displayed waveform (Colman & Krauss, 1999; Kodali, 2013).

As microstream system works at room temperature (25°C), initialization time is smaller than in conventional sidestream. Commercial models display the capnogram in <30 s and devices are fully functional in a few minutes. A pressure transducer coupled to the sampling tubing controls the flow rate (50 ml/min $\pm$ 10 ml/min). The CO_2 measurement range is 0–150 mmHg. The capnograph manufacturers provide the resolution and accuracy values of the measurements according to flow range, e.g., resolution of 1 mmHg in the range 0–70 mmHg and accuracy $\pm$5% from 40 to 70 mmHg. Usually no user calibration routine is required. Special oronasal masks allow nasal and oral breath sampling to CO_2 measurement and also provides O_2 delivery (up to 5 ml/min) without diluting CO_2 sample (Oridion, 2008; Respironics, 2010).

Capnography is a measurement technique that allows to obtain the partial pressure (mmHg) or volume (% vol) of CO_2 in the airway at the end of exhalation. It is a breath-to-breath measurement that provides CO_2 information within seconds, and it is not affected by motion artifact, poor perfusion, or dysrhythmias.

8.4 REVIEW THE LEARNING

1. What are the main information about body functioning obtained from blood oxygen saturation?
2. What are the main information about body functioning obtained from exhaled breath carbon dioxide concentration?
3. What are the main methods to calculate gas concentration in gaseous or liquid solution? Explain briefly how infrared spectrophotometry works.
4. Explain how optical plethysmography technique is applied in pulsatile oximetry. Use Beer–Lambert equation and Figures 8.1 and 8.4 in your answer.
5. Describe the transmittance configuration of pulsatile oximetry. Show a schematic diagram with the components of the transducer and the light interactions with blood. Which are the body regions better suited to place the oximeter? Why?
6. Describe the reflectance configuration of pulsatile oximetry. Show a schematic diagram with the components of the transducer and the light interactions with blood. Which are the body regions better suited to place the oximeter? Why?
7. Show the schematic diagram of a capnography transducer designed to work with mainstream system. Give the name of all components and explain their function. Then explain the overall functioning of the transducer.
8. Show the schematic diagram of a capnography transducer designed to work with sidestream system. Give the name of all components and explain their function. Then explain the overall functioning of the transducer.

9. Show the schematic diagram of a capnography transducer designed to work with microstream system. Give the name of all components and explain their function. Then explain the overall functioning of the transducer.
10. Which are the most important characteristics of microstream system compared to the conventional sidestream system?

REFERENCES

American Society of Anesthesiology (ASA) (2011). Standards for basic anesthetic monitoring.

AMS TSL235R (2014). Light-to-frequency converter. <http://www.ams.com/eng/Products/Light-Sensors/Light-to-Frequency-Sensors> Accessed 10.07.14.

AMS TSL257 (2014). Light to voltage converter. <http://www.ams.com/eng/Products/Light-Sensors/Light-to-Voltage-Sensors/TSL257> Accessed 10.07.14.

AMS TSL267 (2014). Light to voltage converter. <http://www.ams.com/eng/Products/Light-Sensors/Light-to-Voltage-Sensors/TSL267> Accessed 10.07.14.

Aoyagi, T. (2003). Pulse oximetry: Its invention, theory and future. *Journal of Anesthesiology, 17*, 259–266.

Aoyagi, T., Kishi, M., Yamaguchi, K., & Watanabe, S. (1974). Improvement of an earpiece oximeter. In *Abstracts of the Japanese society of medical electronics and biological engineering* (pp. 90–91).

Axetris. Infrared source for gas detection and monitoring. <http://www.axetris.com/en-ch/irs?nr=true> Accessed 16.08.14.

Carlson, K. A., & Jahr, J. S. (1993). A historical overview and update on pulse oximetry. *Anesthesiology Review, 20*, 173–181.

Chan, A. Y. K. (2008). *Biomedical device technology: Principles and design*. Springfield, Ill: Charles C. Thomas.

Colman, Y., & Krauss, B. (1999). Microstream capnography technology: A new approach to an old problem. *Journal of Clinical Monitoring, 15*, 403–409.

Downs, J. B. (2003). Has oxygen administration delayed appropriate respiratory care? Fallacies regarding oxygen therapy. *Respiratory Care, 48*(6), 611–620.

Farish, S. E., & Garcia, P. S. (2013). Capnography primer for oral and maxillofacial surgery: Review and technical considerstions. *Journal of Anesthesia & Clinical Research, 4*(3), 295–320 <http://www.ncbi.nlm.nih.gov/pmc/articles/PMC3897173/pdf/nihms510361.pdf> Accessed 12.08.14.

Fu, E. S., Downs, J. B., Schweiger, J. W., Miguel, R. V., & Smith, R. A. (2004). Supplemental oxygen impairs detection of hypoventilation by pulse oximetry. *Chest, 126*(5), 1552–1558.

Geddes, L. A., & Baker, L. E. (1968). *Principles of applied biomedical instrumentation*. New York, NY: John Wiley & Sons.

Hazinski, M. F., Samson, R., & Schexnayder, S. (2010). *Handbook of emergency cardiovascular care for healthcare providers*. Dallas, TX: American Heart Association.

Jaffe, M. B. (2008). Infrared measurement of carbon dioxide in the human breath: "Breath-through" devices from Tyndall to the present day. *Anesthesia & Analgesia, 107*(3), 890–904.

Kodali, B. S. (2013). Physical method of CO_2 measurement. *Physics of Capnography*, <http://www.capnography.com/new/index.php?option=com_content&view=article&id=216&Itemid=1016> Accessed 10.08.14.

Masimo Sweden, A. B. (2014). Capnography and multigas monitoring solutions. <http://www.masimo.com/capnography/technology.htm> Accessed 10.07.14.

Millikan, G. A. (1942). The oximeter: An instrument for measuring continuously oxygen saturation of arterial blood in man. *Review of Scientific Instruments, 13*, 434–444.

Oridion (2008). Introducing Surestream™ CO_2 sampling lines. <http://www.procamed.ch/pdf/oridion_surestream.pdf> Accessed 15.08.14.

Payne, J. P., & Severinghaus, J. W. (Eds.), (1987). *Pulse oximetry*. New York, NY: Springer-Verlag.

PHASEIN, A. B. (2009). Mainstream gas analyzers. A historical and technological perspective. 1–8. <http://www.masimo.com/pdf/phasein/Mainstream-Gas-Analyzers-A-Historical-and-Technological-Perspective.pdf> Accessed 10.08.14.

Ragg, M. (1994). Transmission of hepatitis C via anaesthetic tubing? *Lancet*, *44*, 367–373.

Respironics (2010). LowFlo Sidestream CO_2 Sensor. <http://oem.respironics.com/Downloads/LoFlo020513.pdf> Accessed 15.08.14.

Severinghaus, J. W., & Aoyagi, T. (2007). Discovery of pulse oximetry. *Anesthesia & Analgesia*, *105*, S1–S4.

Severinghaus, J. W., & Honda, Y. (1987a). History of blood gas analysis. VII. Pulse oximetry. *Journal of Clinical Monitoring*, *3*, 135–138.

Severinghaus, J. W., & Honda, Y. (1987b). Pulse oximetry. *International Anesthesiology Clinics*, *25*, 205–214.

Texas Instrument TMS320C5515 (2010). DSP medical development Kit. Texas instrument application report. <http://www.ti.com/lit/an/sprab37a/sprab37a.pdf> Accessed 13.08.14.

Weaver, J. (2011). The latest ASA mandate: CO_2 monitoring fro moderate and deep sedation. *Anesthesia Progress*, *58*, 111–112.

Webster, J. (Ed.), (2010). *Medical instrumentation. Application and design* (4th ed.). Hoboken, NJ: John Wiley & Sons.

Weinger, M. B., & Lee, L. A. (2011). No patient shall be harmed by opioid-induced respiratory depression. *APSF Newsletter, Fall.*

Whitaker, D. K. (2011). Time for capnography-everywhere. *Anaesthesia*, *66*, 544–549.

Wood, E. H., & Geraci, J. E. (1949). Photoelectric determination of arterial saturation in man. *The Journal of Laboratory and Clinical Medicine*, *34*(3), 387–401.

Yang, J., An, K., Wang, B., & Wang, L. (2010). New mainstream double-end carbon dioxide capnograph for human respiration. *Journal of Biomedical Optics*, *15*(6) 065007-065007-6.

Yoshiya, I., Shimada, Y., & Tanaka, K. (1980). Spectrophotometric monitoring of arterial oxygen saturation in the fingertip. *Medical & Biological Engineering & Computing*, *18*, 27–32.

CHAPTER 9

New Technological Advancements in Biomedical Variables Transducing

Contents

9.1 INTRODUCTION

Chapters 2–8 presented the principle of functioning of basic transducers for main biomedical variables measurement. Most of these principles were discovered more than a century ago and modern transducers are a transcription of the initial knowledge to the technological development achieved in the last decades, mainly in the electronic and material engineering areas. The following text presents some of the new technological advancements that were recently discovered or are being designed and developed for biomedical transducers. New technologies searched by scientists aim to increase the efficiency of biomedical variables measurements, in order to obtain more exact, fast, low-power consumption, and low-cost values. These new technologies can contribute to greater safety, accuracy, and reliability of the use of medical transducers.

9.2 NEW ADVANCES IN BIOMEDICAL VARIABLES TRANSDUCING

Biomedical transducers participation in advanced diagnostic, therapeutic, and monitoring systems is continuously enhanced by the contribution of the advancements in electronic devices, equipment and automation, material sciences and signal and image processing, to register temperature, pressure, concentration of chemical molecules (gases, electrolytes, metabolites, and drugs), position, level, torque, velocity and acceleration, flow (blood, air), electrical activities of body systems (EMG, EEG, and ECG), among other variables. Microsystem technologies, such as MEMS, silicon-based sensors, and microfluidic chips, revolutionized the biomedical electronics segment, resulting in devices of smaller sizes, greater accuracy and precision characteristics, advanced control and low power.

In the last decades, numerous types of medical devices used in medical applications, such as surgical, radiological, physical medicine, orthopedic, ophthalmic, obstetrics,

Principles of Measurement and Transduction of Biomedical Variables.
DOI: http://dx.doi.org/10.1016/B978-0-12-800774-7.00009-X

gynecology, neurological, gastroenterology, urology, cardiovascular, and anesthesia, became more and more dependent of sensors of temperature, pressure, chemical, level, flow, position, etc., due to the increasing seek for greater precision, accuracy and reliability of acquisition and processing of biomedical variables. This "sensing" dependence increased the demand for the development of new transducer technologies, which includes the use of nano and fiber-optic technologies, temperature transducers with several temperature sensing devices, ICT (information and communication technology)-enabled advancements, etc. The development of wireless sensor is one of the major focus areas among novel and upcoming fields of research in biomedical applications. At the same time, several new application fields are continuously emerging for transducers in medical area, for example, in the use of communication technologies for transmission of data acquired through patient home-monitoring.

Technological advancements in microsystem technologies, contributed to MEMS sensors new applications in blood pressure, respiratory and kidney-dialysis monitoring, pacemakers, silicon microphones, micro-actuators and microelectrodes for hearing aids and cochlear implants, micro-pumps for infusion drug delivery, needle-free injection devices, IR ear thermometers, ultrasound sensors, implanted systems for drug delivery, wireless systems for patient monitoring, advanced imaging devices (resolution, miniaturization), sensors for computer-assisted surgery (force feedback, surgery robots), smart pills for drug delivery, closed-loop systems for drug delivery, miniaturized instruments combining sensors and effectors for image-guided therapy and so on.

Blood-sampling sensors, such as glucose and potassium meters, that need only micro-volumetric blood samples, tissue-embedded sensors, such as those used in pacemakers and defibrillators, ingestible sensors embedded in dissolvable pills, that are able to sense temperature, heart and respiration rates, and wireless implantable and wearable physiological monitoring devices attached to the body surface, which also transmit blood chemistry data to an external processor, can provide comfortable (minimally invasive), secure, and low-cost physiological monitoring for a variety of medical applications (computer-assisted physical rehabilitation, arrhythmias monitoring, vital signs monitoring, insulin pump, pain relief pump, etc.).

Immunoassays use antibodies to detect protein biomarkers, with a substantial global market and significant importance for clinical practice. By definition, a biomarker is a characteristic that is objectively measured and evaluated as an indicator of normal biological processes, pathogenic processes, or pharmacologic responses to a therapeutic intervention. Most of the so-called biomarkers are still in an exploratory phase and are thus assayed by research-grade tests, requiring laboratories with highly trained specialists. Immunoaffinity-based assays are the mainstay of testing for proteins and by 2010, commercial tests were available for more than 200 different proteins, using various methodologies. Traditional immunoassays are performed in centralized laboratories using optical detection methods, which means that results can take days (Cummings, Ward,

Greystoke, Ranson, & Dive, 2008; Qoronfleh & Lindpainter, 2010). There have been efforts to develop all-electronic immunoassays through impedance detection method, which is a much faster technology than optical readout. In addition, all-electronic immunoassays have the benefit of increasing the throughput of immunoassays, once measurement on a chip-based microfluidic device with miniaturized reservoirs uses submicroliter volume of blood and can be performed in minutes; the test allows measuring a much higher number of protein biomarkers in a single blood sample. The utilization of common silicon microfabrication technology in the device construction (reservoir, electrodes, etc.) also reduces the cost of the immunoassay (compared to conventional optical technique) and allows integration with other microfluidic components. The concept of an all-electronic biosensor is that the association of antigens to antibodies causes impedance change, and thus, through this impedance change is possible to determine if certain antigens are present in the blood sample (Saleh & Sohn, 2006; Wu & Voldman, 2013).

For a few decades, researchers have been investigating sensing fabrics, wireless microsensor networks, and communication protocols to remote physiological parameters monitoring of soldiers in battlefield, elderly and chronically ill patients during home care, hospitalized children and noncooperative adults or even anesthetized patients in the operating room. The wearable physiological monitoring systems must give reliable recordings of medical data compared to the conventional physiological monitoring systems and they are supposed to monitor continuously the patient for periods long as a few days. Continuous monitoring of chronically ill patients, with early detection of health problems, increases quality of life and allows normal activities of daily life, rather than staying at home or close to specialized medical services (Jovanov, Milenkovic, Otto, & de Groen, 2005; Pandian et al., 2008; Raskovic, Martin, & Jovanov, 2004; Valdastri et al., 2008).

In the last years, patch or epidermal sensor or digital tattoo has gained the interest of scientists in order to develop thin, elastic, transparent, and skin-friendly self-adhesive electrodes. The development of lightweight, foldable, and stretchable formats of electronic circuits with the same performance of rigid semiconductor wafers, would enable their application in medical areas including wearable systems for personal health monitoring and therapeutics. The patch can incorporate multiple sensors including ECG, EMG, and accelerometer, for example, to allow measurement of heart rate and muscle activity, sleep monitoring, and other physiologic metrics. The patch adhesive must be skin-friendly to accommodate different daily activities, such as exercising, sleeping, eating, or taking a shower and remain in place for several days without detaching of the skin or causing irritation and eliminating displacement artifact, electrolyte application and frequent replacement of electrodes. Another example of application of patch sensors, in addition to biopotential monitoring is in the surgical gloves with integrated microelectronic sensors, which could measure directly, during surgical procedures, the flow and pressure of blood, tissue temperature, and thickness of the ventricular wall. These wearable systems integrate inorganic electronic materials, as for example, arrays of nanoribbons of single crystalline silicon used in the digital and analog circuits, with structural ultrathin substrates made from plastic and elastomeric materials (Kim et al., 2008).

Ingestible pills with sensors and even imaging capability are among the newest technology innovations. Among the actual available and most often used medical imaging modalities, tomography (CT), magnetic resonance imaging (MRI), transabdominal ultrasound (TUS), and conventional endoscopy, none can assist in obtaining the image of some body parts, such as the small bowel (Nylund et al., 2009). Recently wireless capsule endoscopy (WCE) technology has been developed to substitute the conventional modality (Given Imaging Inc., 2014). An ingestible pill that can be used for ultrasound imaging of the small bowel, essentially combining the benefits of WCE and TUS was developed. Patients can simply swallow the pill, which will travel through the gastrointestinal tract via peristalsis while ultrasound imaging the surrounding wall. The image data is wirelessly transmitted to an outside sensor belt and the pill is excreted naturally. The overall system is small (around 1 cm in diameter and 3 cm in length) and contains miniaturized 10 MHz ultrasound transducer and related electronics, transmitter, control and power management circuits and a battery (Lee, Anthony, & Boning, 2013).

Today, ingestible sensors are integrated inside inactive pills that dissolve when they are taken. They can also be used to accurate assessment of a patient's adherence to prescribed pharmacotherapy; the sensor is integrated inside the medication pill, which dissolves, then the sensor becomes active and sends the information to an external wireless wearable device. The monitor records ingestion time and date and also collects physiologic data and communicates (e.g., via mobile phone) to a secure server that integrates the data with other wireless devices (e.g., blood pressure, weight) (Au-Yeung et al., 2010; DiCarlo, 2012; Vrijens & Urquhart, 2014). In the future, the ingestible sensor could be integrated directly inside active pharmaceutical pills, in select therapeutic areas, together with drug delivery control circuits (Eisenberger et al., 2013). For example, a sensor to monitor cardiac activity could be taken alongside medication for heartbeat regulation, and the delivered doses of the drug would be adjusted by a control circuit, inside the sensor, according to the heartbeat value sent to a wearable monitor device (wireless) in the outside.

Fifteen-year-old teenage Jack Andraka, became known in whole world, when he created in 2012, a rapid and extremely inexpensive test, which could 1 day enable earlier detection of pancreatic cancer. The test, which is still under development by industry, uses carbon nanotubes combined with an antibody that reacts in the presence of a protein, mesothelin that exists in the blood of people with pancreatic cancer. Embedding the antibody in nanotubes allowed Andraka to create a paper sensor strip that costs only three cents, but is 90% accurate (Tucker, 2012).

One of the biggest challenges of rehabilitation engineering is to recover disrupted nerves in the spinal cord of patients who have suffered spinal injury. Spinal cord injury (SCI) leads to paralysis, decrease in quality of life, and high lifetime medical costs. Direct nerve functional electrical stimulation (FES) induces muscles to contract by electrically stimulating nerves, and it shows promise for clinical applications in restoring muscle function in SCI patients. FES is limited by the lack of graded response in muscle contraction and by high fatigability due to the complexity of the order in which motor units are recruited. Neuromuscular fatigue is difficult to identify and to prevent. Researchers look forward to electrical stimulation strategies to overcome fatigue and to activate specific muscular groups responsible for the development of controlled limbs movement. The design and the fabrication of ion-selective electrodes for *in vitro* intracellular recording (Guenat et al., 2005) led to the development of ion-selective membrane technologies, which can enable *in vivo* measurements. Song et al. (2011) showed that ion-selective membranes could be used to modulate the transmembrane calcium ions (Ca^{2+}) exchange, decreasing the current threshold for nerve stimulation, and eliciting a more graded muscle contraction response; they used planar glass-based electrodes. Khaja and Han (2013) developed flexible, elastic, conductive, and ion-selective polyimide-based cuff electrodes and realized in *in vitro* tests obtaining a decrease in the stimulation current threshold of frog sciatic nerve. Nerve stimulation with the cuff ion-selective electrodes resulted in higher decrease in the current threshold, twitch width, contraction time, and relaxation time than traditional electrical stimulation at all tested contraction force levels. Low-threshold stimulation method obtained with ion-selective electrodes is applicable in current implantable neuroprosthetic devices, whereas the on-demand nerve-blocking mechanism could offer effective clinical intervention in disease states caused by uncontrolled nerve activation, such as epilepsy and chronic pain syndromes (Song et al., 2011). Ion-selective electrodes may in the near future be used in spinal cord implantable devices to restore communication between central nervous system and skeletal muscular system in paralyzed patients.

Temperature measurement and monitoring are important in medical routines to identify any abnormal increase in the body temperature, indicative of the presence of infectious diseases. Temperature transducers are used to monitor the temperature of patients undergoing surgical procedures performed under the effect of volatile anesthetic agents, to identify malignant hyperthermia as soon as it begins. Newborns usually are kept in temperature-controlled environment and baby's skin and circulating air temperatures difference must be null in order to minimize heat loss from the baby's body to the ambient. Medical drugs, blood, and vaccines need to be stored at special environment conditions, among them, specific and narrow temperature ranges. Some biological drugs are damaged if stored at the wrong temperature, even at room temperature. They must be stored at a temperature between 2°C and 8°C. Small pox vaccine should be kept at even below 0°C. Biological products or antibiotics should be kept in refrigerators (2−15°C). Therefore, temperature control is critical, both of patient's body as substances that need to be maintained at specific temperatures.

Examples of devices that store drugs, blood, and other chemical substances and that produces temperature-controlled environment, which need temperature monitoring are refrigerators, ultra-low temperature freezers, cold rooms, liquid N_2 tanks, and incubators. Wireless sensor networks are capable of getting temperature, humidity, or luminosity measurements and transmit data from a storage device to a remote server periodically. Real-time conditions can then be monitored in order to know when a problem in the device happens, avoiding critical situations. Reliable and accurate temperature transducers and monitoring systems are essential in order to keep fragile patients in safety and to store substances in the correct conditions. Adequate temperature transducers must be powered by a durable battery, lightweight, long life, capable of integration with other sensors and equipment and should have high stability precision and linearity. Manufacturers of integrated electronic circuits develop devices with these characteristics to medical temperature sensing. One example is the ADT7420/320 Digital Temperature Sensor (Analog Device Temperature Sensor, 2014), highly accurate (±0.25°C) digital temperature sensors that offer high precision, high-linearity, low-drift and 16-bit resolution over a wide range of temperatures (−20°C to +105°C), which includes the working temperature range of the main biomedical applications. These temperature sensors are plug-in ready devices, requiring no additional signal conditioning or calibration. They have I^2C (ADT7420) or SPI (ADT7320) digital interfaces, which allow easy integration with data acquisition, optical communications, environmental control systems, and medical equipment for temperature monitoring. They also are low-power consumption: 700 μW at 3.3 V/210 μA (typical). ADT7420/7320 are commercialized with 16-lead RoHS-compliant LFCSP package, which allows the development of new temperature transducers as well the replacement of RDT and thermistor of older projects to enhance their characteristics.

Displacement or position transducers (linear and angular), pressure, velocity, acceleration, and torque are used in many medical applications, such as devices that monitor and control the execution of the movement caused by electrical stimulation of paralyzed limbs of patients with cerebral palsy, paraplegia, or tetraplegia. Equipments used in robot-assisted surgery and wearable devices are other examples of use of these transducers. Displacement transducers also work as the primary sensors of different types of pressure transducers, velocity, and acceleration. The development of new materials, light, thin, and flexible to adjust to the shape of the body where they are used, with greater scale of miniaturization, allied to new electronic devices of ultra-low power and high integration scale, and fast software systems for control, information processing and integration between sensors and equipment, are challenges pursued by researchers worldwide.

In the area of prosthesis design, as well in robotics, researches seek for inexpensive, light, flexible, stretchable, and water-and-heat resistant sensors; in addition, sensor areas should be wide and sensible to pressure and shear. These would be the ideal sensors, mainly if mounted in arrays, to be integrated into a skin analog (Lacasse, Duchaine, & Gosselin, 2010; Yamada et al., 2011). Some projects seek to meet these requirements combining the piezoresistive property of composites made from polydimethylsiloxane (PDMS) with carbon black (CB) (Yaul & Lang, 2012). The uncured composite is molded directly into a solid PDMS membrane to form a sensing skin, which can be used to coat an artificial limb (electromechanic or robotic prostheses). D'Asaro, Bulović, and Lang (2013) designed a pressure and shear transducer, which consists of three linearly arranged electrical contacts made from silver/PDMS composite, embedded in PDMS/CB composite. Pure PDMS is used to form the structure of the skin. Each of these materials is extruded onto a plastic membrane, which is removed after curing. Under pressure, the resistances between the center contact and each of the edge contacts are roughly equal. However, when sheared, the resistances between the center contact and the two edge contacts change differently, allowing differentiating between both types of input. D'Asaro et al. transducer prototype still needs some improvements to reduce output drift and to increase the useful pressure-and-shear sensitive area.

Polymer nanocomposites (nanoparticles dispersed in a polymer matrix) have versatile applications in the field of electronic materials, such as integrated decoupling capacitors, acoustic emission sensors, and angular acceleration accelerometers. The addition of nanoparticles to a polymer matrix can enhance mechanical, thermal, barrier, and other properties. Many studies have been done on $BaTiO_3$ due to their remarkable optical and electronic properties. A matrix of PDMS elastomer combined with barium titanate ($BaTiO_3$) nanoparticles results in the PDMS$-$$BaTiO_3$ nanocomposite, which dielectric properties vary according to the concentration of nanobarium titanate. The dielectric constant of the nanocomposite increases significantly with the increase of $BaTiO_3$ concentration, while the volume resistivity decreases (Nayak, Chaki, & Khastgir, 2013).

Optical transducers are important components of pulse oximetry, capnography, and other medical devices. They use photocomponents (emitters and detectors), which work with collimated beams, usually in a narrow range of wavelengths, optical circuits (beam splitters, wavelength filters), and electronic circuits (current and voltage amplifiers). Since the 1990s, researchers seek to develop a new type of component that would allow the construction of various systems/functions within the same optical circuit. The combination of electronics and photonics (capable of carrying information in the form of light) on the same microchip is the goal of the so-called "silicon photonics," which could allow the construction of the same optical circuit several key components such as wavelength filters and beam splitters. The integrated circuit would receive and process information in the form of light.

From the need of obtaining invisibility in various military applications, initially through absorbing electromagnetic waves emitted from radar to minimize the corresponding reflection and scattering, whose optical properties are manipulated in the real permittivity–permeability plane, researchers have been engineering metamaterials, with optical properties designed and manipulated in the complex dielectric-permittivity plane (Leonhardt, 2006; Makris, El-Ganainy, Christodoulides, & Musslimani, 2008; Pendry, Schurig, & Smith, 2006; Rüter et al., 2010).

Recently, an international group of researchers from CalTech (California Institute of Technology, USA), Nanjing University (China), ITA (Instituto de Tecnologia Aeronaútica, Brasil), and IEAv (Instituto de Estudos Avançados, Brasil), created and experimentally demonstrated the operation of a new photonic device, of micrometric scale, compatible with the CMOS manufacturing process used in the semiconductor industry (Feng et al., 2013). The device has the ability to reflect optical waves in one direction and on the same frequencies used today with fiber optics in telecommunications. They showed the experimental realization of chip-scale unidirectional reflectionless optical metamaterials near the spontaneous parity-time symmetry phase transition point, where reflection from one side is significantly suppressed.

The device developed by the international group of researchers is made from silicon, silicon dioxide, germanium, and chromium, all of them passive materials, compatible with the CMOS fabrication process used in the semiconductor industry. The designed passive unidirectional reflectionless parity-time metamaterial has periodically arranged 760-nm-wide sinusoidal shaped combo structures, which were applied on top of 800-nm-wide Si waveguide embedded inside SiO_2 to mimic parity-time optical potentials. A single-mode waveguide directional coupler with ≈ 3 dB of coupling ratio was designed to maximize the detected signal. Prototype width, 20–30 μm, is still subject to optimization, in order to reduce even more dimensions. Numerical simulations and experimental verification consistently exhibit asymmetric reflection with high contrast ratios around a wavelength of 1.550 μm, which is in the near-infrared region of the electromagnetic spectrum (from about 800 to 2,500 nm).

The results obtained by Feng et al. (2013) of the unidirectional phenomenon at the corresponding parity-time exceptional point on-a-chip confirm the feasibility of creating on-chip parity-time (PT) metamaterials and optical devices, of higher complexity, based on their properties. According to Feng and colleagues (2013), the microscopic scale photonic device and its property of reflecting light in only one direction, can have other macroscopic scale uses then the aerospace application and military defense, including the area of sensors and integrated microchip systems based on silicon photonics, in order to assist medical diagnosis, for example, with near-infrared spectroscopy (NIRS). NIRS is a spectroscopic method that uses the near-infrared radiation in applications, such as pharmaceutical, medical diagnostics (blood sugar measurement and pulse oximetry), as well as research in functional neuroimaging, sports medicine and science, ergonomics, rehabilitation, neonatal research, brain computer interface, and urology. This technology is very promising and could revolutionize the field of medical diagnosis in the coming decades, through a multidisciplinary approach.

REFERENCES

Analog Device Temperature Sensor (2014). ADT7420/320 digital temperature sensor. <http://www.analog.com/static/imported-files/data_sheets/ADT7320.pdf> 2012 Initial version; <http://www.silica.com/product/adt7420320-025c-accurate-16-bit-digital-t.html> 2010 preliminary version. Accessed 20.08.14.

Au-Yeung, K. Y., Robertson, T., Hafezi, H., Moon, G., DiCarlo, L., & Zdeblick, M. (2010). A networked system for self-management of drug therapy and wellness. In *Proceedings of the WH'10 wireless health* (pp. 1−9).

Cummings, J., Ward, T. H., Greystoke, A., Ranson, M., & Dive, C. (2008). Biomarker method validation in anticancer drug development. *British Journal of Pharmacology, 153*, 646−656.

D'Asaro, M. E., Bulović, V., & Lang, J. H. (2013). Stretchable pressure- and shear-sensing skin printed from PDMS. MTL (Microsystems Technology Laboratories, Massachusetts Institute of Technology) Annual Research Report 2013. <http://www-mtl.mit.edu/wpmu/ar2013/stretchable-pressure-and-shear-sensing-skin-printed-from-pdms/> Accessed 20.08.14.

DiCarlo, L. A. (2012). Role for direct electronic verification of pharmaceutical ingestion in pharmaceutical development. *Contemporary Clinical Trials, 33*(4), 593−600.

Eisenberger, U., Wüthrich, R. P., Bock, A., Ambühl, P., Steiger, J., Intondi, A., et al. (2013). Medication adherence assessment: High accuracy of the new ingestible sensor system in kidney transplants. *Transplantation, 96*(3), 245−250.

Feng, L., Xu, Y.-L., Fegadolli, W. S., Lu, M.-H., Oliveira, J. E. B., Almeida, V. R., et al. (2013). Experimental demonstration of a unidirectional reflectionless parity-time metamaterial at optical frequencies. *Nature Materials, 12*, 108−113.

Given Imaging Inc. (2014). Capsule endoscopy. PillCam® SB 3. <http://www.givenimaging.com/en-int/Innovative-Solutions/Capsule-Endoscopy/Pillcam-SB/PillCam-SB-3/Pages/default.aspx> Accessed 25.08.14.

Guenat, O. T., Dufour, J. T., van der Wall, P. D., Morf, W. E., Rooij, N.-F., & Koudelka-Heo, M. (2005). Microfabrication and characterization of an ion-selective microelectrode array platform. *Sensors and Actuators B: Chemical, 105*, 65−73.

Jovanov, E., Milenkovic, A., Otto, C., & de Groen, P. C. (2005). A wireless body area network of intelligent motion sensors for computer assisted physical rehabilitation. *Journal of NeuroEngineering and Rehabilitation, 2*, 1−6. <http://www.jneuroengrehab.com/content/2/1/6> Accessed 20.08.14.

Khaja R. E., Han J. (2013). Electro-chemical stimulation of neuromuscular systems using ion-selective membranes. MTL (Microsystems Technology Laboratories, Massachusetts Institute of Technology), Annual Research Report 2013. <http://www-mtl.mit.edu/wpmu/ar2013/electro-chemical-stimulation-of-neuromuscular-systems-using-ion-selective-membranes/> Accessed 20.08.14.

Kim, D. H., Ahn, J.-H., Choi, W. M., Kim, H.-S., Kim, T.-H., Song, J., et al. (2008). Stretchable and foldable silicon integrated circuits. *Science, 320*, 507−511.

Lacasse, M., Duchaine, V., & Gosselin, C. (2010). Characterization of the electrical resistance of carbon-black-filled silicone: Application to a flexible and stretchable robot skin. In *IEEE international conference on robotics and automation (ICRA)*, 2010 (pp. 4842−4848).

Lee, J. H., Anthony, B. W., & Boning, D. S. (2013). An ingestible pill for ultrasound imaging of small intestine. MTL (Microsystems Technology Laboratories, Massachusetts Institute of Technology) Annual Research Report 2013. <http://www-mtl.mit.edu/wpmu/ar2013/an-ingestible-pill-for-ultrasound-imaging-of-small-intestine/> Accessed 18.08.14.

Leonhardt, U. (2006). Optical conformal mapping. *Science, 312*, 1777−1780.

Makris, K. G., El-Ganainy, R., Christodoulides, D. N., & Musslimani, Z. H. (2008). Beam dynamics in PT-symmetric optical lattices. *Physical Review Letters, 100*(3), 103904.

Nayak, S., Chaki, T. K., & Khastgir, D. (2013). Development of poly(dimethylsiloxane)/$BaTiO_3$ nanocomposites as dielectric material. *Advanced Materials Research*, *622–623*, 897–900.

Nylund, K., Ødegaard, S., Hausken, T., Folvik, G., Lied, G. A., Viola, I., et al. (2009). Sonography of the small intestine. *World Journal of Gastroenterology*, *15*(11), 1319–1330.

Pandian, P. S., Safeer, K. P., Gupta, P., Shakunthala, D. T., Sundersheshu, B. S., & Padaki, V. C. (2008). Wireless sensor network for wearable physiological monitoring. *Journal of Networks*, *5*(3), 21–29 <http://ojs.academypublisher.com/index.php/jnw/article/viewPDFInterstitial/1026/732> Accessed 20.08.14

Pendry, J. B., Schurig, D., & Smith, D. R. (2006). Controlling electromagnetic fields. *Science*, *312*, 1780–1782.

Qoronfleh, M. W., & Lindpainter, K. (2010). Protein biomarker immunoassays: Opportunities and challenges Winter 10. <http://www.ddw-online.com/personalised-medicine/p142790-protein-biomarker-immunoassays-:-opportunities-and-challengeswinter-10.html> Accessed 25.08.14.

Raskovic, D., Martin, T., & Jovanov, E. (2004). Medical monitoring applications for wearable computing. *The Computer Journal*, *47*(4), 495–504.

Rüter, C. E., Makris, K. G., El-Ganainy, R., Christodoulides, D. N., Segev, M., & Kip, D. (2010). Observation of parity–time symmetry in optics. *Nature Physics*, *6*, 192–195.

Saleh, O. A., & Sohn, L. L. (2006). An on-chip artificial pore for molecular sensing. In R. Bashir, & S. Wereley (Eds.), *BioMEMS and biomedical nanotechnology: Biomolecular sensing and analysis* (Vol. 4, Chapter 3). New York: Springer.

Song, Y. A., Melik, R., Rabie, A. N., Ibrahim, A. M. S., Moses, D., Tan, A., et al. (2011). Electrochemical activation and inhibition of neuromuscular systems through modulation of ion concentrations with ion-selective membranes. *Nature Materials*, *10*, 980–986.

Tucker, A. (2012). Jack Andraka, the teen prodigy of pancreatic cancer. *Smithsonian Magazine*, <http://www.smithsonianmag.com/science-nature/jack-andraka-the-teen-prodigy-of-pancreatic-cancer-135925809/?no-ist> Accessed 22.08.14.

Valdastri, P., Rossi, S., Menciassi, A., Lionetti, V., Bernini, F., Recchina, F. A., et al. (2008). An implantable ZigBee ready telemetric platform for in vivo monitoring of physiological parameters. *Sensors and Actuators A: Physical*, *142*, 369–378.

Vrijens, B., & Urquhart, J. (2014). Methods for measuring, enhancing, and accounting for medication adherence in clinical trials. *Clinical Pharmacology Therapy*, *95*, 617–626.

Wu, D., & Voldman, J. (2013). Microfluidic electronic detection of protein biomarkers. MTL (Microsystems Technology Laboratories, Massachusetts Institute of Technology) Annual Research Report 2013. <http://www-mtl.mit.edu/wpmu/ar2013/microfluidic-electronic-detection-of-protein-biomarkers/> Accessed 20.08.14.

Yamada, T., Hayamizu, Y., Yamamoto, Y., Yomogida, Y., Izadi-Najafabadi, A., Futaba, D. N., et al. (2011). A stretchable carbon nanotube strain sensor for human-motion detection. *Nature Nanotechnology*, *6*, 296–301.

Yaul, F. M., & Lang, J. H. (2012). A flexible underwater pressure sensor array using a conductive elastomer strain gauge. *Journal of Microelectromechanical Systems*, *21*(4), 897–907.

INDEX

Note: Page numbers followed by "*f*" and "*t*" refer to figures and tables, respectively.

F

G

H

I

U

V

W

Z

Printed in the United States
By Bookmasters